Intimate Interventions in Global Health

When addressing the factors shaping HIV prevention programs in sub-Saharan Africa, it is important to consider the role of family planning programs that preceded the epidemic. In this book, Rachel Robinson argues that both globally and locally, those working to prevent HIV borrowed and adapted resources, discourses, and strategies used for family planning. By combining statistical analysis of all sub-Saharan African countries with comparative case studies of Malawi, Nigeria, and Senegal, Robinson also shows that the nature of countries' interactions with the international community, the strength and composition of civil society, and the existence of technocratic leaders influenced variation in responses to HIV. Specifically, historical and existing relationships with outside actors, the nature of nongovernmental organizations, and perceptions of previous interventions strongly structured later health interventions through processes of path dependence and policy feedback. This book will be of great use to scholars and practitioners interested in global health, international development, African studies and political science.

Rachel Sullivan Robinson is an associate professor in the School of International Service at American University. She holds a PhD in sociology and demography from the University of California, Berkeley and has conducted field research in Nigeria, Senegal, Malawi, and Namibia. She teaches courses on statistics, global health, population studies, development, and nongovernmental organizations.

Intimate Interventions in Global Health

Family Planning and HIV Prevention in Sub-Saharan Africa

RACHEL SULLIVAN ROBINSON
American University

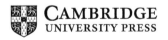

CAMBRIDGE
UNIVERSITY PRESS

University Printing House, Cambridge CB2 8BS, United Kingdom

One Liberty Plaza, 20th Floor, New York, NY 10006, USA

477 Williamstown Road, Port Melbourne, VIC 3207, Australia

4843/24, 2nd Floor, Ansari Road, Daryaganj, Delhi – 110002, India

79 Anson Road, #06–04/06, Singapore 079906

Cambridge University Press is part of the University of Cambridge.

It furthers the University's mission by disseminating knowledge in the pursuit of education, learning, and research at the highest international levels of excellence.

www.cambridge.org
Information on this title: www.cambridge.org/9781107090729

First published 2017

A catalogue record for this publication is available from the British Library.

Library of Congress Cataloging-in-Publication Data
Names: Robinson, Rachel Sullivan, author.
Title: Intimate interventions in global health : family planning and HIV prevention in sub-Saharan Africa / Rachel Sullivan Robinson.
Description: Cambridge, United Kingdom; New York, NY : Cambridge University Press, [2017] | Includes bibliographical references.
Identifiers: LCCN 2016056470 | ISBN 9781107090729 (hardback)
Subjects: | MESH: HIV Infections – prevention & control | Family Planning Services – methods | Sexual Behavior | Behavior Control – methods | Public Policy | Global Health | Africa South of the Sahara
Classification: LCC RA643.86.A357 | NLM WC 503.6 | DDC 614.5/9939200967–dc23
LC record available at https://lccn.loc.gov/2016056470

ISBN 978-1-107-09072-9 Hardback

To my respondents and all those who strive to make pregnancy wanted and HIV obsolete

Contents

Tables and Figures

Tables

Figures

Acknowledgments

This book would not have been possible without the assistance, contributions, and good will of many, many people. First and foremost, I thank my respondents, the people doing the day-to-day work of managing programs for family planning, HIV prevention, and reproductive health provision in Malawi, Nigeria, and Senegal. For their contributions both large and small, this book is dedicated to them. Their willingness to share time with a stranger and patiently answer her questions also made the analysis in the case study chapters possible.

In addition to my respondents, numerous people facilitated the process of field research both before and after I arrived in country. In Malawi, these included Nicole Angotti, Crystal Biruk, Peter Fleming, Emily Freeman, Monica Grant, Frank and Thandi Honde, Hans-Peter Kohler, Rage Majamanda, Ann Swidler, Frank Taulo, Jeff Thindwa, and Susan Cotts Watkins. The staff at the Centre for Social Research at Chancellor College and at the Malawi National Archives kindly granted me access to their materials.

In Nigeria, Ben Agande, Lou Goodman, Jasmine Jones, Carl LeVan, Peter Lewis, Cynthia Ticao, and Patrick Ukata supplied contacts, help with logistics, and practical advice. Kole Shettima opened the MacArthur Foundation's library in Abuja to me, which contained numerous resources unavailable elsewhere, as did the library at the Yar'Adua Centre.

In Senegal, I would have been lost without the assistance of the Centre de Recherche Ouest-Africain, the Dakar outpost of the Boston-based Center for West African Research. There, Ousmane Sène, Mame Coumba, Abdoulaye Niang, and many others created a home away from home as well as gave much practical research support for each of my research trips to Dakar, starting from 2004. Gary Engleberg at Africa Consultants International shared a number of helpful contacts, as did Ellen Foley. The Sarr and Sow families have graciously hosted me on different trips. Chris Ansari, Jennifer Browning, and Ivy Mills offered numerous tips and insights about visiting and doing research in Dakar. The staff at the Association Sénégalaise pour le Bien-être Familial and Africa Consultants International granted me access to their libraries and the wealth of gray literature therein, and the Senegalese National Archives helped me locate relevant, and dusty, files.

I am also grateful to the population experts who I interviewed for the book, who served both as respondents as well as sounding boards for the overall argument. These included Stan Bernstein, John Bongaarts, John Cleland, Duff Gillespie, Tom Merrick, and Malcolm Potts.

Funding for the fieldwork and time spent writing this book came from American University's Faculty Research Award program and the Council of American Overseas Research Center's Multi-Country Fellowship. The University of Washington's Center for Studies in Demography and Ecology provided a desk and intellectual community during my 2015 sabbatical, most of which was spent revising the text.

A number of people were instrumental to the writing process. Two writing groups at American University read drafts of chapters and gave criticism as well as encouragement. The first – the SoHos – included Kristin Diwan, Kate Haulman, Adrea Lawrence, Susan Shepler, Brenda Werth, and Elizabeth Anderson Worden. The second included jimi adams, Nicole Angotti, Michael Bader, Ernesto Castaneda, Taryn Morrissey, Randa Serhan, and Nina Yamanis. I also received immensely helpful feedback on drafts of chapters from a number of other people: Stan Bernstein, Kim Yi Dionne, Gary Engelberg, Anne Esacove, Ellen Foley, Amy Kaler, Amy Patterson, Daniel Jordan Smith, Ann Swidler, and Susan Cotts Watkins.

A book incubator at American University proved invaluable prior to the revisions that preceded submission of the manuscript for review. Participants included Jason Beckfield, Evan Lieberman, Naomi Rutenberg, Jeremy Shiffman, and Paul Wapner. Funding for the incubator came from Dean Jim Goldgeier of the School of International Service and the Institute for International Affairs Research (including Maya Barak, Holly Bennett Christiansen, Jon Gould, Shannon Looney, and Mana Zarinejad) as well as Kim Blankenship of the Center on Health, Risk, and Society and Clarence Lusane of the Comparative and Regional Studies Program.

I also have benefitted greatly from audience comments at presentations I have given on the book at Cornell University, University of California Irvine, University of California Los Angeles,

University of Texas Austin, and University of Washington; at the annual meetings of the African Studies Association, American Sociological Association, and Population Association of America; and at the Center on Health, Risk, and Society and the School of Education, Teaching, and Health at American University.

Numerous colleagues at American University mentored me throughout the writing of this book including: Kim Blankenship, Deborah Brautigam, Ken Conca, Carole Gallaher, Jim Goldgeier, Jeremy Shiffman, and Sharon Weiner. Other colleagues who have advised me on a number of dimensions include Jeff Colgan, Peggy Eskow, Adrienne LeBas, Adrienne Pine, Dan Schneider, and Jordan Tama. Derrick Cogburn shared access to QDA Miner qualitative data analysis software through COTELCO. Meagan Snow gave me a crash course in ArcGIS that produced the maps in Chapter 3. Also at American University, a number of students have supplied expert research assistance through the life course of writing the book: Yolande Bouka, Julia Fischer-Mackey, Dorothy Fort, Alana McGinty, Kate Tennis, Jennifer Vanderburgh, Christine Yelibi, and Yang Zhang.

The *Journal of the International AIDS Society* published an early version of the argument for this book in a special issue entitled, "Bridging the Social and the Biomedical: Engaging the Social and Political Sciences in HIV Research," edited by Susan C. Kippax, Martin Holt, and Samuel R. Friedman. The Population Reference Bureau opened their Washington, DC library to me, and the Center for Global Development and Rachel Nugent invited me to contribute a background paper on the UNFPA to a working group that helped form the background for Chapter 3. Deborah Barrett kindly shared data from her and Amy Tsui's article on population policy impacts that I used in Chapter 3. Sean Stewart at the Center for Communication Programs at Johns Hopkins University and Maria Dieter at Population Services International helped with granting image permissions.

At Cambridge University Press, I thank my current editor, Maria Marsh, and content managers, Ian McIver and Claire Sissen, as well as the previous two editors who also supported the project, William Hammel and Eric Crahan. Two anonymous reviewers gave valuable feedback on the initial submission. I also thank Sri Hari Kumar at Integra Software Services and the other staff who copyedited and helped move the book to final production.

As part of this book grew out of my dissertation, I yet again extend my gratitude to my committee for all of their support, insight, and guidance: Jennifer Johnson-Hanks (chair), Neil Fligstein, Ann Swidler, and Ken Wachter. A number of units at the University of California, Berkeley provided funding for the dissertation, which included some of the interviews used for the analysis in the book, including the Department of Demography, the Rocca Center for African Studies, and the Institute for Business and Economics Research. I also received funding from a National Science Foundation Graduate Research Fellowship and a training grant through the National Institute for Child Health and Human Development. My dissertation writing group also helped immensely in many ways: Shannon Gleeson, Damon Mayrl, Ben Moodie, Aliya Saperstein, and Laurel Westbrook.

Finally, I am forever grateful for the encouragement and love from my family and friends throughout the creation of this book and more broadly. Molly Moeser and Darragh Paradiso have been the best of friends since college. My Seattle family – my parents Barbara and Woody, my sister Sarah and brother-in-law Virtaj – made a sabbatical at the University of Washington possible and have been at my side for many more years. My in-laws, Bill and Rita, and Josh and Amy Robinson, have been supportive of my endeavors large and small. Finally, for their unconditional love and simple act of being there at the end of the day, I thank my husband Jeremy, who has been to Africa more times than he ever bargained for, and my daughters Olivia and Annabel, both of whom beat this book to the finish line.

1 | Introduction: Understanding the Links between Family Planning and HIV Prevention

Intimate interventions are programs, policies, and organizational actions that aim to change sexual behavior in the name of the individual or collective good. This book examines two intimate interventions across sub-Saharan Africa and in Malawi, Nigeria, and Senegal: efforts to prevent pregnancy and efforts to prevent the heterosexual transmission of HIV. Existing research on the implementation and effectiveness of HIV prevention programs has failed to account for the prior history of family planning programs. By accounting for this history, we can better explain why some countries successfully prevent HIV and others do not. By recognizing the similarities between preventing pregnancy and preventing HIV, we are able to reach broader conclusions about why and how countries respond to health problems.

The book considers intimate interventions implemented in sub-Saharan Africa from the late 1970s onwards, focusing primarily on the 1980s and 1990s, the years prior to the mid-2000s when affordable treatment for HIV became widely available. This was a period of intensive action among donors, governments, and nongovernmental organizations (NGOs) to first prevent pregnancy, and then to prevent HIV. Significant numbers of sub-Saharan African governments began to implement family planning programs and adopt national population policies to slow population growth in the late 1970s. Soon thereafter, in the mid-1980s, most countries reported the first cases of AIDS, but the extent and nature of the response within countries varied. With both family planning and HIV programs, international actors played a significant role. The book thus follows the transfer of resources, discourses, and strategies associated with intimate interventions from the prevention of pregnancy to the prevention of HIV. In so doing, it shows that knowing the history of health interventions in a country increases our understanding of how and to what extent countries respond to new health threats. The conclusion addresses this last point specifically, with a short examination of responses to high maternal mortality in Malawi, Nigeria, and Senegal.

There are two main reasons why research on responses to HIV has not taken into account the historical context. First, the vast majority of HIV research is biomedical, and the doctors and epidemiologists who lead prevention programs have little reason or training to examine how social relations and norms shape policy and programs. Social scientists seeking to find patterns in HIV transmission and responses across historical time and social space are a minority of those studying HIV (Adam 2011; Kippax and Holt 2009). Although a small group, they have made important contributions, particularly in emphasizing structural factors driving HIV transmission as well as resilience to HIV among communities and individuals, but even then, their attention has rarely been to history (Auerbach, Parkhurst, and Cáceres 2011; Blankenship, Bray, and Merson 2000; Gupta et al. 2008; Seeley et al. 2012). Second, scholars, policymakers, and activists alike have viewed AIDS as an exceptional health event, unlike anything seen in modern times (see discussions in Benton 2015; Foley and Hendrixson 2011; Forman 2011; Seckinelgin 2012; Smith and Whiteside 2010). This framing of AIDS initially helped activists and public health policymakers raise awareness and galvanize action to prevent HIV. But treating AIDS as an exceptional and unprecedented disease obscured how responses to it would come from actors – local activists, NGOs, state ministries of health, and donor agencies – that brought their experience from other public health programs with them. And, as I will show, many of these actors had familiarity with designing and implementing intimate interventions for family planning. Because heterosexual sex causes almost all pregnancy and most HIV transmission, both intimate interventions have aimed to affect the very same behavior, particularly in sub-Saharan Africa.

Making contraception available to all who desire it and preventing HIV are quite literally matters of life and death. High maternal mortality in sub-Saharan Africa stems from high fertility – women on average bear five children in their lifetimes – in the context of inadequate health systems, gender inequality, and other factors (Population Reference Bureau 2015). Maternal mortality accounts for 9 percent of deaths to women aged 15–49 globally, almost half of which occur in sub-Saharan Africa (Hogan et al. 2010; Sepúlveda and Murray 2014). Close to a quarter of maternal mortality globally could be prevented if women wanting to avoid pregnancy but not using contraception did so, which averages approximately one quarter of married women in sub-Saharan African countries (Bradley et al. 2012; Singh, Darroch and Ashford 2014). While maternal mortality is a major preventable cause of death, so is HIV. HIV is the sixth-leading cause of death globally, and theoretically could be completely avoided through prevention (Lozano et al. 2012). HIV first emerged in Central Africa in the 1950s; today, slightly more than two thirds of those who are HIV-positive globally live in sub-Saharan Africa (Kaiser Family Foundation and UNAIDS 2016).

High fertility and high HIV prevalence have, among other factors, led to significant foreign aid commitments towards family planning and HIV programs. Donor expenditure for population assistance *not* including HIV and sexually transmitted infections was US$4.4 billion in 2012, the most recent data available (UNFPA 2014). In comparison, donor government disbursements for all AIDS activities in 2015 reached US$7.5 billion, and total investments in the global AIDS response in 2015 were estimated to be US$19 billion (Kaiser Family Foundation and UNAIDS 2016). That both unintended pregnancy and HIV are preventable in almost all cases, and yet thousands of deaths due to each occur every day, demands an explanation for why some countries have been more successful than others in providing contraception and HIV prevention services to their citizens. The volume of resources, both domestic and global, going towards addressing both issues only heightens the urgency.

Organized efforts to prevent pregnancy in developing countries have primarily taken the form of family planning programs designed to introduce and supply modern contraceptive techniques in order to reduce fertility, lower maternal mortality, and improve infant wellbeing. These efforts have also sought to change norms about family size among both women and men, promoting a small family with two or three children. Donor organizations have funded such programs, while African governments have managed and implemented them alongside local NGOs. In addition to family planning programs, in the 1980s and 1990s many sub-Saharan African governments also adopted population policies, explicit policies targeted at slowing population growth as well as altering other elements of population dynamics, such as mortality and migration.

HIV interventions have sought to prevent and treat HIV, while also caring for those affected by it. The chapters that follow focus primarily on HIV prevention because the parallels with pregnancy prevention are strongest, but do reference interventions to provide treatment that now has the capacity to greatly extend the lives of people who are HIV-positive, and can also help prevent HIV. HIV prevention programs have revolved around messages of abstinence, faithfulness to one partner, condom usage during sex (the "ABC" approach), and testing for the virus. Generally speaking, these programs have encouraged change in the number and/or type of sexual partners, as well as promoted the use of technology (condoms) during sex.

In the analysis of intimate interventions that follows, I refer frequently to the population and AIDS fields. A field consists of the set of individual and collective actors who interact with one another with a shared understanding of the purposes, relationships within, and rules of the field (Fligstein and McAdam 2011). The population field within a particular country thus subsumes all activities around pregnancy prevention and family planning and consists of all of the actors engaged in providing contraception and generating discourse about it: women and men using contraception; local and national organizations that participate in provision of and advocacy around reproductive health; the government, including relevant ministries such as health, finance, women, and youth, as well as legislators and executive leaders; multilateral, bilateral, and nongovernmental international organizations that provide aid and services; and religious institutions and their leaders. The AIDS field consists of a largely parallel, and often overlapping, set of actors that includes people living with HIV and those who care for them as well as global, national, and local organizations that participate in prevention, treatment, care, and advocacy around HIV/AIDS. The population and AIDS fields are "global assemblages," spanning different elements (actors, ideas, treaties, government structures, etc.) and the relationships among them across the global-local scale (Browner and Sargent 2011; Campbell, Cornish and Skovdal 2012; Ong and Collier 2005). Each field encompasses different social movements, some of which overlap, and which attend either directly or indirectly to the focal activity of the field. Actors within each field have differential capacities and ability to influence outcomes, which depend on their position in the field as well as their resources. For example, international donors have massive financial resources, which mean that their opinions and desires carry great weight, but the programs funded by these resources may ultimately have no impact because the position of the donors is so culturally different than those of the people targeted by interventions. Fields cut across levels of analysis, containing both international and local organizations, with local organizations and actors often playing a mediating and interpretive role for the messages from international organizations (e.g., Browner and Sargent 2011; Ferguson 2006; Li 2007; Merry 2006).

Fields are not isolated entities, but are instead densely connected to one another. These connections span space, as well as time. Understanding how a new field emerges requires considering the fields that preceded it, and indeed, Fligstein and McAdam (2011: 12) note that "New [fields] are likely to emerge nearby existing [fields]. They are likely to be populated by existing groups who 'migrate' or by offshoots of existing groups." This book's emphasis on the linkages between population interventions and HIV interventions invites the investigation of how exactly the AIDS field globally as well as in individual sub-Saharan African countries grew out of extant fields, in particular the population field.

The fields involved in intimate interventions define the scope of relevant actors, purposes, relationships, and rules. With that understanding of fields as a backdrop, I draw from both the sociological and political science literature to develop a model that specifies transnational, political, sociocultural, and economic factors as driving the extent and contours of intimate interventions within countries. The chapters that follow combine cross-country statistical analysis of all sub-Saharan African countries with detailed case studies of Malawi, Nigeria, and Senegal, countries that vary in terms of their experiences with family planning and HIV programs. The statistical analysis facilitates making generalizable claims, while the case studies reveal mechanisms and nuances invisible to macro-level analyses.

The remainder of the introduction provides core background for the chapters that follow. First, I present an argument about the connections between family planning programs and HIV prevention interventions in order to motivate examination of pregnancy prevention within the context of understanding responses to HIV in sub-Saharan Africa. I then develop a model for why countries "do what they do" that structures both the cross-country statistical analysis as well as the individual case studies around transnational, political, sociocultural, and economic factors. Following that, I explain the logic of case selection and introduce the three cases – Malawi, Nigeria, and Senegal – as well as details on data collection and analysis. I conclude with summaries of the book's remaining chapters.

Connecting Pregnancy Prevention to HIV Prevention

Pregnancy and HIV transmission in sub-Saharan Africa occur mostly through the same mechanism: sex between a man and a woman. The use of assisted reproductive technologies is extremely limited in sub-Saharan Africa, meaning almost all pregnancies occur through sexual intercourse, and the vast majority of the approximately 25 million women and men who are HIV-positive in sub-Saharan Africa acquired HIV through heterosexual intercourse (UNAIDS 2014). The remaining cases are the result of mother-to-child transmission during pregnancy, delivery, and breastfeeding;[1] homosexual male sex; injection drug use; or unsafe medical practices. In the sub-Saharan African context, then, any program to change the number of children people bear, or their risk for contracting HIV, almost certainly requires engaging in the intimate arena of sex. In this section, I note a number of similarities between these two types of intimate interventions, and also discuss some important ways in which pregnancy and HIV, and the prevention of each, differ. These similarities provide the basis for the argument that the experience donors, governments, and NGOs gained through family planning programs should be considered when studying responses to HIV. The argument does not, however, depend on family planning programs being successful. Family planning programs can influence HIV interventions regardless of whether they increased contraceptive prevalence or lowered fertility.

Family planning programs and HIV interventions both draw on the same resources: donors, country-level organizations, and human capital. Specifically, external nongovernmental and governmental organizations with deep pockets have strongly shaped the contours of both interventions. Within countries, the same federal ministries of health, women, and youth as well as many of the same local NGOs have been involved in both types of interventions. Across organizations at all levels, it is often the very same people who first

---

[1] Sometimes referred to as "vertical transmission."

worked on family planning who then came to work on HIV. For both intimate interventions there are "layers of local brokers who mediate between international donors and the poor villagers whose lives are seen as requiring transformation," facilitating the flow of money from a global to a local level (Swidler and Watkins 2017; Watkins and Swidler 2013: 212). Put in another way, both family planning and HIV interventions represent well "the global-to-local supply chain of interventions to improve the human condition" (Dionne 2012: 2475).

Intimate interventions introduce new ideas about the rationalities of sex, including sex for purposes other than procreation and the concomitant safe sex practices that prevent HIV and other sexually transmitted infections. The goal of family planning programs has been to lower fertility by limiting the overall number of births, as well as spacing them further apart, through the use of contraception. Contraception greatly reduces the risk of pregnancy and distances the risk of pregnancy from decisions about when to have sex and with whom. HIV prevention interventions have encouraged people to have "safe" sex, meaning avoiding sex with those believed to elevate the risk for HIV transmission, like extramarital partners, sex workers, or multiple partners. HIV prevention programs have also promoted condoms, particularly with partners deemed "risky," but even within relationships, adding a decision about condom use to any sexual interaction. Changing rationalities of sex, whether for family planning or HIV, takes time and so reductions in fertility and HIV transmission rarely occur rapidly (Cleland and Watkins 2006b; Merson et al. 2008).

Family planning programs and HIV interventions have both developed and then applied the same templates for action to wildly different cultural, demographic, and epidemiological settings, including the same technologies, logics, and target populations. Contraception is the primary technology of family planning programs, and sub-Saharan African programs have tended to emphasize long-lasting and female-controlled, hormonal forms (Zaba, Boerma and Marchant 1998). The main technology associated with HIV prevention has been the condom, but other technologies include the kits used to test for HIV and now even antiretroviral medication. Condoms can, of course, prevent both pregnancy and HIV. As one long-time observer of family planning and HIV programs put it, "What brings family

planning and HIV together is our old friend the condom."[2]
As I describe in Chapter 3 on sub-Saharan Africa, while programmers
have generally not promoted condoms as a means of family planning in
the region, the associated social marketing programs that include condoms in their arsenal of technologies *have* been a link between intimate
interventions.

Both family planning and HIV prevention have relied on the logic
that the provision of information and technology will change the
calculus of sexual decision making and facilitate implementation of
those decisions. In fact, many family planning programmers assumed
that supplying technology (pills, injections, and other contraceptive
devices) would, in and of itself, lower desired family size and ultimately, fertility. Similarly, HIV programs have admonished people to
use condoms and handed them out en masse, presuming that availability would increase use. In both cases, practitioners have been sur-
prised that these templates have not produced the desired behavior
change, even though such an outcome is predictable given the importance of context to program implementation and success (Pritchett and
Woolcock 2004).

Both interventions have also disproportionately targeted women.
With family planning, such a focus is because most contraceptive
methods are female-controlled. But with HIV prevention in sub-
Saharan Africa, intimate interventions have targeted women
because women have more interactions with the health system,
creating more opportunities to communicate behavior change messages and to test for HIV. Indeed, much of women's interaction with
the health system is centered around fertility. In addition, HIV
prevention programs have also targeted female sex workers,
a group particularly at risk for HIV. Intervention programs have
sought to arm these women with male condoms, regardless of their
actual ability to negotiate condom use with clients. Such strategies
have worked best in instances where there is regulation and monitoring of sex work, such as in Thailand and Senegal (Hearst and
Chen 2004; Phoolcharoen 1998; Pisani 1999). In parallel, men have
frequently been "blamed" for both high fertility and the transmission of HIV. Academics and policymakers have given great weight

[2] Expert 5 – see the "methods" section of this chapter for discussion of population
experts interviewed for this book.

to male preferences for large families in explaining high fertility, and men's extramarital relationships in explaining the spread of HIV (see the thoughtful discussion and critique in Dodoo and Frost 2008; Greene and Biddlecom 2000).

Intimate interventions challenge the status quo regarding relationships between sex partners, between generations, and between citizens and the state. They intersect with the socially prescribed arena of sex and create moral reactions about appropriate behavior, and who even has the authority to define what counts as "appropriate." While sex within marriage is less contested than other forms of sex, even contraception within marriage raises questions: who has the right to manage an individual woman's fertility? Does she, her partner, her mother-in-law, her spiritual counselor? Sex *outside* of marriage raises moral objections across a wide variety of contexts as it more strongly disassociates sex from procreation and is often explicitly forbidden by religious and legal dictates. As a result, intimate interventions have high potential to invoke the approbation of a variety of social groups, requiring their proponents to go to great lengths to depoliticize them. Contraception has thus turned into "family planning," and HIV treatment has superseded HIV prevention. Such depoliticization has, I will show, complicated what might have otherwise been productive linkages between intimate interventions.

Intimate interventions, *par excellence*, broadcast, reflect, and reinforce biopower, or the management of the population through a variety of techniques and practices that act on individual bodies (Foucault 1978). Separated from directive state power in the form of force, biopower operates through the agents of the state – such as schools, hospitals, and public health programs – that train people to discipline themselves through engaging in appropriate behaviors. Sexuality is thus a dense transfer point for relations of power between the state and individual. From this perspective many authors have examined the state's intervention into reproductive life as well into sexuality more broadly in the name of HIV prevention (e.g., Ginsburg and Rapp 1991; Greenhalgh 2003; Kaler 2003; Newland 2001; Nguyen 2010; Pigg and Adams 2005; Richey 2004; Richey 2008; Thomas 2003). Programs and policies related to family planning and HIV deploy disciplinary tactics, including the close monitoring of populations "at risk" for pregnancy or HIV transmission. Such monitoring requires the collection of detailed data from women of childbearing age, sex workers, and men who have sex with men,[3] thus bringing these populations under the gaze of the state. These are ultimately mechanisms of biopower, which tie individual sexual and reproductive behavior directly to national power (Gordon 1991).

Though preventing pregnancy and preventing HIV bear many similarities, becoming pregnant and becoming HIV-positive are nonetheless very different transitions with different outcomes. Thus policymakers and programmers addressing HIV, while at times building on the history of family planning, have also required new approaches. Pregnancy does not lead to death with the certainty that HIV did in the era before effective treatment and still does in many contexts where treatment is not readily accessible. As a result, much of the activism around HIV, particularly in the early years of the epidemic, centered on access to treatment and was spearheaded by organizations representing gay men in relatively wealthy countries. Pregnancy is not a disease, and in many instances is a celebrated state. Women's groups promoting reproductive health and rights have been the primary activists associated with pregnancy prevention. Although women can purchase, carry, and in theory demand that male sex partners use a condom, their technological ability to protect themselves from HIV is significantly less than with pregnancy. Trials of female-controlled microbicide gels that would kill the HIV virus have proven overwhelmingly disappointing (Karim, Baxter and Karim 2013) and female condoms cannot be used as clandestinely as can hormonal contraception, an intrauterine device, a cervical cap, or diaphragm. While these differences are important to remember, the similarities between pregnancy prevention and HIV prevention nonetheless motivate investigating how the history of family planning globally as well as within countries has shaped the HIV interventions that followed.

---

[3] "Men who have sex with men" is the term used in the public health field, preferred because it focuses on the behavior that puts individuals at risk for HIV, as opposed to terms like "gay" or "homosexual" that describe a sexual identity that many men are unlikely to espouse in the context of sub-Saharan Africa and elsewhere.

The Relationship of History to Social Policies and Programs

Scholars have as of yet rarely studied HIV interventions with an eye to the sex-related health interventions that preceded them. As described above, this lack of connection results from disciplinary particularities and AIDS exceptionalism. The literature on HIV which does take into account history tends to consider sexually transmitted infections, rather than family planning. For example, Brandt (1988) as well as many of the contributions in the volume edited by Setel, Lewis, and Lyons (1999) considered the history of sexually transmitted infections in sub-Saharan African countries in order to better understand the response to HIV, including a chapter on Malawi (Chirwa 1999). Packard and Epstein (1991) noted that a lack of epidemiological evidence about both syphilis and AIDS led to racist interpretations of disease transmission in sub-Saharan Africa, while Patton (2002: xxvi) emphasized how "the legacies of colonialism and modernization allow for the spectacular and insidious recycling of racist, sexist, xenophobic, and homophobic ideas as though they were 'scientific'." Baldwin has argued that approaches to HIV in France, Germany, Sweden, and the US "broadly corresponded to the preventive tactics they had adopted during the nineteenth century when dealing with earlier epidemics of contagious disease" and formed as the result of a "deep historical public health memory" (Baldwin 2005: 1). This scholarship on the history of sexually transmitted infections also reflects the many brilliant analyses of the colonial obsession with subjects' sexuality (e.g., Ngalamulume 2004; Stoler 1995; Stoler 2002; Thomas 2003).

The importance of history to understanding social and political processes is in part due to path dependence. As a country follows a particular course of action, the costs of leaving the chosen path rise and so the benefits to staying on the path also rise (Pierson 2000). Thus complex systems that are expensive to establish and require extensive knowledge and coordination on the part of involved actors are difficult to change, even if they are not the most efficient means of achieving a desired outcome (Arthur 1994). Furthermore, as earlier events weigh disproportionately on ultimate outcomes, the sequencing of events becomes an important point of inquiry (Pierson 2000). Privileging path-dependent processes does not, however, mean that events are set in stone, that outcomes are one hundred percent predictable, or that outcomes are even necessarily suboptimal (Torfing 2009). Instead, path dependence "operates through the provision of distinct materials – either policy precedents or institutional arrangements – that can then be adapted to new purposes" (Clemens 2007: 538, citing Thelen 2004). The complexity of the global-local field of actors involved in the development process writ large as well as of national and local public health structures makes them both systems where path-dependent processes are very likely to explain action (and inaction) across contexts. Path dependence in conjunction with the parallels between different types of intimate interventions thus promotes examining how the history of family planning programs influenced later HIV interventions. Path dependence does not imply, however, that nothing came before family planning or that family planning programs were the sole determinant of responses to HIV, simply that responses to HIV bear the mark of the family planning programs that preceded them.

More broadly, the analysis presented in the book heeds the call of some social scientists for greater incorporation of history into the study of policy and programs. Woolcock, Szreter and Rao (2011) argued for a serious and non-superficial attention to history, both as method but also because of its attention to process and context. Related to history and policy, as Theda Skocpol so clearly articulated, "Policies transform or expand the capacities of the state. They therefore change the administrative possibilities for official initiatives in the future, and affect later prospects for policy implementation... new policies [also] affect the social identities, goals, and capabilities of groups that subsequently struggle or ally in politics" (Skocpol 1992: 58). As a result, when studying social policy, we need to consider how processes emerge over time, and in particular how the effects of previous policies as well as preceding events might influence current policies (Clemens 2007; Skocpol and Amenta 1986). Such historical attention raises the possibility of both positive and negative policy feedbacks that can "'spill over' from one policy to influence the fate of another policy proposal that seems analogous in the eyes of relevant officials and groups" (Skocpol 1992: 59). Understanding when such policy feedback is most likely to occur, and when either positive or negative learning from policies occurs, are important research questions that the analysis of Malawi, Nigeria, and Senegal helps to answer (Pierson 1993).

In much the same spirit as these broader investigations of policy feedback and path dependence, a small body of literature exists on the connection between family planning programs and HIV prevention interventions. Cleland and Watkins (2006a; 2006b) considered the history of behavior change associated with modern contraceptive technology to understand the length of time likely required to observe the similarly extensive behavior change necessary to reduce HIV transmission. They concluded that such behavior change will occur, but that it will be slow and will require the domestication of foreign techniques. While acknowledging some of the differences between pregnancy and HIV described above, Cleland and Watkins concluded, "The ambitions, assumptions and implementation of both [population and AIDS] movements are strikingly similar and the social processes by which the AIDS crisis is ultimately resolved are likely to be similar to the processes that earlier led to the widespread adoption of fertility control" (Cleland and Watkins 2006a: 208). Watkins and Swidler (2013) echoed the similarities between the global population movement and what they call the AIDS enterprise.

Others who have linked population and HIV interventions have done so while critiquing both interventions. Relatively early in the epidemic, Elizabeth Reid (1995), the director of the HIV and Development Programme at the United Nations Development Programme, noted that both population and HIV interventions applied the same simplistic, technological interventions everywhere, rather than addressing the complex social realities that put women in particular at risk for both pregnancy and HIV. Stillwaggon (2006) found fault with both HIV interventions and population interventions for failing to address larger issues driving population growth and HIV transmission, specifically poverty, and in particular blamed fertility researchers' understandings of sexuality for leading to inappropriate responses to AIDS (Stillwaggon 2003). Similarly, Richey (2003; 2005) pointed to the continued narrow focus of population interventions on family planning, which comes at the expense of an integrated approach that incorporates HIV into broader reproductive health care. Gisselquist et al. (2003) surmised that the consensus reached in the late 1980s that HIV was sexually transmitted in sub-Saharan Africa, rather than through unhygienic health care practices (their argument), may well have emerged because doing so allowed for an emphasis on condom promotion, which matched the goals of pre-existing population programs. Others have noted that the treatment of population and

HIV as crises resulted in technical interventions (Foley and Hendrixson 2011) that failed to take into account the context or larger social and structural factors driving the problem at hand, part of a broader critique of both family planning and AIDS programs (Ahlberg 1991; Mhloyi 1995). Relatedly, there is a large body of literature debating the benefits and drawbacks of integrating family planning and HIV prevention, revolving particularly around prevention of mother-to-child transmission, which I discuss in the following chapter.

The importance of path dependence combined with the similarities – be they good or bad – between intimate interventions drives the argument of the book, namely that understanding the history of family planning programs both globally and locally helps to understand how countries responded to HIV, and to a certain extent, how successful those interventions have been. In the chapters that follow, I investigate how the resources, discourses, and strategies developed to support one intimate intervention (family planning) did and did not transfer to the next intimate intervention (HIV prevention). First, I consider the question globally, then across sub-Saharan Africa, and finally with the specific case studies of Malawi, Nigeria, and Senegal. To prepare for the analysis of individual countries, the following section places the history of intimate interventions within the context of the transnational, political, sociocultural, and economic factors likely to influence the response to HIV within a given country.

A Model to Understand Variation in Responses to HIV across Countries

Understanding why countries respond to health and development issues in particular ways requires a multidisciplinary perspective because the range of actors and variables involved is so extensive: political executives, policymakers, and government bureaucracies, but also civil society groups, religious leaders, and international donors, all operating within different economic and social contexts. I thus draw from both sociology and political science in order to build a model that structures the analyses that follow. While limited numbers of sociologists or political scientists have explicitly studied country-level responses to HIV, each discipline provides broader theories of why countries behave the way they do. Within sociology, those working from a world-culture paradigm have developed a set of explanations for country-level behavior that rests on the ties countries have to intergovernmental and nongovernmental organizations. Political scientists, on the other hand, have focused more specifically on either domestic politics as enacted by executives and interest groups within particular election systems, or on the positioning of states within the global system. Across both disciplines, scholars who have conducted cross-national, macro analyses have rarely carried out case studies within countries, while those who have looked at specific cases often have not tried to generalize further. The analyses presented in the following chapters thus bring together the perspectives of both disciplines and combine macro and micro approaches.

To provide a framework to approach the nature and extent of HIV prevention interventions, I identify four sets of factors that influence responses to HIV: transnational, political, sociocultural, and economic. This typology draws from Shiffman and Garcés del Valle's (2006) analysis of differential responses to high maternal mortality in Honduras and Guatemala. I describe each set of factors in the sections that follow with reference to theoretical work as well as specifics from the existing literature on variation in responses to HIV across countries. There is, however, not much research that examines responses to HIV across large numbers of countries, and so to the extent possible, I draw from studies of individual countries. In the analyses presented in the following chapters, I then consider what transferred from family planning to HIV within each category of factors, focusing in particular on resources, discourses, and strategies. Resources include funding, organizations, and human capital. Discourses refer to the framing and interpretation of particular elements of intimate interventions. Strategies are the technologies and techniques deployed primarily by organizational actors to carry out intimate interventions. The model provides guidance as to the areas to investigate for direct connections between family planning and HIV prevention, and for similar patterns in responses, all as a means to better understand country responses to HIV in particular, but also to other health issues. As the chapters that follow demonstrate, the links between intimate interventions are most visible when considering transnational and political factors.

Transnational Factors

The extent and nature of countries' responses to HIV is strongly influenced by countries' relationships with external actors, most notably the international organizations that have promoted intimate interventions as well as other health, development, and economic programs. International organizations, both governmental and non-governmental, can force countries to take particular actions because of power and resource differentials, and can also transmit norms that, once embraced by country-level elites and others, lead to the adoption of policies and programs. A country's overall relationship with, and interpretation of, the international community thus influences the extent to which ideas and programs developed externally are welcomed or rejected.

Sociologists in particular have understood patterns in country-level policy adoption, bureaucratic structure, and programs as dependent on the number of ties countries have to international governmental and nongovernmental organizations. These organizations transmit messages about the appropriate ways for countries to behave. For example, countries should have three-tiered education systems and ministries of the environment, demonstrate respect for human rights and women, and follow neoliberal economic policies. The general conclusion of such research – described variously as being about the world polity, world culture, or policy diffusion – is that largely independent of national characteristics, ties to international organizations explain the remarkably homogenous nature of policies, programs, and structures across a diverse set of nations (cf. Boli and Thomas 1997; Meyer 2004; Meyer et al. 1997).

We should thus expect that sub-Saharan African countries with more extensive ties (be it in strength or number) to international organizations will be more likely to adopt the behaviors of the wealthy countries of the Global North that most international organizations represent, or the policies and programs that such countries and organizations promote. Compliance with global norms among poorer countries of the Global South can then result from a genuine embrace of norms, or from coercion by wealthy countries and organizations. Research that has specifically attended to mechanisms of transfer between international organizations and poorer countries has identified connections at the level of the technocrat through international conference attendance or academic training (Barrett 1995; Barrett and Frank 1999; Macpherson and Weymouth 2012). Scholars have also shown that power differentials between countries can lead to differential policy outcomes (Dobbin, Simmons and Garrett 2007; Henisz, Zelner and Guillen

2005). In sub-Saharan Africa, most countries are severely indebted to international financial institutions that can make policies or programs conditions of loans, and even in the absence of explicit loan conditionality simply make policy and programmatic suggestions difficult to refuse. The case studies in this book contribute to a greater understanding of how exactly organizations representing global interests influence outcomes at the national level.

Despite the recognized importance of transnational factors across multiple disciplines and topics, most research has not explicitly examined how transnational factors explain *variation* in country-level responses to HIV. It has simply presented the various transnational actors involved as an important piece of the puzzle. For example, there is as of yet minimal research on country-level responses to HIV that explicitly comes from the sociological world polity/culture perspective. The lack of such research is striking given that poorer countries have directly borrowed wealthy countries' AIDS interventions more than they did family planning programs, a subject well studied within the sociological policy diffusion literature (e.g., Barrett 1995; Barrett and Frank 1999; Barrett, Kurzman, and Shanahan 2010). One of the most important statistical analyses of cross-national outcomes in HIV responses largely excluded transnational measures (Lieberman 2007).[4] Among the (small) quantitative literature on the topic, Bor (2007) found a significant (but negative) relationship between foreign direct investment and overseas development assistance and political support for AIDS, while Clark (2009; 2013) showed that more multilateral aid from development banks was associated with earlier responses to AIDS. Those who consider provision of antiretroviral therapy as the measure of response to HIV have found a positive relationship between external funding and antiretroviral therapy coverage (Nattrass 2008; Robinson 2011).

Beyond ties to international organizations, the tenor of a country's relationships with these organizations and the more powerful countries they represent is another transnational factor that drives country-level behavior. In sub-Saharan Africa, as in other regions, explicit anti-Western discourse can strongly influence the course of country-level action. To the extent that such discourse references and relies on

---

[4] Lieberman's book (2009) does, however, include extensive discussion of transnational factors.

sexuality to exemplify what is bad about the "Western" and contrary to what is good about the "African," it greatly complicates intimate interventions. Such discourse frequently occurs in sub-Saharan Africa and in African Islamist movements in particular (Trinitapoli and Weinreb 2012). For example, many scholars understand South Africa's initial refusal to provide antiretroviral therapy to citizens as partially driven by President Mbeki's *negative* response to pressure from transnational donors and pharmaceutical companies (e.g., Decoteau 2013). In The Gambia, President Jammeh framed his supposed AIDS cure with "appeals to tradition, ethnicity, religion, nation and pan-Africanism" (Cassidy and Leach 2009: 561). Both cases exemplify what Fox (2014) has called a "pan-African" response to HIV, in opposition to the recommendations of international organizations, and drawing from constructions of authentic Africanness.

Perspectives from sociology and international relations in conjunction with the volume of funding for AIDS from transnational actors indicate the importance of looking for variation in the extent and nature of ties between countries and global actors when explaining variation in country responses to HIV. As the following chapters demonstrate, transfers between family planning and HIV prevention within the resources, discourses, and strategies of transnational actors have formed an important part of global and local responses to HIV.

Political Factors

The majority of existing research on why countries have responded differentially to AIDS has focused on political factors, particularly the strength of civil society and the extent and quality of political leadership and commitment. These factors matter on their own, and there is a powerful interaction between them, with states structuring the space for civil society and collective action (Nathanson 2007) while civil society holds the state accountable. I describe this research below and add a discussion of a third political factor important to intimate interventions, what I call "technocratic leadership."

Many authors have argued that a strong and proactive civil society, and in particular government interaction with such a civil society, is both necessary for an effective response to HIV, and a key explanation for variation between countries' responses (Boone and Batsell 2001; ECA 2004; Kalipeni and Mbugua 2005; Moran 2004;

Parkhurst and Lush 2004; Putzel 2004; United Nations Population Division 2003; World Health Organization 2000). Here, civil society is broadly understood to include NGOs, community-based organizations, and religious organizations, among others. State and donor coordination with such groups creates the conduits through which messages about prevention are spread, as well as increases the perceived legitimacy of messages about sensitive issues relating to sex, morality, and religion. Civil society can also serve as the originating source of messages related to behavior change that the government or other actors then may adopt, or can pressure recalcitrant governments to take action. Much of the research that has identified civil society as an important driver of variation in responses to HIV is based on case studies, particularly of Uganda and Senegal, countries with strong civil societies that predated the HIV epidemic. But examples exist in other countries, such as in South Africa, where the Treatment Action Campaign lobbied the government and successfully used the judicial system to increase access to antiretroviral treatment (Grebe 2011). Clearly, civil society has played a role in successful HIV responses, but knowing which types of civil society matter, and why some countries have a more effective civil society than others, is crucial for understanding more broadly how civil society explains variation in HIV prevention efforts.

Political commitment and leadership can galvanize action around HIV/AIDS, organize those efforts, and provide high-level legitimacy to messages promoting behavior change (Boone and Batsell 2001; ECA 2004; Gow 2002; Kalipeni and Mbugua 2005; Moran 2004; Parkhurst and Lush 2004; Putzel 2004; United Nations Population Division 2003; World Health Organization 2000). The evidence for the importance of political leadership in addressing HIV/AIDS stems primarily from outlier cases: President Mbeki of South Africa's denial that HIV leads to AIDS and President Museveni of Uganda's active promotion of monogamy as an HIV prevention strategy. Scholars and other commentators also frequently reference political leadership as important to Senegal's response to HIV, but with much less detail about President Diouf's actions. Looking cross-nationally, countries with global reputations for "good" leadership provide more of their HIV-positive citizens with antiretroviral therapy than would otherwise be expected given financial, institutional, and demographic constraints (Nattrass 2008).

Political commitment as a key element of good leadership is, however, difficult to measure (Daly 2001; Fox et al. 2011; Goldberg et al. 2012; Gore et al. 2014; Moran 2004; Putzel 2004; United Nations Population Division 2003). Although extreme examples of "good" and "bad" leadership are easy to pinpoint, it is challenging to position the remaining, vast majority of examples between those two poles. Pisani has referred to the experiences of Senegal and Uganda, described in greater detail later, as having "spawned a messianic belief in 'Leadership'" as the key to successful responses to AIDS (Pisani 2008: 147). That leadership influences responses to HIV is unsurprising, so the key becomes identifying the contextual factors that make good leadership possible, as well as interrogating the exact characteristics of leadership that particularly influence HIV interventions. The analysis in the chapters that follow addresses these elements of leadership, situating it within a broader set of transnational relationships, and developing the concept of technocratic leadership, described further below.

Scholars have argued that other political characteristics of countries influence responses to HIV, but the findings are somewhat varied. Dionne (2011) has shown that executives in sub-Saharan African countries hard-hit by AIDS with shorter expected tenure in office were more likely to adopt policies but take little action to actually address HIV, while those with longer expected time in office were more likely to actually invest in health programs. Bor (2007) found that political support for HIV was higher in countries with greater press freedoms, suggesting that in those contexts, democracy functioned to hold political leaders accountable. But other research shows surprisingly little relationship between democracy and responses to HIV, perhaps because HIV and health more broadly have not become major issues in elections (Patterson 2006: 91), and also likely because most sub-Saharan African countries did not "become" democracies until the 1990s. And even though institutional capacity should leave countries better able to respond to health threats, some of the most capable countries in sub-Saharan Africa – Botswana and South Africa – initially had miserable responses to HIV, while Uganda marshaled a strong response despite low institutional capacity (Allen and Heald 2004; Patterson 2006).

Another political factor may explain positive responses to HIV across countries: what I call "technocratic leadership." A technocrat is someone in a managerial or administrative position who has expertise in a particular technology, such as science, engineering, economics, health, or any other specialized discipline. Government bureaucracies are filled with technocrats whose expertise gives them legitimacy and the potential to provide leadership towards progressive action. When they do so, technocrats become policy entrepreneurs, or people with access to the policymaking process who desire change and who have the skills, creativity, and energy to bring about that change (Kingdon 1995; Mintrom 1997; Mintrom and Norman 2009). In developing the importance of technocratic leadership, I draw inspiration from Thailand and Mechai Viravaidya. Mechai (as he is known) started the key Thai family planning NGO Population and Community Development Association in 1974, and then ultimately became the country's AIDS "czar." Thanks in large part to his creativity, entrepreneurial spirt, and political access – he served as a senator, Deputy Ministry of Industry, Cabinet Spokesman, and has connections to the Thai royal family – Thailand experienced major declines in fertility as well as HIV prevalence (Hanenberg et al. 1994; McNicoll 2006; Mechai Viravaidya Foundation n.d.; Rosenfield and Min 2007). Mechai's position and access to those with power allowed his creative ideas for reducing fertility and HIV prevalence to gain traction. He is thus a prime example of technocratic leadership and also illustrates how human capital developed in association with family planning can come to facilitate HIV interventions.

Technocratic leaders, as policy entrepreneurs, are able to define problems as well as frame them in ways that are meaningful to those with the political power to enact the necessary change. Technocrats who are involved in research in their own countries are particularly important potential policy entrepreneurs as policymakers are more likely to pay attention to research that is locally produced, particularly when scholars and policymakers are able to interact (Hutchinson et al. 2011). As the examples discussed in the following chapters show, technocratic leaders may not always engage directly in the policymaking process, but can advise or legitimate the actions of those who do. While the ultimate source of technocratic leaders' authority is their expertise, the case studies that follow demonstrate that just as charisma can justify the authority of a political leader (Weber 1978), it can also facilitate the conversion of technocrats into policy entrepreneurs.

Intimate interventions cut across many of the political factors described in this section. In particular, the cross-national analysis and case studies below show that civil society organizations founded to facilitate pregnancy prevention frequently went on to engage in HIV prevention activities. In addition, many technocrats who began their careers working in pregnancy prevention also went on to do work with HIV prevention. Political factors, along with transnational factors, thus serve as a core point of transfer between pregnancy prevention and HIV prevention at the country level.

Sociocultural and Economic Factors

Transnational and political factors are the primary focus of the analyses that follow, but there are certainly other characteristics of countries that can affect the contours of intimate interventions. Cultural and social factors influence responses to HIV, and particularly how the larger population perceives intimate interventions, but are vexingly difficult to measure, and thus hard to use to explain overall patterns. While economic factors are easier to measure, they are arguably more distal to the study of intimate interventions in sub-Saharan Africa given the generally high levels of poverty across countries. I discuss these factors briefly below in order to preface the places in the following chapters where they reappear.

Culture matters to all development interventions, and particularly to intimate interventions, but generalizations are nearly impossible. Scholars have noted the lack of specificity given to the idea of "culture" in HIV research as well as to the negative stereotypes it received, particularly early on (Preston-Whyte 2008; Schoepf 2001). For example, erroneous assumptions about Africans' differing sexual cultures have been particularly detrimental to the response to AIDS (Patton 1990), a point to which I return in Chapter 3. Similarly, many scholars and practitioners have automatically presumed religion inhibits HIV prevention efforts, but here the picture is also complex, belying any broad generalizations and showing improvement over time (Burchardt, Patterson and Rasmussen 2013; Patterson 2011; Trinitapoli and Weinreb 2012). One Muslim country may act very differently from another, and one Christian organization may be quite unlike the next. Ultimately religious organizations large and small have been instrumental in caring for those affected by HIV, and as with all other factors, the participation of churches and religious leaders in the response to AIDS is always moderated by political and social factors (Patterson 2010; Patterson 2013).

Of those who have focused on sociocultural variables outside of religion, Evan Lieberman's work on ethnic fractionalization stands out (Gauri and Lieberman 2006; Lieberman 2007; Lieberman 2009). Ethnic fractionalization is a measure of ethnic diversity, specifically the odds that any two people drawn randomly from a population will be from different ethnic groups. Lieberman convincingly showed across a number of states globally that countries with high levels of ethnic fractionalization have had weaker responses to HIV, measured either as government spending on HIV/AIDS, or mentions of HIV/ AIDS in budget speeches. He interpreted this outcome as a result of the competition between ethnic groups common in contexts of high fractionalization that then leads to dominant ethnic groups (who are also often in charge of the government) blaming minority ethnic groups for AIDS, rather than investing in strong government responses. In other words, ethnically divided societies are more likely to interpret problems like AIDS in terms of group differences, even if those problems do not vary systematically by group, thus leading to weaker responses. In contrast, in places with minimal fractionaliza- tion, elites face less risk of their own group being stigmatized should they advocate for governmental resources to go towards HIV. As case studies supporting this argument, Lieberman (2009) considered Brazil, India, and South Africa, with Brazil's lack of politicized racial categories allowing for a "national" response to the epidemic, and ethnically/racially charged politics in both India and South Africa preventing such a strong and organized response. Similarly, Bor found that greater income inequality leads to lower levels of political commitment to HIV/AIDS, suggesting that in societies where the distinction between "us" and "them" is more apparent and accepta- ble, government interventions for the good of the collective are less tenable (Bor 2007). This research on inequality and HIV responses parallels broader findings that ethnically divided societies do a poorer job in general of supplying public goods (Easterly and Levine 1997). Thus in the analyses that follow, I attend to how ethnic fractionaliza- tion has influenced responses to HIV.

Economic factors are a final set of country-level characteristics to consider in the response to HIV. Economic factors capture the government's fiscal capacity to enact programs, as well as its likely overall dependence on external donors. While strong responses to HIV need not be expensive, they often are, particularly if many people are in need of antiretroviral therapy. GDP (gross domestic product) per capita and public health expenditure thus tend to be positively associated with government commitment to HIV/AIDS, as well as the level and extent of services provided (Lieberman 2007; Nattrass 2006; Robinson 2011). I include such factors in the cross-national analyses presented in Chapter 3, but they are harder to weigh in the comparison of the cases of Malawi, Nigeria, and Senegal which, although varying in their economic capacity, are all overwhelmingly poor. Furthermore, just because a government has resources that it could spend on intimate interventions does not mean that it chooses to spend them, again pointing to the importance of political factors.

As this section lays out, the dominant focus of the chapters that follow is the transnational and political factors that are associated with the transfers between intimate interventions at the country level. While I consider sociocultural and economic factors where relevant, transnational and political factors drive the majority of the variation in intimate interventions that can be measured and observed. In particular, the organizational actors most important to the stories of family planning and HIV prevention operate primarily within the transnational and political realms.

Case Selection

This book argues that taking into account the history of pregnancy prevention interventions in a country helps us better understand the response to HIV, both because of direct connections between the two intimate interventions, but also because observing both intimate interventions reveals patterns in transnational and political factors that drive country-level action. The analyses that follow are thus *not* a test of the hypothesis that pregnancy prevention interventions are the sole driver of variation in responses to HIV. Indeed, as the above discussion demonstrates, there are many factors that are associated with responses to HIV. Taking this approach reflects calls by historical and comparative sociologists to consider process and mechanism in a quest to identify broad patterns, as opposed to testing narrow hypotheses (Clemens 2007; Tilly 2001). While countries' pregnancy prevention histories motivated case selection, the cases ultimately reflect different combinations of experiences with both family planning and HIV prevention, and do not rely on the supposition that pregnancy prevention interventions had to be successful in order to influence HIV prevention interventions.

I based case selection on two dimensions of the history of pregnancy prevention in a country, both of which reflect transnational and political factors from the model described above. The first dimension captures political commitment to reducing population growth: whether and when a country adopted a national population policy designed to slow population growth. The second dimension reflects civil society: the date of founding of a country's affiliate of the International Planned Parenthood Federation. These measures are preferable to the Family Planning Effort Index (Ross and Smith 2011) as they exist for all countries and better capture the actions of both government and civil society, as well as their relationship with international actors. While there are few sub-Saharan African countries that stand out as early and strong promoters of family planning,[5] sufficient variation exists in the timing of population policy adoption and the family planning organization foundation date to make these meaningful variables on which to select cases.

At the national level, starting in the late 1980s and continuing through the 1990s, two thirds of sub-Saharan African governments adopted national population policies (Robinson 2015). These policies served as a means to express national goals related to health, development, and wellbeing, and provided a framework for family planning programs (Robinson 2012; 2016). In addition, international organizations, particularly the World Bank and USAID, the United States Agency for International Development, promoted these policies. Chapter 3 describes these policies in greater detail, including their antecedents and some of their impacts. In addition to population policies, almost all sub-Saharan African countries came to have an NGO focused on providing family planning. In many cases, this

---

[5] Zimbabwe is likely an exception. There, modern contraceptive prevalence doubled between the early 1980s and late 1990s, from approximately 25 to 50 percent, accompanied by a strong family planning program (Boohene and Dow 1987; Zimbabwe National Statistics Agency and ICF International 2012). The political deterioration that occurred from the late 1990s onwards, however, would have made it a difficult case to consider for the book.

NGO ultimately affiliated with the International Planned Parenthood Federation, and in some cases was even started by the International Planned Parenthood Federation. At the time of case selection in 2009, all but four countries (Equatorial Guinea, Sao Tomé and Principe, Somalia, and Zimbabwe) had an affiliate of the International Planned Parenthood Federation (IPPF 2009). The earliest affiliate was founded in 1932 (South Africa) and the latest in 1999 (Malawi).

In order to identify those countries that had shown particularly strong commitment to family planning and that had family planning organizations on the ground prior to the beginning of the AIDS epidemic, Table 1.1 arrays countries based on the timing of their population policy and of the founding of their International Planned Parenthood Federation affiliate relative to two key dates. In 1994, the United Nations hosted the International Conference on Population and Development in Cairo, which promoted population policy and made adoption of such a policy a way to show commitment to global norms about reproductive health (Robinson 2015). Countries that adopted a population policy before that date were more committed to pregnancy prevention, or at least willing or wanting to give the impression that was the case. In 1986, most sub-Saharan African countries identified their first cases of AIDS, so countries with an International Planned Parenthood Federation affiliate prior to that year had at least one organization on the ground with skills related to intimate interventions that could be applied in response to HIV.

Table 1.1 shows possible cases for the analyses that follow: countries with early commitment to, and organizations for, family planning (the first column), those with mixed commitment and organizational founding dates (the second column), and those with late commitment and organizations (the third column). To generate the most contrast, cases came from the first and third columns: Nigeria and Senegal because they were among the first three countries (along with Liberia) to adopt national population policies in 1988, thus starting a "wave" of population policy adoption across sub-Saharan Africa (Robinson 2015), and Malawi because its national population policy and International Planned Parenthood Federation affiliate came late, and because of the high-quality secondary literature on family planning and population policy there (e.g., Chimbwete, Watkins, and Zulu 2005; Kaler 2004). The three countries' family planning effort scores in both 1982 and 1989 support these choices: Nigeria and Senegal had among the highest

Table 1.1 *Sub-Saharan African Countries by Timing of Population Policy and Founding Date of Major Family Planning NGO*

Population Policy before 1994 and Family Planning NGO before 1986	Population Policy before 1994 or Family Planning NGO before 1986	No Population Policy before 1994 and No Family Planning NGO before 1986	No Population Policy
Burkina Faso	Benin	Botswana	Angola
Ethiopia	Cameroon	Cape Verde	Burundi
Gambia	Central African Republic	Chad	Comoros
Ghana	Cote d'Ivoire	**Malawi**	Congo
Guinea	Lesotho	Mauritania	Dem. Rep. of the Congo
Kenya	Niger	Mozambique	Djibouti
Liberia	South Africa	Namibia	Equatorial Guinea*
Madagascar	Togo		Eritrea
Mali	Uganda		Gabon
Nigeria	Zimbabwe		Guinea-Bissau
Rwanda			Mauritius
Senegal			Sao Tomé and Principe*
Sierra Leone			Somalia*
Tanzania			Sudan
Zambia			Swaziland

Note: "Family planning NGO" refers to the affiliate of the International Planned Parenthood Federation. Bolded countries are case studies in Chapters 4–6. Countries with asterisks in the fourth column did not have affiliates of the International Planned Parenthood Federation as of 2009.

(in the top half or third) family planning effort scores of sub-Saharan African countries, while Malawi ranked in the bottom third (Mauldin and Ross 1991).

Malawi, Nigeria, and Senegal have also had very different experiences with HIV/AIDS, reflecting the continent-wide variation described in greater detail in Chapter 3. Malawi has had the worst epidemic of the three countries, with 9.1 percent of the adult population HIV-positive in 2015, and prevalence peaking somewhat higher in the late 1990s (UNAIDS 2016a; UNAIDS and World Health Organization 2008). The epidemic is generalized, meaning that it extends throughout the whole population, although there are a number of at-risk populations that have higher prevalence, such as sex workers and men who have sex with men. Approximately one million Malawians were HIV-positive in 2015, of which 61 percent received antiretroviral drugs (UNAIDS 2016a). Nigeria has a moderate epidemic, with 3.2 percent of the adult population HIV-positive in 2013 (the most recent data available), and only a slight decline in prevalence (from probably about 5 percent) since the mid-1990s. The epidemic is technically generalized as prevalence is above 1 percent, but remains highly concentrated in at-risk groups, as well as particular states that encompass a belt running north-south through the country. Because of Nigeria's large population, this low prevalence still translates into 3.2 million HIV-positive people, only 21 percent of whom received antiretroviral drugs in 2013 (UNAIDS 2014). Finally, in Senegal HIV prevalence has remained below 1 percent since the discovery of the first cases in the 1980s, leaving a relatively small population of 46,000 people HIV-positive in 2015 (UNAIDS 2016b). The epidemic is almost entirely concentrated among sex workers and men who have sex with men, and both groups in the capital of Dakar have prevalence rates near 20 percent (UNAIDS 2010). Of those who are HIV-positive, 40 percent are receiving antiretroviral drugs (UNAIDS 2016b).

Although the HIV epidemics in Nigeria and Senegal have been moderate compared to that in Malawi and in other countries in southern and eastern Africa, this outcome was unknown during the 1980s and 1990s, the period of focus for the book. For example, a 1995 article noted "HIV/AIDS is spreading rapidly through the Sahel" (*AIDS Analysis Africa* 1995: 1), and many scholars and activists at the time assumed that West African countries were on a path to develop epidemics like those of southern Africa. Of the three cases, the global AIDS field has identified Senegal as the most "successful" in addressing HIV because of continued low HIV prevalence and because many country-level actors have readily engaged in the "best practices" identified by the field. Malawi has come to be seen as a treatment success in recent years, while international organizations have increasingly singled out Nigeria for its large contribution to the total number of people who are HIV-positive globally, as well as to the total number of cases of mother-to-child transmission of HIV.

These three cases thus represent a variety of experiences with family planning and HIV prevention that are, broadly speaking, representative of the range of experiences of sub-Saharan African countries overall. Although Nigeria is much larger than either Malawi or Senegal and has devolved considerable authority and responsibility to its thirty-six states, in all three countries the federal government maintains a strong degree of control over national policy and is the primary locus of donor intervention. While there are certainly many other factors that vary between these three countries, the goal of the comparison is not to create causal leverage, but to explore how the history of intimate interventions is associated with HIV responses across varied contexts, which these three countries provide.

Methods

The book relies on a number of analytic techniques. The analysis of intimate interventions globally (Chapter 2) is based primarily on a review of primary and secondary documents, supplemented by a small number of interviews (six) conducted in 2014 with global experts from the population field. Experts represented a range of major organizations – nongovernmental, multilateral, bilateral, and academic – involved in family planning globally at the time of the emergence of the HIV epidemic. They provided information about how they, their organizations, and the population field more broadly approached HIV when it first emerged.

The analysis of intimate interventions across all sub-Saharan African countries (Chapter 3) derives from the same sources as Chapter 2, supplemented by two statistical analyses. The first examines how donor funding for family planning received at the country level was associated with funding received later for HIV, while the second measures how a variety of factors – including the history of family planning interventions but also the transnational, political, sociocultural, and economic factors described above – influenced a variety of HIV responses.

The analysis of the three cases (Chapters 4–6) is based primarily on over 130 semi-structured interviews I conducted in Malawi, Nigeria, and Senegal with individuals from the federal ministries, national and local NGOs, and donor organizations providing family planning services and helping to curb the spread of HIV. The goal of these interviews was to elicit local descriptions of governmental and organizational activities related to the history of intimate interventions in each country. Almost all respondents were natives of the country in question, and the interviews were divided evenly among government, nongovernmental, and donor organizations. I conducted one fifth of these interviews in 2006 as part of an initial research project on population policy adoption in Nigeria and Senegal (Robinson 2015; Sullivan 2007). I completed the remainder of these interviews in all three countries during 2009–10 specifically for the analysis for this book. I conducted all interviews in Malawi and Nigeria in English, and the majority of interviews in Senegal in French. Almost all of the interviews were recorded and then transcribed in the US by myself and research assistants. The Institutional Review Boards of the University of California, Berkeley (for research conducted in 2006) and American University (for research conducted in 2009–10) approved all research involving human subjects, and all respondents gave informed consent to be interviewed. The research was also approved by Malawi's National Health Sciences Research Committee and Senegal's Ministre de l'Enseignement Supérieur.[6]

The interviews are supplemented with analysis of documents from nongovernmental, governmental, and donor organizations, a valuable source of data on the evolving attitudes towards health problems over time. Many of these documents are available online and through libraries in the US (e.g., from the Library of Congress, USAID's Development Experience Clearinghouse, and the Population Reference Bureau's library in Washington, DC). I also gathered approximately 4,000 pages from archives and document depositories in the three case study countries. These included the national archives in Malawi and Senegal, and the libraries of the Centre for Social Research at Chancellor College (Zomba, Malawi), the MacArthur Foundation (Abuja), the Yar'Adua Centre (Abuja), Africa Consultants International (Dakar), and the Association Sénégalaise pour le Bien-être Familial (Dakar). Many of these documents dated from the early years of the HIV epidemic and made it possible to

---

[6] No parallel body for evaluating social science research existed at the time in Nigeria.

identify when and how knowledge gained from family planning programs shaped HIV prevention activities.

The diversity of data analyzed in the chapters that follow facilitates the construction of a rich account of both family planning and HIV interventions across sub-Saharan African countries, as well as of the links between intimate interventions.

A Note on Terminology

Throughout the book, I have tried to limit the use of acronyms given the alphabet soup associated with both the population and AIDS fields and its capacity to confuse even experts. As there are a number of technical terms specific to each field, I give definitions upon first use, so readers looking for a definition may refer to the index to find when a term is first used. I most frequently use "family planning" to refer to contraception to prevent pregnancy, primarily because this is the term used by practitioners in the field and is relatively neutral. I do not use "birth control" as it is infrequently used in sub-Saharan Africa. I also do not use the phrase "population control" as it implies that the goal of efforts is indeed to control the population, which is not always case, and because it tends to be used by scholars who are particularly critical of intimate interventions (cf. Connelly 2008; Hartmann 1995), which is not my ultimate aim. Where relevant, I make the distinction between HIV, the virus that causes AIDS, and AIDS, the syndrome/condition/ disease that ultimately occurs if HIV remains untreated, but often use the combined "HIV/AIDS" to capture the broad range of activities occurring in a field that addresses both HIV and AIDS. In the chapter on Senegal, I refer to organizations by English names wherever possible and give the original French for the benefit of those already familiar with the context. Finally, the book focuses exclusively on the experiences of sub-Saharan African countries and uses the term "sub-Saharan Africa" repeatedly, but does at times use the adjective "African" for stylistic ease.

Summary of Remainder of Book

Chapter 2 provides background on population interventions and HIV interventions globally, focusing primarily on donor organizations. These organizations, by virtue of the levels of aid they provide to sub-Saharan African countries, have profoundly shaped the discursive and structural possibilities for interventions at the country level. The population field's interest in slowing population growth in developing countries began in the late 1960s, with the United Nations Population Fund (UNFPA), USAID, and a number of private foundations taking the lead. The first cases of AIDS were diagnosed in most sub-Saharan African countries by the mid-1980s, with key global actors including the World Health Organization from the late-1980s, and then the Joint United Nations Program on AIDS (UNAIDS) from the mid-1990s onwards. Other key organizations emerged in the early 2000s following advances in treatment options, including the Global Fund to Fight AIDS, Tuberculosis and Malaria (the Global Fund), the US President's Emergency Plan for AIDS Relief (PEPFAR), and the Gates Foundation.

Resources, discourses, and strategies transferred from pregnancy prevention to HIV prevention. Not only did HIV become *the* focus of global aid and take priority (and funding) away from family planning, but many of the same people who began careers in family planning switched to working in HIV prevention, and many organizations that had originally focused on family planning expanded their emphasis to include HIV. Discourses associated first with family planning reappeared in conjunction with HIV, while international organizations implementing HIV programs also borrowed strategies from family planning, including social marketing, entertainment-education, and community-based distribution schemes. Global HIV prevention efforts did not, however, borrow full cloth from family planning programs. In particular, the population field resisted incorporation of HIV in the early days of the epidemic, fearing that gains towards their own politically sensitive agenda might be lost with the incorporation of another hot-button issue.

Chapter 3 presents a brief history of population and HIV/AIDS interventions specifically in sub-Saharan Africa in order to situate the three case studies that follow as well as to identify the points of transfer between intimate interventions across a broad set of countries. Based on statistical analysis, it shows that countries that were the site of a major population intervention spearheaded by USAID in the 1980s went on to receive far more funding from the Global Fund in the 2000s, even after controlling for the severity of the HIV epidemic. It also demonstrates that countries with an affiliate of the International

Planned Parenthood Federation that predated the AIDS epidemic experienced greater declines in HIV prevalence than other countries. In addition, countries with a population policy provided antiretroviral therapy to a greater percentage of their citizens than those without such a policy. Taken together, these findings exemplify the relevance of path dependence and histories of intimate interventions to HIV responses, particularly transnational and political factors, the details of which I explore in the case study chapters that follow.

In Malawi (Chapter 4), the long-time post-independence president, Hastings Kamuzu Banda, drove the nature of both intimate interventions, producing relatively poor family planning and HIV prevention programs. Banda saw contraception as Western and thus anti-Malawian, and so family planning programs began only slowly in the 1980s and did not really pick up until after he left office in 1994. Malawians' negative perceptions of the family planning program and its coincidental implementation as AIDS deaths became visible led to the history of family planning casting a "long shadow" over HIV prevention (Kaler 2004). In addition, Banda's authoritarian rule drove intellectuals from the country who could have provided technocratic leadership, and left civil society weak. Nonetheless, some elements of the family planning program positively influenced the response to HIV, including Banja la Mtsogolo, the family planning organization that emerged soon after the HIV epidemic began and ultimately provided HIV testing and treatment. Community-based distribution and social marketing programs initially set up for family planning also came to incorporate elements of HIV prevention. Overall, the intersection of transnational (Malawi's relationship with the West) and political factors (Banda's leadership) in large part explains Malawi's response to HIV, with resources, discourses, and strategies from family planning both negatively and positively influencing HIV prevention.

In Nigeria (Chapter 5), family planning programs in the 1980s were the result of transnational factors, including strong pressure from the World Bank to adopt a population policy, as well as political factors, including technocratic leadership by the charismatic Minister of Health Olikoye Ransome-Kuti and savvy political maneuvering on the part of President Babangida. Resources in the form of local NGOs as well as ties with international donors flowed from family planning to HIV interventions, but the political upheaval during the 1990s that distracted the government, limited the reach of civil society, and led to loss of donor funding ultimately produced relatively unremarkable HIV prevention efforts. As with family planning, Nigeria's response to HIV has always been strongly conditioned by transnational factors, and by the time the country transitioned to democracy in 1999, global focus had shifted towards treatment, and Nigeria followed suit.

The global AIDS field has hailed Senegal (Chapter 6) as an HIV prevention "success" story because HIV prevalence has never exceeded 1 percent, and because government and civil society have engaged actively in the response. Almost universal male circumcision has protected much of the population against HIV, making it difficult to identify whether HIV outcomes can be causally attributed to the actions taken by the Senegalese government and organizations. At the same time, a unique historical element, the legality of sex work, has allowed unparalleled access to one of the populations most at risk for HIV. Transnational factors driving Senegal's response include the country's generally cosmopolitan and outward-oriented perspective, resulting from a long history of connections to Europe and beyond. A strong civil society that predated both family planning and HIV and remarkable technocratic leadership are political factors that have facilitated both intimate interventions. As in the other two cases, the transfer from pregnancy prevention to HIV prevention occurred through transnational and political factors. Multiple Senegalese civil society organizations predated the epidemic, including a strong family planning NGO that then engaged in AIDS-related work. In addition, through promoting family planning, the government and NGOs gained experience interacting with religious leaders that may have facilitated later conversations with those same leaders regarding HIV.

The conclusion (Chapter 7) synthesizes the findings from the examination of the transfer of resources, discourses, and strategies from pregnancy prevention to HIV prevention at the global level, the analysis of variation in HIV prevention across all sub-Saharan African countries, and the experiences of the three case study countries. To demonstrate the applicability of the book's argument to other, less intimate health realms, the conclusion also briefly presents how each of the three case study countries have responded to high levels of maternal mortality. Despite being a very different health problem, the patterns of response to maternal mortality in Malawi,

Nigeria, and Senegal bore striking similarity to each country's experiences with family planning and HIV prevention.

Transnational and political factors explain much of the variation across cases in responses to HIV. So, funding relationships with donors persisted across interventions and relationships between individual countries and external actors influenced outcomes. Political factors, including the strength of civil society and the existence of technocratic leadership, also structured intimate interventions. In all three countries, NGOs created to provide contraception went on to do HIV prevention work. Technocratic leadership facilitated the availability of contraception, particularly in Nigeria and Senegal, while a paucity of technocratic leaders in Malawi may explain delayed family planning and HIV interventions. Ethnic fractionalization, a sociocultural factor, complicated male circumcision programs in Malawi and hampered implementation of family planning in Nigeria, while its relative absence facilitated intimate interventions in Senegal. Finally, all three countries' marginal economic position helped bring them under the gaze of international financial institutions, with associated effects on transnational relationships.

Based on the transfers that occurred at the global level, the cross-national analysis of all sub-Saharan African countries, and the three cases, I draw several broad conclusions in the final chapter. First, relationships with global actors in addition to local organizations and histories are important to understanding responses to HIV. Thus both transnational factors – the nature of countries' interactions with the international community – as well as political factors – including the strength and composition of civil society and the existence of technocratic leaders – influenced variation in HIV prevention. Furthermore, resources, discourses, and strategies from family planning transferred to HIV via both transnational and political factors, often but not always bolstering responses to HIV.

Second, a country's history of health interventions influences outcomes associated with later health issues. Existing relationships with outside actors, NGOs, and perceptions of previous interventions structure the path of later interventions through path dependence and policy feedback. Those who wish to understand why a country seems to be a "success" or why interventions are inexplicably not leading to change must consider how history has influenced the resources, discourses, and strategies available to actors, global or local, working to address health and other development problems. The concluding chapter's brief examination of efforts to address maternal mortality in Malawi, Nigeria, and Senegal only strengthens this second point.

Third, and coming directly from the first two conclusions, it is clear that more money will not "solve" the problem of AIDS in Africa. While such a conclusion does not imply that less aid should be given, it should be understood that any aid that *is* given will be filtered through relationships that have histories and are more or less promoted by individual actors operating in federal ministries and national NGOs. For example, technocratic leaders who have risen as a result of AIDS and are still in positions of power when the next public health threat emerges will, all other things held equal, have a disproportionate effect on their countries' response to that new threat. Their experience may benefit that response, particularly if the new threat resembles HIV in any way, but it is also possible that their experience will leave them blind to solutions to new problems. Similarly, organizations that exist in a country because of either family planning or HIV that can retool to address a new threat will benefit the response more extensively. Countries lacking organizations will be at a disadvantage.

Fourth, and finally, despite weak states and extreme poverty, African organizations and institutions persist, function, and can have profound positive effects. The grounded analysis presented in *Intimate Interventions* puts the book in the company of others who insist on the importance of local institutions, often with deep historical roots, to achieving a diverse set of goals ranging from democracy to development (Acemoglu, Johnson, and Robinson 2001; Pritchett and Woolcock 2004; Woodberry 2012). Scholars and practitioners alike thus must remember that health interventions have histories when addressing the newest health threat, be it Ebola or noncommunicable diseases.

2 | The Intersection of the Global Population and AIDS Fields

This chapter[1] examines how and when the resources, discourses, and strategies of pregnancy prevention were translated into HIV prevention at the global level. Primarily it will focus on multilateral, bilateral, and nongovernmental donor organizations. These organizations, by virtue of the levels of aid they provide, have profoundly shaped the realm of possible interventions within African countries, and so this background sets the stage for the chapters that follow on sub-Saharan Africa as a whole, and the individual case studies of Malawi, Nigeria, and Senegal. This chapter thus describes the transnational factors from the model presented in the previous chapter so important to the analyses that follow.

Following an abbreviated history of global funding for HIV prevention, I discuss the resources, discourses, and strategies that transferred between pregnancy prevention and HIV prevention, integrating the history of population interventions where relevant. The resources – including donor funding, organizational activities, and human capital – shifted from one intimate intervention to the other. The population and AIDS fields have used remarkably similar discursive frames stressing development, security, and personal responsibility. And strategies originally developed for family planning, including social marketing, entertainment-education, and community-based programs to distribute commodities and information, were ultimately applied to HIV. Despite these connections, however, there were major barriers between the population and AIDS fields that complicated collaboration and inhibited learning, somewhat ironically because of the political and cultural sensitivities that could have brought the fields together. To make this point, I draw particularly on interviews with global population experts.[2]

---

[1] Short portions of this chapter were published in a working paper for the Center for Global Development (Robinson 2010b).
[2] References to interviews are denoted by "E" for expert and a number.

As this chapter is not intended to provide an exhaustive history of either the population or AIDS fields, I refer the reader to one of the many histories written by others, including *International Discord on Population and Development* (Kantner and Kantner 2006); *Fatal Misconception: The Struggle to Control World Population* (Connelly 2008);[3] *World Population Policies: Their Origin, Evolution, and Impact* (May 2012); *The Origins of AIDS* (Pepin 2011); *No Time to Lose: A Life in Pursuit of Deadly Viruses* (Piot 2012); and *HIV/AIDS: A Very Short Introduction* (Whiteside 2008).

HIV Prevention

The first official report of AIDS was in 1981, although the disease existed in sub-Saharan Africa before then (Chin 2007; Pepin 2011). Despite the gravity and severity of HIV, the global response to the disease was slow for several reasons. First, the absence of a cure or vaccine left health practitioners without any of the standard biomedical tools for addressing disease (Heller 2008). Second, and more importantly, HIV was highly stigmatized through its association with a number of marginalized groups, particularly homosexuals, injection drug users, and sex workers. In the US, Ronald Reagan did not mention the word "AIDS" in public until 1986 (Kaiser Family Foundation 2015a).

The World Health Organization was the first international organization to "claim" HIV. The World Health Organization, and the donors who funded it, saw the organization as the proper home for HIV in the United Nations system as it was the agency that dealt with disease. But even the World Health Organization did not immediately respond. According to Peter Piot, the first executive director of UNAIDS, at the time of the first organized meeting on AIDS in Africa in 1985, "the Africa office of [the World Health Organization] desperately did not want to get involved in anything to do with AIDS," both because they thought there were bigger health issues in sub-Saharan Africa, but also because the organization had recently shifted its emphasis towards primary health care and away from single diseases (Piot 2012: 149). The World Health Organization's response to AIDS began in 1986

---

[3] See, though, important critiques of this work by population experts John Cleland, Dennis Hodgson, and Malcolm Potts in the September 2008 issue of *Population and Development Review*.

with the Control Programme on AIDS, which morphed into the Special Programme on AIDS in 1987, and then ultimately became the Global Programme on AIDS in 1988 (Knight 2008). Under the charismatic leadership of Jonathan Mann, who convinced Director General Halfden Mahler that the organization needed to respond to AIDS, the Global Programme on AIDS emphasized a human rights approach to the epidemic that has fundamentally shaped HIV interventions to this day, particularly the emphasis on strictly confidential voluntary testing (Bayer and Edington 2009; De Cock and Johnson 1998; Gellman 2000; Merson et al. 2008; Smith and Whiteside 2010). As the staff and budget of the Global Programme on AIDS grew, however, so too did discord. Donors criticized the program for being overly medical and following a one-size-fits-all approach, most national leaders remained unwilling to commit to tackling HIV, and experts fought over whether the best strategy for addressing HIV drew from public health paradigms related to health behavior communication or should instead address the structural factors driving transmission, such as poverty, inequality, and gender discrimination (Knight 2008; Merson et al. 2008).

These criticisms, along with donor concern about infighting between the World Health Organization, the United Nations Development Programme, the United Nations Children's Fund, and the World Bank over management of HIV, resulted in a donor review of the Global Programme on AIDS in 1989 (Knight 2008). Donors wanted not only greater coordination across United Nations agencies, but also hoped for a more efficient and thus less expensive program that, if unencumbered from other mandates, might be more willing and able to address the complicated and sensitive nature of HIV/AIDS (Merson et al. 2008; UNAIDS Leadership Transition Working Group 2009). The resulting 1992 report led to a task force that proposed a new entity to coordinate the United Nations' response to AIDS, which ultimately became UNAIDS (Knight 2008). The United Nations Economic and Social Council approved a resolution for the creation of such an entity in 1994 and selected the six agencies that at the time were members of the management committee for the Global Programme on AIDS to develop a proposal for the joint program (UNAIDS Leadership Transition Working Group 2009). These organizations ultimately became the cosponsors for UNAIDS: the World Health Organization, the United Nations Children's Fund, the United Nations Development

Programme, UNFPA, the United Nations Educational, Scientific and Cultural Organization, and the World Bank (Knight 2008).[4] Peter Piot, a medical doctor and charismatic technocrat who had been the associate director of the Global Programme on AIDS, served as UNAIDS' first executive director from 1995 to 2008, when Michel Sidibé assumed the post. Despite the creation of a separate United Nations agency to address HIV, the 1990s represented a low point for the response to the global AIDS epidemic. As it became clear that no rich country was going to suffer an epidemic of monumental proportion, development assistance waned, the AIDS field struggled to organize itself, and HIV epidemics worsened in many poor countries (Merson et al. 2008).

Unlike with pregnancy prevention, where the biomedical understanding of how to prevent pregnancy existed by the time of large-scale, donor-funded interventions, HIV interventions grew up alongside the techniques for preventing HIV. It took three years after the first AIDS cases were reported in 1981 until the HIV virus was identified in 1984 (Kaiser Family Foundation 2015a). The immediate hope was that a vaccine would soon be produced, but as HIV is prone to mutation and capable of making itself unrecognizable to the body's own immune system, a successful vaccine has yet to emerge. The US Food and Drug Administration did not approve the first HIV test until 1985, the same year that a study showed definitively that male condoms were effective in preventing HIV transmission (Brier 2009; Whiteside 2008). The package of HIV interventions developed in the US in response to its own epidemic in the early 1980s thus consisted of messages about reducing risky behaviors – including anal sex, sex with prostitutes, and injection drug use – combined with voluntary, confidential counseling and testing, which emerged out of the rights-oriented perspective of the gay community in the US, and was reflected at the global level by the World Health Organization's Global Programme on AIDS. Additional steps taken in the US and other wealthy countries included securing the blood supply, as well as setting up national bodies to coordinate the response to the epidemic.

The US Food and Drug Administration approved the first antiretroviral drug to treat HIV in 1987, azidothymidine, or AZT. But it was not until

[4] There are now five additional cosponsors of UNAIDS: the Office of the United Nations High Commissioner for Refugees, the World Food Programme, the United Nations Office on Drugs and Crime, the International Labor Organization, and UN Women.

1996, fifteen years after the first AIDS diagnoses, that an antiretroviral regimen sufficiently effective to halt the progression of HIV to AIDS among the majority of patients was identified. Progress in drug research and increasing availability came in large part thanks to the activism of groups working across the globe. Even at this point, the treatment was prohibitively expensive for those living in wealthy countries, let alone the many who were HIV-positive in developing countries. Within a relatively short period of time, however, drug companies located in places like India, Brazil, and Thailand developed and began manufacturing generic antiretroviral drugs such that by the early 2000s, the cost of therapy had dramatically lowered. The availability of affordable antiretroviral therapy had a profound effect on the global response to HIV. Before such therapy, the only possible HIV interventions were either to prevent the transmission of infection, or to care for the secondary conditions of those infected with HIV. Affordable antiretroviral therapy opened up a third path: treatment.

At the same time that antiretroviral therapy options expanded and decreased in price, many began to frame AIDS as a threat to security (Elbe 2006; Prins 2004; Rushton 2010). In 1999, the US National Intelligence Council produced a National Intelligence Estimate on infectious disease, which linked infectious disease, and particularly HIV, to political, economic, and social instability in developing countries (National Intelligence Council 2000). The Estimate did not clearly state how exactly HIV/AIDS threatened US security, but the National Intelligence Council's authorship of such a report drew significant political attention to HIV. Then, in 2000, HIV became the first health issue discussed by the United Nations Security Council and resulted in a resolution that stated with very little evidentiary base that AIDS was likely both the result of violence and insecurity, and a threat to stability and security (McInnes 2006; Merson et al. 2008).

The increased availability of antiretroviral therapy and the securitization of AIDS, in the presence of a growing epidemic, ultimately led to massive global funding for AIDS through the multilateral Global Fund to Fight AIDS, Tuberculosis, and Malaria in 2002, and the US bilateral PEPFAR program in 2003.[5] The Global Fund evolved under the watch of United Nations Secretary General Kofi Annan via discussions at the

---

[5] The growth in funding for treatment and for AIDS more broadly also led to a rise in the volume of research on HIV conducted by scientists from the global North within African countries, as interrogated by Crane (2013).

2000 Group of 8 (G8) summit in Japan; the 2001 African Union Summit in Abuja; a 2001 United Nations General Assembly special session on AIDS; and the 2001 G8 summit (The Global Fund n.d.-b). The Global Fund became operational in 2002 and serves only as a fundraising and distributing mechanism; it does not actually implement any programs. It relies on voluntary contributions, with the majority coming bilaterally, and the US contributing the largest portion, ranging from one-fifth to a third of all contributions (IHME 2014). Developed in response to concerns about top-down programs and lack of transparency, to acquire a grant from the Global Fund, countries must put together a Country Coordinating Mechanism, a steering committee that consists of representatives from government, donors, civil society, and populations living with HIV/AIDS. Although the Global Fund targets three major diseases, the majority of grants have funded HIV/AIDS. Total disbursements from 2002 through 2015 summed up to US$29.03 billion, of which HIV/AIDS made up 53 percent (The Global Fund n.d.-a). Although HIV-related Global Fund grants can fund prevention, treatment, or care, a large percentage have gone to treatment, particularly in countries not receiving PEPFAR funds. Despite (or perhaps because of) its commitment to transparency, the Global Fund has been closely scrutinized and has sometimes come up lacking. For example, in Uganda, millions of dollars of Global Fund grants ended up in the personal accounts of government elites (Richey and Ponte 2011).

President George W. Bush announced PEPFAR during his 2003 State of the Union Address, stating, "Seldom has history offered a greater opportunity to do so much for so many ... To meet a severe and urgent crisis abroad tonight I propose the Emergency Plan for AIDS Relief, a work of mercy beyond all current international efforts to help the people of Africa" (*The Washington Post* 2003). A number of factors brought PEPFAR into being, including moral arguments promoted by prominent Christian leaders such as Franklin Graham (the son of Billy Graham), security concerns described above, and the need to offset the global image of a belligerent US in the post-September 11 context (Busby 2010; Donnelly 2012; Ingram 2010; Merson et al. 2012; Susser 2009). In addition, PEPFAR's focus on treatment delinked HIV from sex, and thus from the politically sensitive issue of condoms that would have complicated Congressional support, even among conservatives otherwise likely to follow the president (Dickinson 2010).

The US$15 billion program initially targeted fifteen so-called "focus" countries, chosen because of their high HIV prevalence, limited availability of funding for HIV, and extant experience with US government programs (Donnelly 2012). Thus some countries with relatively low levels of HIV but great import to US security concerns became focus countries (Ethiopia, Nigeria) and others with high levels of HIV but minimal US security import did not (Lesotho, Malawi, Swaziland). Indeed, a 2002 Intelligence Community Assessment entitled *The Next Wave of HIV/AIDS* identified Ethiopia and Nigeria (along with India, Russia, and China) as "countries of strategic importance to the United States that have large populations at risk for HIV infection" (Gordon 2002: 1). The Assessment made no distinction, however, between these two very different countries or their unique HIV epidemics. Indicating the speed with which the PEPFAR program was put together, Mozambique did not even know it had been selected as a focus country until after the fact (Timberg and Halperin 2012).

Twelve of the original fifteen PEPFAR focus countries are in sub-Saharan Africa, although when PEPFAR was reauthorized in 2008, it moved away from the focal country framework and began funding initiatives in a broader set of countries. The bulk of PEPFAR money has funded treatment – at least half since the original authorization (Kaiser Family Foundation 2015b) – while the dollars that have gone towards prevention have overwhelmingly adhered to the ABC approach: abstain, be faithful, or use a condom. Abstinence was in line with the sexual health policies promoted in the US by President Bush and conservative supporters at the time of PEPFAR's creation, and faithfulness was understood as part of Uganda's successful reduction in HIV prevalence. PEFPAR also initially included restrictions on the provision of support to sex workers, although the US Supreme Court overturned this provision in 2013. PEPFAR was reauthorized in 2008 for US$48 billion for five years with fewer restrictions placed on how the money could be spent, and extended for an additional five years in 2013. During the fiscal year 2013, PEPFAR provided antiretroviral therapy to 6.7 million people, support for HIV testing and counseling for 57.7 million people, and prevention of HIV transmission to 240,000 infants (PEPFAR 2014). PEPFAR's impact on HIV prevention is hard to discern, but there is strong cross-country and within-country evidence that it has reduced both all-cause mortality and HIV mortality (Bendavid et al. 2012; Merson et al. 2008).

The history of the global effort to combat HIV/AIDS, and the major organizations involved with it, influences the story told in the rest of this book in two related ways. First, following relative inaction in the early years of the epidemic, HIV/AIDS ultimately has come to make up the largest single piece of development assistance for health (IHME 2014). Second, and relatedly, starting in the early 2000s, the tide of HIV interventions turned very sharply towards treating, rather than preventing, HIV. In turn, the global preferences for the scope of HIV interventions have profoundly shaped what happens at the national level, and those preferences have heavily emphasized treatment for more than a decade. The following section describes how, at the global level, the resources, discourses, and strategies associated with pregnancy prevention did, and did not, transfer to HIV prevention, particularly in the years that preceded the widespread availability of affordable antiretroviral therapy.

From Pregnancy Prevention to HIV Prevention

This book argues that knowing about the history of family planning programs globally and nationally helps us understand variation in HIV interventions across countries. In analyzing the transfer between pregnancy prevention and HIV prevention at the global level, I consider the resources, discourses, and strategies associated with each intimate intervention. Although HIV interventions borrowed from family planning programs, interviews with global experts as well as analysis of United Nations documents show that divisions prevented strong collaboration between the population and AIDS fields.

Resources

Resources for pregnancy prevention and HIV prevention, broadly defined, include donor funding, organizations, and human capital. Transfers between intimate interventions occurred across all three types of resources.

Today, global donor disbursements for HIV/AIDS are approximately twice as much as those for family planning: in 2012, the most recent year for which comparable figures are available, US\$7.9 billion for AIDS and US\$4.4 billion for family planning (Kaiser Family Foundation and UNAIDS 2016; UNFPA 2014). Such was not the case in the early years of the epidemic: in 1995 only US$250 million was available for HIV globally (Pisani 2008). Analysis of funding trends over time suggests that HIV crowded out funding for other areas, such as family planning, even as it dramatically increased the overall amount of funding available for health (Lordan, Tang and Carmignani 2011; Shiffman 2008; Shiffman, Berlan, and Hafner 2009). As Figure 2.1 shows, since at least the mid-1990s, the share of donor funding for family planning services has decreased as the share for combating HIV/AIDS has increased, particularly in sub-Saharan Africa. Many have noted that the proportion of global funding directed towards AIDS far exceeds the proportion of morbidity and mortality due to AIDS (England 2007; Shiffman 2008), and the body of evidence suggests that resources *did* flow from pregnancy prevention to HIV prevention.

The transfer of these resources created divisions between the population and AIDS fields. In one population expert's words, "Neither community has been able to share the bounty when they have it."[6] At its peak resource point, each field controlled vast funds that created resentment among those from the other field,[7] and led to suspicion (partially founded) that any interest expressed by the other side in working together was motivated solely by a desire for resources.[8] Many insiders within the population field cited HIV/AIDS as a competing priority that had detracted attention from family planning (Blanc and Tsui 2005).

Many organizations that existed prior to the advent of AIDS and did work in the area of pregnancy prevention shifted to take on HIV prevention activities. Some did so early, when AIDS emerged in the 1980s, while others waited until later. HIV programs funded by US foreign aid followed the same strategy as those that preceded in population, with US NGOs implementing programs, often through local NGO partners (Merson et al. 2008). In the early days of the AIDS epidemic, family planning organizations became the "go-to" destination for donors, including faith-based ones, that could not convince developing country governments, particularly in sub-Saharan Africa, to accept their HIV money.[9] Many existing international nongovernmental organizations that had worked in health more broadly also added HIV to their agendas, such as CARE, World Vision, and

[6] E3.   [7] E5.   [8] E4.   [9] E4.

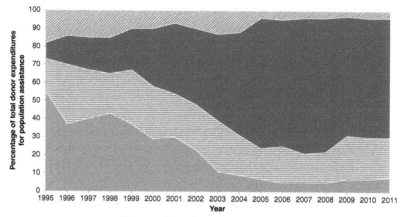

Figure 2.1. Distribution of Donor Expenditures for Population Assistance, 1995–2011
Source: UNFPA (2006; 2013).

Save the Children. The rise of HIV also created completely new organizations: the Global Fund, UNAIDS, and PEPFAR as described above, but also NGOs such as the International AIDS Alliance, the Elizabeth Glaser Pediatric AIDS Foundation, and the International Council of AIDS Service Organizations. Strikingly, however, more new AIDS NGOs formed at the national and local levels, rather than globally.

Below, I discuss the resource transfers that occurred between family planning and HIV within major international organizations, focusing on USAID, the World Bank, and UNFPA as well as the International Planned Parenthood Federation, Population Council, Ford Foundation, and Family Health International. This chapter, as well as those that follow, is biased towards the experiences of US-based organizations. While such a bias is on the one hand warranted given the overwhelming contributions these organizations have made to both family planning and HIV prevention, on the other hand it certainly excludes the important activities of a number of other organizations, including the UK's Department for International Development (DFID), the Scandinavian/Nordic bilateral aid agencies, and Marie Stopes International.

Between 1965 (when USAID was founded) and 1980, the US government provided half of all population assistance globally, with much of that money going through USAID (Donaldson 1990). Much of USAID's early focus on population can be credited to Rei Ravenholt, the director of the Office of Population from 1966–79, who strongly, and some would say overzealously, promoted population-related interventions around the world (Donaldson 1990; Hartmann 1995). USAID in particular believed that slowing population growth was a necessary precursor to economic development, and in the 1980s it funded the Futures Group to develop multiple country-specific presentations detailing the negative impacts of population growth on the economy, health care system, schools, and beyond. These presentations, called Resources for the Awareness of Population Impact on Development (RAPID), were given to policymakers and other leaders (Hartmann 1995) and are still used today, in many cases updated to PowerPoint. In addition to RAPID, USAID also operated a project called OPTIONS, which ran from 1986 to 1991 and emphasized population reduction through the promotion of family planning (Liagin 1996). Since the 1980s, USAID has also funded the Demographic and Health Surveys, the evolution of the World Fertility Survey of the 1970s and early 1980s, and the core source of demographic information for developing countries.

USAID began work on HIV/AIDS in 1986 with a US$2 million project, and funding levels quickly increased to more than US$16 million the following year when the contracts for AIDSTECH (AIDS Technical Support) and AIDSCOM (AIDS Control and Prevention) were awarded (USAID 2013). AIDSTECH ran from 1987 to 1992 with a total contract price of US$40 million and focused on prevention, including secure blood supplies, in fourteen countries, half of which were in sub-Saharan Africa (Family Health International 1997). AIDSCAP followed from 1992 to 1997 and had programs in a total of thirty-five countries, roughly half of which covered both pregnancy prevention and HIV prevention, the majority of which were in sub-Saharan Africa (Family Health International 1997). AIDSCAP was a prevention-oriented program and focused on behavior change, condom usage, and diagnosis and treatment of sexually transmitted infections. In addition to funding HIV interventions, starting in the late 1980s, the USAID-funded Demographic and Health Surveys began to collect HIV data, and today provide much of the population-based data for calculating national HIV prevalence.

Those critical of USAID's emphasis on condoms in the fight against AIDS have seen the roots of that strategy in the history of family planning or as the result of AIDS prevention money disproportionately going through family planning organizations (Green 2011; Timberg and Halperin 2012). Family Health International instead saw benefits from the connections to family planning, noting in their final report for AIDSCAP that behavior change communication for HIV drew from experiences with family planning and that "The use of social marketing to promote and deliver condoms for the prevention of HIV and other [sexually transmitted infections] has not differed fundamentally in technique from the family planning efforts, especially in its basic, mass marketing approach" (Family Health International 1997: 90).

USAID's experience with family planning strongly shaped the organization's perception of AIDS. In the early days of AIDS, the head of USAID's HIV/AIDS office, Jeffrey Harris, reached out to the family planning bureau believing that their experience with sexual behavior would be relevant to AIDS. He received little support, however, because the family planning bureau was contending with the challenges of the Mexico City Policy[10] and did not want another controversial issue like AIDS (Behrman 2004). In the 1990s USAID lobbied *against* Congressional earmarks for AIDS, which some have interpreted as USAID protecting its family planning turf (Piot 2012), and others have seen as due to fatigue from battling Congress over foreign aid, particularly for family planning (Gellman 2000). At the same time, many of those working at USAID felt that problems such as population growth and diseases leading to infant and child mortality in sub-Saharan Africa should be prioritized given they affected more people and had known interventions, unlike AIDS, which had no vaccine or cure (Gellman 2000; Piot 2012). In addition, those in a position to address AIDS at USAID knew that the portfolio would come with no

---

[10] Also referred to as the Global Gag Rule, the Mexico City Policy restricts foreign nongovernmental organizations receiving US funds from engaging in any activities related to abortion, including education or referral, even with funds received from non-US sources. President Reagan put the policy in place in 1984 at the United Nations population conference in Mexico City, it was lifted in 1993, reinstated in 2001, lifted in 2009, and then reinstated in 2017.

money and no staff, and was very politically and culturally sensitive in the US and elsewhere.[11] Thus while characteristics of USAID's family planning programs strongly influenced early HIV interventions, the history of family planning kept the organization from strongly embracing HIV.

The World Bank most emphasized the impact of population growth on economic development during the 1970s and early 1980s (Fair 2008). Robert McNamara, president from 1968 to 1981, promoted this emphasis as did the findings from the Pearson Commission, which made recommendations for the Bank's activities for the 1970s (Gibbon 1992; McNamara 1984). McNamara sought out and was influenced by the advice of Bernard Berelson, president of the Population Council, regarding the positive role of population planning and contraceptive use in reducing population growth (Gibbon 1992). In 1972, the Bank created a Population Projects Department, but its population activities in the mid-1970s were ultimately not very extensive because its lending focused on infrastructure and because it doubted that developing country governments would accept interest-bearing, repayable loans to provide family planning services (Johnson 1987; Kantner and Kantner 2006). By the 1980s, however, the Bank's involvement in population-related activities accelerated, particularly in sub-Saharan Africa (Gibbon 1992; Mosley and Branic 1989; Sinding 1991). The 1984 *World Development Report* emphasized the relationship between population and development, and in 1986 the Bank published, *Population Growth and Policies in Sub-Saharan Africa* (World Bank 1986), which specifically highlighted the negative relationship between population growth and socioeconomic development on the continent. During these years, President Conable and Vice-Presidents Stern and Jaycox promoted population concerns with African and other developing country leaders (Conly and Epp 1997). Simultaneously, the Bank's use of structural adjustment programs the world over, and particularly in sub-Saharan Africa, gave it (and the International Monetary Fund) a high degree of leverage to promote reduction in population growth for socioeconomic development. The Bank also supported production and distribution of many of the RAPID presentations described above.[12]

[11] E4.
[12] The Bank's position on the relationship between population growth and socioeconomic development has gone through several further iterations, first with a de-emphasis following the 1986 publication of the National Academies of

The Bank's first AIDS project was in the Democratic Republic of the Congo, then Zaire, in 1988 (Fair 2008). This was also the Bank's first free-standing project for a single disease. That same year, the Africa Technical Department prepared a report on AIDS and the Bank. For the most part, though, with the exception of being one of the co-sponsors of UNAIDS in 1996, the Bank remained relatively unengaged in HIV activities until the late 1990s. By that point, the Bank had become the largest financier of development assistance for health globally (Fair 2008) and had begun to emphasize the negative impacts of HIV/AIDS on development, particularly in sub-Saharan Africa (Ruger 2005). In those intervening years, the Bank had also shifted its focus away from explicit family planning programs and more towards health systems and health more broadly (Conly and Epp 1997). Thus in 1997 the Bank published *Confronting AIDS: Public Priorities in a Global Epidemic* (Ainsworth and Over 1997). Due to the lobbying of two Bank employees committed to AIDS, Debrework Zewdie and Hans Binswanger, in 1999 the Bank formed The AIDS Campaign Team for Africa, ACT*Africa*, to coordinate its response to HIV in sub-Saharan Africa (Harman 2010). In 2000, the Bank made a US$500 million commitment to AIDS through the first phase of the Multi-Country AIDS Program, and again gave the same amount for the second phase in 2002 (Fair 2008). Relevant to individual-country responses to AIDS, the Bank made the creation of a national AIDS commission, a centralized national body to coordinate the country's response to HIV, a condition for receiving Multi-Country AIDS Program funding (Harman 2010). Thus while some early Bank-led AIDS interventions were part of the Bank's work on family planning, other forces motivated most of the Bank's AIDS work, such as the good governance agenda of the 1990s and the conviction that HIV negatively impacted development (Harman 2010).

UNFPA became operational in 1969, reflecting the emergence of the global population field as well as particular interest from the US in slowing population growth globally. As a fund reliant on voluntary contributions, as opposed to a specialized agency that could depend on assessed contributions, UNFPA made it possible to sidestep

Science report finding some, but not extensive, evidence of a link between the two (National Research Council 1986), and then with a re-emphasis in the 2000s related to greater interest in the demographic dividend (e.g., Canning, Raja, and Yazbeck 2015).

controversy related to family planning and population issues in countries' general contributions to the United Nations (Johnson 1987). The US ambassador to the United Nations at the time, future US president George H.W. Bush, pushed hard for the creation of a strong population program (Donaldson 1990). President Nixon identified the United Nations as *the* organization to provide leadership in population issues (Hartmann 1995). The World Health Organization, however, felt that it had a claim to family planning that superseded the other United Nations agencies and would have preferred to incorporate family planning into its larger health mandate (Donaldson 1990; Johnson 1987). With UNFPA's support, the number of family planning programs grew from the 1950s onwards, first in Asia, then Latin America, and finally in sub-Saharan Africa in the 1980s (Sadik 2002; Singh 2002). During the 1970s and 1980s, UNFPA also funded the World Fertility Survey in slightly more than forty countries as well as the African census program (Mousky 2002).

UNFPA's involvement in HIV activities in the early years of the epidemic was minimal. UNFPA did contribute to the creation of the World Health Organization's Global Programme on AIDS by "seconding" a staff member to it (Mousky 2002) and was one of the original cosponsors of UNAIDS. But accounts of the process of UNAIDS' creation do not specifically discuss UNFPA (e.g., Knight 2008; Merson et al. 2008; Piot 2012; UNAIDS Leadership Transition Working Group 2009), and the UNFPA never really laid claim to HIV at any point. One population expert noted that UNFPA kept AIDS at "arm's length," much like USAID,[13] and another that UNFPA saw AIDS as competition for the organization's work in family planning.[14] Indeed, UNFPA publications from the late 1980s onwards mentioned HIV fairly peripherally. The UNFPA annual report first referenced AIDS in 1987, in the family planning section of the "Programme Priority Areas," which noted UNFPA was a part of the World Health Organization's Special Programme on AIDS. The 1988 and 1989 annual reports mentioned AIDS in a similar fashion – in conjunction with the World Health Organization's programs. Similarly, discussions of UNFPA's activities in the 1990s in the secondary literature authored by UNFPA staff (for example, Sadik's edited volume (2002) for the thirtieth anniversary of UNFPA) rarely mentioned AIDS. Only starting in the 1990 annual

---

[13] E4.   [14] E1.

report did UNFPA separate discussion of AIDS from the World Health Organization, and list it as a "Special Programme Interest," along with topics such as aging and youth.

As time passed, UNFPA incorporated AIDS into its work more and more. In 1992, UNFPA began producing an annual publication called *AIDS Update* that described the organization's HIV prevention activities (UNFPA n.d.). In 1993, AIDS appeared in the table of contents of the annual report for the first time, and then starting in 1995 the "Programme Priorities" section of the report included HIV. By the late 1990s and following the establishment of reproductive health as the concept orienting the population field, UNFPA's work fully incorporated HIV. A 2004 UNFPA publication even linked UNFPA's broader experience with family planning and related topics to its capacity to address HIV: "UNFPA's efforts to prevent HIV infection are built on three decades of programme experience in addressing sensitive issues such as family planning, gender and sexuality in various socio-cultural settings" (UNFPA 2004: 19). Thus UNFPA ultimately incorporated HIV throughout its work, as part of the organization's adaptation to the broader concept of reproductive health.

In addition to bilateral and intergovernmental organizations, NGOs working in family planning also incorporated AIDS into their activities in the late 1980s. The International Planned Parenthood Federation encouraged affiliate organizations around the world to add AIDS education to their family planning activities (Finger 1991) and in 1989 published a volume entitled *Preventing a Crisis: AIDS and Family Planning Work* (Gordon and Klouda 1989). Dr. Fred Sai, the organization's president from 1989 to 1995 noted in the mid-1990s that "family planning expertise is a crucial element to AIDS prevention work" (Sai 1994: 57). In 2002, the organization published *Learning from the Field: Experiences in HIV Prevention from Family Planning Associations Worldwide* (International Planned Parenthood Federation 2002).

Founded in 1952 by John D. Rockefeller III, the Population Council from the beginning played a pivotal role in the population field by promoting the importance of slowing global population growth to both US and global leaders. In addition to social demographic research on the drivers of high fertility, early on the Population Council also engaged in evaluation research of family planning programs as well as basic medical research on contraceptive devices, including the Copper

T IUD and the injectable hormonal contraception Norplant. The Population Council also funded population research centers at a number of US universities, including Princeton and the Universities of Michigan and Pennsylvania, and was closely involved in the creation of Kenya's 1967 population policy (Chimbwete, Watkins, and Zulu 2005; Sending and Neumann 2006; Warwick 1982). The Population Council's earliest HIV activities centered around research on microbicides, following a commitment to clinical research that the Council had pioneered with the development of contraceptive technologies. The Population Council's HIV prevention activities were initially focused through the Horizons project, which ran from 1997 to 2008, and was financed by USAID, a long-time funder of the Council (Crane 1993; Hartmann 1995; Rutenberg and Weiss 2010). A reorganization in the mid-2000s led to the creation of a separate HIV division, and by 2013, 28 percent of the Council's funds were used for HIV/AIDS (Population Council 2013).

The population-related work of the Ford Foundation also flowed into HIV activities, albeit somewhat slowly. Like the Population Council, the Ford Foundation at first provided support for demographic research as well as the training of demographers, and Ford was the largest source of population resources in the 1950s and 1960s (Sending and Neumann 2006; Warwick 1982). Ford's limited experience with single diseases and with health more broadly initially kept the foundation from AIDS grant making, but the AIDS-related deaths of six employees in the 1980s prompted action (Brier 2009). Ford became the second American organization to give an international AIDS-related grant (after Rockefeller) in 1987–88 (Brier 2009). In 1988, Ford gave thirteen AIDS grants to Brazil, Haiti, Thailand, Senegal, and Mexico; all but Haiti were places where Ford already had field offices working on population activities (Brier 2009).

Family Health International[15] started in 1971 as the International Fertility Research Program, a group of scholars from the University of North Carolina, Chapel Hill, studying family planning around the world (Family Health International 2010). The program became a nonprofit in 1975 with the financial support of USAID and then

---

[15] In 2011 Family Health International bought the Academy for Educational Development and became FHI 360. I refer to the organization as Family Health International given it was known as such during the period covered by the book.

changed its name to Family Health International in 1982 (Family Health International 2010; Timbs 2011). Like the Population Council, Family Health International's early work was both clinical and operational. For example, in 1984 its research showed that breast-feeding women could safely use progestin-only birth control pills (Family Health International 2010). Family Health International was already working in a number of sub-Saharan African countries when AIDS emerged, and had HIV pilot programs in Cameroon, Ghana, and Mali as early as 1986 (FHI 360 2012). Family Health International received the first contract from USAID to address HIV, AIDSTECH, that was followed by a series of multi-million dollar USAID-funded projects, including AIDSCAP and IMPACT (Implementing AIDS Prevention and Care, 1998–2007). Family Health International's experience with family planning clearly shaped how they addressed HIV. The organization justified its capacity to carry out the contract for AIDSTECH based on its experience with family planning and the similarities between family planning and HIV interventions regarding behavior change and technology distribution (Timbs 2011). A 1990 handbook on AIDS prevention in sub-Saharan Africa published by Family Health International included a chapter entitled "AIDS Prevention in Family Planning Programs" (Williamson and Boohene 1990). The chapter noted that family planning services were generally not well developed in sub-Saharan African countries, but argued for the ways in which family planning programs could facilitate HIV prevention, concluding that: "Family planning managers have already demonstrated their willingness to take on one highly controversial issue, namely family planning in Africa. With financial and technical assistance, the same people can apply their experience to AIDS preven-tion, an even more controversial area, while ensuring that family plan-ning programs fulfill their important mission of delivering family planning services" (Williamson and Boohene 1990: 208). In its AIDS work, Family Health International even used a family planning manual produced by the NGO PATH and ultimately worked with PATH to formally adapt the manual for HIV (Zimmerman et al. 2002).

The examples above demonstrate greater flexibility, and perhaps willingness, on the part of nongovernmental organizations than gov-ernmental and intergovernmental organizations in adding HIV pre-vention to their portfolios. That neither the World Bank nor UNFPA immediately began work on HIV, despite opportunities for doing so, could well be due to both organizations being part of the United Nations system and so ceding the management of AIDS first to the World Health Organization, and then to UNAIDS. In particular, given that UNFPA had had to fight regular battles about family planning and abortion, avoiding a stigmatized disease with no cure and no vaccine was perhaps not surprising. In contrast, the World Health Organization tried to hold on to both family planning and HIV, believing each to be integral parts of the broader public health agenda it promoted, and thus published a manual connecting family planning and HIV, *Family Planning and AIDS Prevention: Technical and Managerial Guidelines* (World Health Organization 1989).

In interviews, global population experts described how those involved with family planning often distanced themselves from HIV for fear that the hard-fought ground they had won regarding family planning and abortion would be lost via association with a highly stigmatized disease. As one expert described the context, "The history of family planning and HIV is a bizarre ping pong game of who or what is most stigmatized. They are two communities that should be natural allies by virtue of both dealing with people having sex, but have more frequently been competitors."[16] Gruskin (2009) confirmed these patterns and has described the two fields as running parallel to one another. In particular, she noted that "HIV shed light on many thorny issues around sexual behavior and sexuality that the reproductive health community had been more than happy to keep off the table in order to engage more easily with governments and other conservative forces" (Gruskin 2009: 126). In particular, in the absence of extensive demand for family planning, the population field focused on creating a positive environment for family planning and thought that inclusion of a sexually transmitted infection would stigmatize their other activities. At the same time, actors in the AIDS field kept their own distance because they felt family planning and fertility reduction brought stigma and sensitivities in target countries, particularly with policymakers, while simultaneously de-emphasizing male reproductive decision-making and the needs of adolescents not yet focused on "family" planning.[17]

Population experts noted other factors that prevented greater collaboration between the population and AIDS fields. At the beginning

[16] E3.   [17] E3.

of the HIV epidemic, HIV was seen as a disease of gay men, a distinctly different population from the women on whom the population field so closely focused.[18] According to one expert, "The last thing family planners wanted in the late 1980s/early 1990s was to get involved in extramarital, premarital, same-sex, or transactional sex."[19] The initial response to HIV also drew heavily from public health approaches, which had never been the population field's strategy.[20] The Millennium Development Goals, which separated reproductive health and HIV/AIDS between goals five and six, only reflected and magnified these distinctions.[21]

As a result of these divisions, individuals and organizations involved with HIV were minimally present at the United Nations International Conference on Population and Development in Cairo in 1994 despite the fact that the umbrella term "reproductive health" institutionalized by the conference included HIV (O'Malley 2004). As one expert explained, "HIV was hardly on the agenda at the conference."[22] Divisions that existed at the global level among academics and donors trickled down to the local level (Gruskin 2009). For example, at one point, UNFPA said that condoms designated for family planning could not be used for HIV prevention, while UNAIDS said that AIDS condoms could not be used for family planning.[23] Similarly, the widespread provision of free condoms for HIV prevention threatened the population field's greater embrace of social marketing of condoms for pregnancy prevention (described in greater detail below).[24] At the local level, those providing sexual and reproductive health services were concerned that HIV would stigmatize their work, while those providing HIV care wanted to focus on populations beyond married women and feared that those who worked in family planning were ill-equipped to address questions of sexuality and marginalized populations associated with HIV (Gruskin 2009). So while the organizations in the population field influenced the AIDS field, a number of factors kept the two fields further apart than might otherwise have been expected, given the centrality of human sexuality to both.

Human capital is the final resource that transferred from pregnancy prevention to HIV prevention. Much of this human capital worked for the organizations described above, first in family planning and then either incorporating HIV into their agendas as their organizations

[18] E3.   [19] E5.   [20] E2.   [21] E3.   [22] E1.   [23] E1.   [24] E3.

changed, or shifting almost entirely to HIV. Individuals such as John Bongaarts (Population Council), Peter Lamptey (Family Health International), and Malcolm Potts (International Planned Parenthood Federation, Family Health International) all had exceptionally strong family planning credentials, but then also worked on HIV. John Bongaarts is a demographer whose research has focused primarily on topics related to fertility and mortality, but published work on the demographic impact of HIV from 1988 through the mid-1990s, conducted early work on the connection between male circumcision and HIV, and then again published on HIV in the 2000s. As a vice president at the Population Council, his background has had the capacity to influence the organization's work. Peter Lamptey has been a major player at Family Health International since the 1980s, serving as the director of all three HIV programs that USAID funded through the organization (AIDSTECH, AIDSCAP, and IMPACT). Prior to that, however, he worked for a USAID-funded family planning project in his native Ghana (Center for Strategic and International Studies n.d.). Malcolm Potts, the former medical director of the International Planned Parenthood Federation and a key global advocate for safe abortion, has described himself as helping "initiate the first HIV prevention initiatives in Africa" while the CEO of Family Health International from 1978 to 1990 (Potts et al. 2013: 2) and has published on HIV as well (e.g., Potts et al. 2008). Jyoti Shankar Singh, a division director at UNFPA, lobbied to be the first head of UNAIDS and was interviewed for the post.[25] A combination of overlapping interests between fertility studies and HIV alongside increasing resources for HIV meant that many of the best people in family planning also came to work on HIV.[26] While such shifts are easiest to observe among organizational leadership, they certainly also occurred at lower ranks within organizations.

Within academia, research on AIDS by demographers initially focused primarily on technical aspects of the disease, such as its influence on population size and thus population projections (Gregson 2003). But ultimately transfer between pregnancy prevention and HIV prevention occurred in academia, as many prominent demographers

[25] E3. The selection of Peter Piot instead led to a sense among those within UNFPA that UNAIDS was not supportive of family planning and reproductive health, which further increased divisions between the two fields.

[26] E2, E3.

who had studied fertility and contraceptive use began to study HIV, including its social aspects. John Caldwell, Pat Caldwell, John Knodel, and Susan Cotts Watkins were all well-respected demographers study-ing fertility who then prominently incorporated HIV into their research agendas.

Across many dimensions the resources built up to provide family planning were deployed to help prevent HIV. To the dismay of the population field, funding did shift from pregnancy prevention to HIV prevention, and then to HIV treatment. The vast majority of organiza-tions that worked in pregnancy prevention went on to do work in HIV prevention. Shifting funding patterns drove at least part of this transi-tion – organizations need resources to survive – but organizations also actively applied their family planning expertise gained globally and in countries to HIV. Finally, valuable human capital in the form of people working both for organizations but also doing research directed their skills and know-how gained from family planning to the new problem of AIDS. In the following chapter, I turn to addressing how these shifts in resources influenced changes in HIV prevalence and incidence as well as antiretroviral coverage within the context of sub-Saharan Africa.

Discourses

A number of discursive similarities exist between population and HIV interventions, in particular regarding how proponents have framed the issues to generate political priority (McInnes and Lee 2012; Shiffman and Smith 2007). Both population growth and HIV have been treated as emergencies, the causes of underdevelopment, problems with rights-based solutions, and drivers of insecurity. In considering individual outcomes, scholars and programmers have assumed individual respon-sibility as the cause and solution to unwanted fertility and HIV trans-mission, often ignoring the structural drivers of each.

The population and AIDS fields have each successfully framed their issue as an emergency (Cleland and Watkins 2006b; Foley and Hendrixson 2011). The population field in the 1960s used the threat of a population "bomb" (Ehrlich 1969) to generate support for family planning and large-scale intimate interventions, while from the earliest years of the epidemic activists and public health programmers loudly argued that AIDS was an emergency. The emergency frame for AIDS gained the most attention once a biomedical intervention –

antiretroviral therapy – became available, providing a politically palatable solution. Coupling a sense of emergency with a discourse of moral obligation in the presence of affordable treatment made AIDS difficult for policymakers and funders to ignore (Busby 2010). Indeed, President Bush's reference to PEPFAR as an "act of mercy" drew on moral obligation, which had strong roots in the compassionate conservatism and evangelical Christianity of his base.

Those advocating for intimate interventions have blamed both population growth and the HIV epidemic for negative development outcomes. A belief that population growth would slow or hinder socioeconomic development motivated family planning programs starting from the late 1950s and still does today. Similarly, in the 1990s concern arose about the negative impact of HIV on development, and some saw the solution to AIDS through participatory development. The position was championed by Elizabeth Reid, who founded and directed the United Nations Development Programme's HIV and Development Programme from 1992 to 1997. The HIV and Development Programme was in part a corrective to what was viewed as an overly medicalized response to HIV from the World Health Organization.[27] The perceived (negative) effects of AIDS on development grew through the 1990s, in part prompting the World Bank's greater involvement with the disease (Ruger 2005). More recently, UNAIDS and the United Nations Development Programme have again promoted the links between HIV and development within the context of the Millennium Development Goals as a means to maintain priority for HIV (Woodling, Williams, and Rushton 2012).

The population and AIDS fields have also both made extensive use of rights discourse. The population field has long promoted the right of individual couples to freely determine the number of children they bear, and rights discourse reached a peak in the 1990s. At this point, in conjunction with the 1994 United Nations International Conference on Population and Development, reproductive health became a right. Proponents of access to HIV prevention, care and treatment have also tapped into macro-level rights discourses (Rushton 2010; Seidel 1993),

---

[27] The World Health Organization had however partnered with the United Nations Development Programme in 1988 to form the World Health Organization -UNDP Alliance to Combat AIDS in order to have some point of access other than weak health ministries for its programs in developing countries (Jönsson and Söderholm 1995).

starting from Jonathan Mann and producing an emphasis on the voluntariness and confidentiality of HIV testing that pervades the response to the epidemic globally.

Finally, in an effort to generate support, actors in the population and AIDS fields have linked their issues to (in)security. In the early era of the population movement, fears about large, poor populations becoming communist motivated and justified interventions (Wilmoth and Ball 1992), and have resurfaced more recently as concerns have grown about the impact of youth "bulges" in conflict and other forms of instability (Goldstone 2010; Goldstone, Kaufmann, and Toft 2012; Leahy 2007). Turning HIV into a security issue through the National Intelligence Council's 1999 report and the United Nations Security Council's 2000 resolution helped garner support for action on HIV from the highest levels, even though there is much academic debate about the actual relationship between HIV and security (Barnett and Prins 2006; McInnes 2006; Paxton 2012). Somewhat ironically, in the late 1980s sub-Saharan Africa's rapid population growth served as justification for the Central Intelligence Agency to *avoid* investigating AIDS. Some within the agency believed that AIDS would help solve overpopulation, and that it was unlikely to weaken African militaries that could be replenished by large populations (Gellman 2000).

Discourse about individual responsibility permeates both pregnancy prevention and HIV prevention, and treats the avoidance of pregnancy and HIV as the unquestionable primary goal of individual sexual behavior. The discourse about pregnancy prevention has focused primarily on women, and on the need for individual women to adopt contraceptive technologies in order to reduce their overall number of children, as well as to space their births further apart. A substantial component of this discourse must work to explain women's non-use of contraception in situations where they do not want more children, a so-called "unmet need" for contraception. This discourse of individual responsibility fails to treat women, and people more broadly, as members of families, communities, and markets who can simultaneously hold conflicting desires, who may be pulled in different directions at the same time, and who often have imperfect access to services and technology.

In parallel, the discourses of safe sex and abstinence make staying HIV-negative, and not transmitting HIV if HIV-positive, the responsibility of the individual, a responsibility which can be achieved through abstinence, condom usage, or faithfulness to an HIV-negative partner (Esacove 2013). It is assumed that staying HIV-negative through condom usage will trump all other goals and objectives, such as intimacy, pregnancy, continued trust in the relationship, or even health itself (Smith 2004b; Tavory and Swidler 2009). There are twinges of racism and patriarchy in the discourse about both family planning and HIV, where the solution to overproducing (African) female bodies is long-lasting contraceptive methods that are difficult to individually control. Similarly, the "problem" of HIV is attributed to the differential, even hyper-, sexuality of Africans, and in particular to the multiple concurrent sexual partnerships believed to be driving HIV transmission (Epstein and Morris 2011).

A key discursive element that likely inhibited transfer from pregnancy prevention to HIV prevention is the extent to which programmers divorced pregnancy prevention from sex. Such a divorce has been necessary to win support for family planning at the global level as well as in individual countries, and as a result, contraceptive technology has been described euphemistically. As a synonym for contraception, "family planning" makes technologies and techniques to prevent pregnancy – concrete actions to make an outcome *not* occur – sound as if though they are instead actions to create a family. The very direct term "birth control" has long been out of favor with the population field because it has not always been clear whether the people doing the "controlling" are the women in question, or the external actors interested in slowing population growth. "Child spacing" has been particularly popular in countries with strong opposition to contraception, as will be seen in particular in the chapter on Malawi that follows, and its usage has facilitated the provision of services by connecting traditional concepts to modern technology (Kaler 2003). "Reproductive health" is a much broader concept than family planning, but to the extent that it is treated as a synonym for family planning in many developing countries, it also distances pregnancy prevention from sex. Such euphemisms emerged in large part to depoliticize pregnancy prevention. This depoliticization comes at the cost of potentially reducing emphasis on contraception (Cleland et al. 2006; Luke and Watkins 2002), while simultaneously minimalizing discussion of sex. The separation of pregnancy prevention interventions from sex has surely hampered the transfer of lessons learned to HIV prevention, which is more difficult to disentangle from sex (Pigg and Adams 2005). Indeed, those writing on the topic at the beginning of the epidemic were keenly aware of sexuality's more explicit connection with HIV prevention than with family planning (Pachauri 1994; Williamson and Boohene 1990). Demonstrating the need to delink health interventions from sex in order to generate broad support, it was only with HIV treatment, which takes sex off the table, that major donor funding became available for HIV. As Duff Gillespie, a long-time USAID administrator, put it: "What happened [with treatment] is that it took sex out of AIDS" (as quoted in Boseley 2011).

While the discourses associated with HIV could have emerged regardless of those used by the population field, it is nonetheless striking that both fields have used essentially the same discourses to justify both intimate interventions. Looking at both sets of discourse in tandem reveals overly simplistic interpretations of both high fertility and HIV transmission on the part of programmers, academics, and even sometimes activists. These interpretations have limited the reach of social programs that otherwise have the potential to empower people and prevent both unwanted pregnancy and disease. At the same time, the divorce of pregnancy prevention from sex made it more difficult to transfer resources and strategies from one intimate intervention to the other.

Strategies

Programmers from the global to the local levels have used similar strategies across intimate interventions in order to try to change the ways in which people have sex and to deliver the technology to facilitate their doing so. Condoms, stand-alone vertical programs, social marketing, entertainment-education, and community-based distribution are all examples of technical strategies that the AIDS field borrowed from the population field.

The male condom prevents both pregnancy and HIV with approximately equivalent effectiveness of about 85–90 percent (Hearst and Chen 2004; Trussell 2011). Prior to HIV, the condom was, however, rarely promoted as a pregnancy prevention technique among married women, particularly in sub-Saharan Africa, where long-lasting, female-controlled methods were stressed instead (Zaba, Boerma, and Marchant 1998). The dual function of condoms has, however, been consistently promoted to sex workers, and to some extent adolescents, with the capacity of condoms to protect against sexually transmitted infections often emphasized more than their ability to prevent pregnancy. Unlike married women, it has been socially and politically acceptable to assume that sex workers do not want to father children with their clients, that unmarried adolescents would be ashamed to become pregnant, and that both groups are at risk for sexually transmitted infections.

Both family planning and HIV programs have frequently run parallel to general health programs. Vertical family planning programs, so called because they were unintegrated with other, related health areas or broader programs to improve primary health care, offered two potential advantages. First, they created a means to provide family planning in a context where programmers believed overall health systems to be too weak to incorporate family planning programs. Second, they highlighted the importance of family planning in a way that some believed necessary in order to garner sufficient political and financial support (Singh 2002). Vertical HIV programs offered the same benefits, a strategy for ensuring resources that people responding to HIV had seen work earlier for family planning.[28]

Social marketing, which uses techniques from commercial marketing in order to promote positive behavior change (Grier and Bryant 2005), is a strategy used heavily in pregnancy prevention programs, and which transferred to HIV prevention programs. Within social marketing, the item to be consumed can be a thing (pills or condoms), a behavior (safe sex), or a belief (people should only have two children) (Walsh et al. 1993). Social marketing in most developing countries, including in sub-Saharan Africa, takes the form of organizations selling highly subsidized, branded commodities, such as condoms, pills, and injectables, as well as bed nets and water purification tablets. The presumption behind social marketing is that people will value, and be more likely to use, a product for which they have paid something, even if it is only a small amount. Social marketing campaigns related to family planning began in developing countries in the 1970s, in part because of the rise of popularity of the idea of social marketing, but also because programmers were trying to increase contraceptive usage beyond the low levels achieved by clinic-based distribution programs (Walsh et al. 1993).

[28] E1.

When AIDS emerged, donors then rapidly expanded social marketing of condoms (Sweat et al. 2012). As one population expert explained, social marketing of condoms was a relatively "easy" program for donors to enact, and so it became popular practically overnight.[29] Social marketing campaigns are appealing to donors because they are relatively cost efficient to implement, and they reflect a neoliberal preference for market solutions to health problems (Pfeiffer 2004). Today, most countries in sub-Saharan Africa have one or more country-specific condom brands that are socially marketed. Rigorous studies on the effectiveness of condom social marketing programs are few, but suggest significant positive effects on both condom sales and condom usage (Sweat et al. 2012). Cleland and Ali (2006) attribute increased condom usage among young women in sub-Saharan Africa in part to such programs. The key international NGOs engaged in social marketing activities for HIV all started as family planning organizations and include Population Services International, Marie Stopes International, and DKT International (Pfeiffer 2004). For example, Population Services International was founded in 1970 as a social marketing organization for family planning products, has partner organizations on the ground in numerous countries, and implemented their first AIDS project in 1988 (Population Services International n.d.-b).

Pregnancy prevention and HIV prevention interventions have also both relied on entertainment-education, or "edutainment," a cousin of social marketing that combines education with entertainment to increase the audience's retention of the educational message, and thus to promote behavior change. The most effective form of edutainment relies on serialized dramas for either radio or television that contain specific types of characters to serve as role models. The serial drama aspect of edutainment is particularly important to producing behavior change because it allows for the development of characters, as well as the attachment of the audience to those characters, such that when characters change, it is believable, and replicable, by audience members (Barker 2009). The so-called Sabido methodology was first used in Mexico in the 1970s by Miguel Sabido, the vice president for research at the Mexican national television network. Sabido produced a series of soap operas to "sell" a variety of positive behavior changes (rather than soap), including the use of family planning (Barker 2009).

---

[29] E4.

Randomized control studies have shown the effectiveness of such programs (Vaughan and Rogers 2000) and indicate that programs that follow the Sabido methodology are more effective than simple entertainment-education, most likely because they do the best job of increasing self-efficacy (Barker 2009). Although the exact contribution of Sabido's dramas to Mexican fertility decline is impossible to measure, between 1976 and 1985, Mexico's population growth rate decreased by a third, and as a result, Mexico received the United Nations Population Prize in 1986 (Barker 2009). Even in cases where the Sabido methodology has not been strictly followed, soap operas promoting small families through the usage of contraception (as well as "modern" lifestyles with ample consumption) have been credited with facilitating fertility decline, particularly in Brazil (La Ferrara, Chong and Duryea 2008). Two organizations in particular have facilitated the spread of dramas deploying the Sabido methodology: the US-based NGO Population Communications International and the Johns Hopkins Center for Communication Programs. Both organizations started with family planning, and then expanded their work to include HIV. Notable examples of Sabido-style dramas focusing on AIDS include *Soul City* in South Africa (1994–present) and *Twende na Wakati* (Let's Go with the Times, 1993–2002) in Tanzania, with almost a third of the educational content focused on family planning (Vaughan et al. 2000).

Community-based distribution is a final technique that began with pregnancy prevention, and then was adopted as an HIV intervention. It refers to the use of community organizations and members to distribute health information and supplies as well as to refer clients to clinics. Community-based distribution has been promoted both as a means to compensate for minimal health resources (often in rural areas) and to motivate new or continuing users. The technique assumes that people will be more likely to change their behavior if urged to do so by someone from their community, and if they do not have to go to a clinic to obtain the necessary supplies. Most often the distributors volunteer all or part of their time, but are sometimes compensated with items like bicycles or radios. Community-based distribution of contraception began in the 1960s in Asia and soon spread to Latin America. In both regions, programmers believed the technique increased contraceptive use, so then applied it to sub-Saharan Africa (Janowitz et al. 2000; Phillips, Greene and Jackson 1999). USAID, UNFPA, and the German bilateral aid agency have all been strong promoters of community-based distribution programs for contraception (Janowitz et al. 2000). Despite a lack of strong evidence that community-based distribution was actually an effective means for increasing contraceptive usage in sub-Saharan Africa (Phillips, Greene, and Jackson 1999), the technique was adopted as an HIV intervention. Specifically, such programs have included information and condom distribution, as well as testing and counseling. Analysis of these interventions has found that people are much more likely to be tested for HIV when it is convenient, including in their homes (Angotti et al. 2009; McKenna et al. 1997; Menzies et al. 2009).

Social marketing programs, entertainment-education, and community-based distribution programs have frequently addressed pregnancy prevention and HIV prevention simultaneously. In addition, there have been concerted attempts at several key points to directly integrate pregnancy prevention and HIV prevention interventions within health systems and clinics under the logic that because family planning is frequently the only way that African women interact with the health care system, this integration will expose women to other services, increase efficiency, and reduce costs (Lush et al. 2001; Stover, Dougherty, and Ham 2006). Discussion about integration of family planning and HIV interventions within health systems emerged in particular following the 1994 United Nations International Conference on Population and Development. The Programme of Action promoted the integration of family planning with services for sexually transmitted infections and HIV (Lush et al. 2001). At the time, those espousing integration pointed to all that had been learned from family planning programs about changing sexual behavior and that could be applied to integrated programs (Pachauri 1994). As a result of the conference, some donor countries (although not the US) integrated their until-then independent HIV/AIDS activities into broader reproductive health mandates (Merson et al. 2008). Similarly, following the conference, many countries attempted to integrate HIV and family planning services. Results have, however, been mixed because of the challenges associated with merging two vertical programs, overcoming resistance to coordination and cooperation among staff, training workers to provide the additional services, and carrying out the integration in the context of general donor preference for HIV/AIDS over family planning (Adeokun et al. 2002;

Blanc and Tsui 2005; Lush et al. 2001; Stover, Dougherty, and Ham 2006; Strachan et al. 2004; Zaba, Boerma, and Marchant 1998).

Some years after the 1994 United Nations International Conference on Population and Development and the overwhelming shift in funding towards HIV, a new wave of research has appeared that focuses on integrating family planning services into HIV programs. This research has identified increased usage of family planning and referrals to family planning when those services are integrated into HIV services, as well as generally positive benefits to integration overall (Johnson, Varallyay, and Ametepi 2012; Wilcher et al. 2013). Renewed interest in integration was in part tied to the drive to achieve the Millennium Development Goals by 2015, which required both reducing HIV prevalence and maternal mortality, and to meeting UNAIDS' goal of zero new infections, targets which persist in the post-2015 Sustainable Development Goals. One of the four pillars of the prevention of mother-to-child transmission of HIV is contraception to prevent unwanted pregnancies among HIV-positive women. In addition, as the volume of funding available for AIDS has grown, attempts to leverage that funding to achieve outcomes beyond AIDS have increased. In particular, the Global Fund's Round 9 funding focused specifically on health systems strengthening, which countries could link to any of the Fund's three primary diseases. Many of the programmers I interviewed in Malawi, Nigeria, and Senegal for the case studies that follow saw the potential to increase family planning services through linking them to HIV.

Pregnancy prevention and HIV prevention thus share many technologies and techniques, most of which emerged alongside contraceptive promotion, and some of which have been used in tandem to promote both contraceptive use and HIV prevention.

Conclusion

Resources, discourses, and strategies transferred from pregnancy prevention to HIV prevention at the global level. Such transfers were facilitated in large part by the organizations that worked on family planning, many of which had connections with countries in sub-Saharan Africa that were hit first and hardest by HIV. I conclude the chapter with some thoughts on whether the transfers were beneficial or not to HIV prevention.

The resources that came from pregnancy prevention – including funding, organizations, and people – have benefitted HIV prevention insofar as they provided resources and expertise on the ground when HIV first emerged. I return to this question more specifically in the following chapter on sub-Saharan Africa, but at the global level, it is clear that after a short period of hesitation, USAID in particular picked up with HIV activities from where they had been working both conceptually and geographically on pregnancy prevention. The same is true for the Population Council and Ford Foundation, as well as for major international NGOs such as Family Health International, International Planned Parenthood Federation, and Population Services International. The notable absence of transfer is within the United Nations system, where both the UNFPA and the World Bank did not engage deeply with HIV prevention until the late 1990s. One interpretation for the lack of engagement is that first the World Health Organization and then UNAIDS served as the agencies responsible for AIDS within the United Nations division of labor, thus relieving UNFPA and the World Bank of responsibility. In addition, as member organizations accountable to all countries in the world, the political risk to taking on a stigmatized issue like HIV was likely formidable, particularly to UNFPA. Such concerns were minimalized in nongovernmental organizations and foundations that did not have to answer to as wide of a constituency.

The process of transfers of resources, discourses, and strategies has not come without cost. For example, most research suggests that even though HIV increased the volume of funding available for health, family planning lost attention and funding. Whether family planning might now benefit from increased emphasis on integration and health systems strengthening achieved through funding for HIV is an open question. Discourses common to both family planning and HIV prevention stressing individual responsibility are problematic given that both pregnancy and HIV transmission at the bare minimum require an interaction between two people, but more broadly, are situated within the context of families, communities, and markets. Some have argued that the emphasis of the population field on reducing fertility and population growth, rather than on lowering infant mortality and improving women's and children's health overall, hampered its success, and that the same mistakes were repeated with HIV interventions (Mhloyi 1995; Stillwaggon

2006). Many critique HIV interventions for being overly individualistic and insufficiently focused on the structural drivers of the epidemic, but without blaming the history of pregnancy prevention (e.g., Auerbach, Parkhurst, and Cáceres 2011).

In sum, the global response to HIV bears the imprint of the population interventions that preceded it. Many of the international organizations important to HIV interventions began their work with pregnancy prevention and brought with them strategies from their earlier activities. The impacts of these transfers were, however, both positive and negative. As much as they provided resources for a stigmatized disease that was otherwise neglected for many years, such connections provided easy opportunities for the flaws of pregnancy prevention programs to repeat themselves with HIV prevention. In addition, the divorce of pregnancy prevention from sex, a framing technique used by the population field to win support for family planning, made linking it to HIV prevention all the more complicated, as HIV was even harder to distance from sex than contraception. With these global trends in mind, in the following chapter, I begin to analyze how these relationships between pregnancy prevention and HIV prevention played out in the context of sub-Saharan Africa.

3 | From Family Planning to HIV Prevention in Sub-Saharan Africa

While the previous chapter focused on intimate interventions globally, this chapter discusses trends in intimate interventions across sub-Saharan Africa. I return to the model developed in Chapter 1, focusing on how the transnational factors elaborated in the previous chapter along with domestic political, sociocultural, and economic factors influenced intimate interventions across countries. After a brief discussion of political, sociocultural, and economic factors across sub-Saharan African countries, I present background on trends in fertility and HIV prevalence, as well as on the general contours of intimate interventions. Most sub-Saharan African countries did not begin offering family planning programs until the late 1970s or early 1980s, and HIV prevention dates exclusively from the mid-1980s, after the first cases of AIDS were diagnosed. The chapter then addresses the book's overall question about the links between family planning and HIV interventions through statistical analyses of all sub-Saharan African countries, thus setting the stage for the case study chapters that follow. These analyses support the argument that the history of family planning helps explain variation in responses to HIV across countries.

Political, Sociocultural, and Economic Factors in Sub-Saharan Africa

Generally speaking, sub-Saharan African countries share a number of characteristics that have made them vulnerable to the development prescriptions, including intimate interventions, promoted by transnational actors. They are some of the newest, and most fragile, states in the world, most having gained independence only in the 1960s and many having experienced significant and/or consistent conflict in the intervening years. NGOs, a political factor, have increased in number in all countries since the 1990s, in many instances spearheading interventions, or taking up duties that would be carried out by the state in a higher resource context. The arbitrary boundaries of sub-Saharan African countries have left most countries highly diverse, and religion in its many variants figures heavily in the lives of the majority of people, rendering sociocultural factors salient to a number of outcomes. As a result, the state is but one source of authority that must compete with other voices. Economic characteristics also matter to intimate interventions, as sub-Saharan African countries are some of the poorest in the world, and remain indebted to a variety of external actors, further increasing the capacity of these actors to influence domestic outcomes.

Particularly from the 1990s onwards, domestic NGOs increased in number and prominence across sub-Saharan African countries. Their numbers grew because the second wave of democratization created new space for such organizations, donors sought aid recipients other than the state, and states that were already relatively weak retreated in response to structural adjustment policies and other neoliberal reforms (Clapham 1996; Fisher 1997; Grown 2008; Holmen 2010; Igoe and Kelsall 2005; Lewis 1992; Manji and O'Coill 2002; Nugent 2004; Silliman 1999). While NGOs abound across sectors and countries, the ability of NGOs to enact positive social change remains an open question, with many of their impacts registering through service provision and its governance (Brass 2016; Bratton 1989; Fisher 1997). Donors have used NGOs for a number of reasons: as a way around corrupt states, to avoid some of the politics of foreign aid, to gain knowledge of or access to local populations, and to provide legitimacy to foreign interventions by endowing them with the authenticity of the local (Chabal and Daloz 1999; Fisher 1997; Forbes 1999; Watkins, Swidler, and Hannan 2012). As the analysis below demonstrates, they are an integral part of the population and AIDS fields within African countries.

Sub-Saharan African governments face many competing sources of authority, in particular from the leaders of different religious and ethnic groups, which can make it difficult to implement programs of any sort (Herbst 2000; Hyden 1980; Lund 2006; Migdal 2001). Sub-Saharan African countries also have extraordinarily high ethnic, religious, and linguistic diversity. Based on one measure of ethnic diversity, on average sub-Saharan African countries are twice as diverse as countries outside the region, with a nearly two-third chance that two random people selected will be from *different* ethnic groups (calculation from Alesina et al. 2003). Similarly, the populations of sub-Saharan African countries rarely all adhere to the same faith. Religion drives much of social identity, organizes social life, and often overlaps with ethnicity (Trinitapoli and Weinreb 2012). Diversity across a number of dimensions results in large part from the relatively arbitrary state borders that colonialism produced. First drawn by European powers at the Berlin Conference in 1885, African countries disproportionately have borders that are straight lines, as opposed to following the contours of geography or social groups. Indeed, 44 percent of African borders are astronomical lines (e.g., of latitude or longitude), 30 percent are mathematical lines (e.g., curves), only 26 percent are geographical features, and none are cultural or linguistic boundaries (Englebert 2000: 88, citing Sautter 1982). Thus national identity has tended to follow state creation, rather than preceding it as in much of Europe, and because of global norms about border fixity, borders set by colonialists have remained largely the same over time (Anderson 1991; Atzili 2012). As a result, ethnic diversity is a reality for most sub-Saharan African countries, and in cases where it translates into fractionalization, can complicate program implementation for the same reasons that it challenges the provision of public goods more broadly (Easterly and Levine 1997).

Africa is the poorest continent in the world: based on the United Nations 2014 human development index, only two of the least developed twenty-five countries in the world were not in sub-Saharan Africa (United Nations Development Programme 2014).[1] Poverty leaves sub-Saharan African governments with few resources to implement programs as well as exposes them to the gaze of international organizations. Colonialism institutionalized sub-Saharan Africa's marginal position in the global economy, leaving national economies dependent on primary commodity exports. Although the post-independence period was a time of immense hope for better living standards, by the 1970s the future became bleaker as military rulers replaced democratically elected leaders and economies, although growing rapidly, failed to lift populations out of poverty. The oil boom of the 1970s helped countries with oil reserves, such as Nigeria, but in other countries just made life more expensive, and combined with a concurrent decrease in

---

[1]   Afghanistan and Haiti.

the availability of foreign exchange, caused poverty to worsen. When the world economic recession hit in the 1980s, and the prices fell for the primary goods on which so many sub-Saharan African countries relied for foreign exchange, countries slipped into extreme debt and became even more beholden to international financial institutions. Structural adjustment loans, first disbursed from international financial institutions in 1981, came with the expectation that states would pursue neoliberal economic policies in return. Although sub-Saharan African countries continue to face deep poverty, seventeen countries have rapidly growing economies and decreasing poverty levels (Radelet 2010).

This brief background introduces the variety of political, sociocultural, and economic factors across sub-Saharan African states likely to influence intimate interventions. First, there are a number of actors other than the state: NGOs, but also traditional and religious leaders. These organizations and individuals can greatly facilitate or complicate intimate interventions. Second, poverty has been driven by, as well as opened, sub-Saharan African countries to the meddling of international organizations. While countries can and do develop their own solutions to problems, sub-Saharan African governments often have to involve donors in domestic affairs more than they might like. That said, some use their country's disadvantageous global status to procure resources from foreign donors in a process of extraversion (Bayart 1993; Bayart 2000). Donors' interest in intimate interventions, as outlined in the previous chapter, has thus heavily influenced outcomes in sub-Saharan African countries.

Fertility, Contraceptive Use, and Pregnancy Prevention Interventions

Sub-Saharan Africa has the highest fertility of any region in the world, with women on average bearing five children in their lifetimes (Population Reference Bureau 2015). As Figure 3.1 shows, this average masks a great deal of variation: fertility is above five children per woman in West and particularly Central Africa, and lowest in southern Africa at only 2.7 children per woman (Population Reference Bureau 2015). In the past, average fertility rates hovered closer to seven children per woman. Causes for declining fertility include increased female education and participation in the formal labor market, the cost of

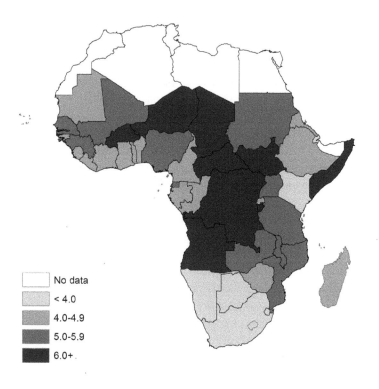

Figure 3.1. Total Fertility Rates, Sub-Saharan Africa, 2014
Source: Population Reference Bureau (2015).

schooling, and urbanization, all facilitated by greater availability and use of contraception. Desired fertility, however, remains high in many countries, in part because infant and child mortality are also still high, but also because of links between childbearing and social status, particularly for women.

Policies and programs designed to lower fertility have focused on trying to increase contraceptive use. Contraceptive prevalence rates among married women across sub-Saharan Africa vary inversely with fertility rates. The lowest rates of contraceptive prevalence are in West and Central Africa, where only 10–12 percent of married women use modern contraception on average, while the highest rates are in southern Africa, where almost 60 percent of married women use modern contraception (Population Reference Bureau 2015). Variation in contraceptive use also exists within countries, where more educated and urban women have the highest rates. Many countries also have high percentages of women who indicate they would have liked to delay or avoid their last birth, but were not using contraception.

Outsiders first tried to control Africans' fertility during the colonial era in the late nineteenth and early twentieth centuries, also the period of peak European concern with the management of sexual behavior in order to improve population quality (Thomas 2003). In some cases, colonial efforts were directed towards preventing pregnancy, but in others the goal was to increase the size of the African population in order to create more subjects and soldiers. In Rhodesia (current-day Zimbabwe), the white, ruling class's concern about the potentially destabilizing effects of rapid population growth among black Africans led settlers to justify the provision of family planning both as a means to maintain racial hierarchy and as part of a paternalistic care regime (Kaler 2003). The sub-Saharan African countries with the earliest family planning associations were thus those with larger white settler populations, including South Africa (1932), Zimbabwe (1953), Uganda (1957), Tanzania (1959), and Kenya (1961) (International Planned Parenthood Federation 2009).

Following independence in the 1960s, most sub-Saharan African governments were not interested in preventing pregnancy. In particular, most governments saw large populations as either valuable assets or not as cause for concern, most cultures supported high fertility norms, and most families and individuals benefitted from large numbers of children as they provided social insurance as well as access to social status and networks. In addition, most sub-Saharan African countries had low relative and absolute population density, and still had populations concentrated in rural areas. In addition to limited desire for reducing fertility, discourse about family planning as a form of "biological colonialism" circulated to differing degrees, supported by the Vatican (Kissling 2010; Tarnoff 1994).

Post-colonial efforts by the global population field to prevent pregnancy began in sub-Saharan Africa in the 1960s, primarily in Kenya and Ghana. As described in the previous chapter, wealthy countries were concerned about the potential ecological and political impact of rapidly growing populations in poor countries. Kenya adopted a population policy designed to limit fertility, and thus population growth, in 1967, making it the first country in sub-Saharan Africa to do so. Kenya adopted the policy because of international pressure and a desire among Kenyan policy elites to signal to outsiders that Kenya was committed to forward-progressing development and not "backward" because of its high fertility rate. At the same time, the international organizations promoting the policy, in particular the Population Council, sought a case to demonstrate the benefits to family planning programs (Chimbwete, Watkins, and Zulu 2005). The government adopted the policy following a visit by the Population Council, a near copy of the international organization's trip report (Chimbwete et al. 2005; Frank and McNicoll 1987; Warwick 1982). President Kenyatta put aside his personal objection to family planning and facilitated the adoption of the policy in part because it brought resources that the government could redirect towards maternal and child health care, and because it also promised greater donor financing (Chimbwete et al. 2005; Hodgson and Watkins 1997). Kenyatta walked a narrow line between the desire to attract donor resources and the risk of being perceived by Kenyans as un-African, and so failed to vigorously support the population policy and associated family planning programs, which ultimately lessened their impact (Thomas 2003).

The story of Ghana's 1969 population policy parallels that of Kenya in many ways. Prior to independence, contraceptive supplies were readily available to Europeans living in the colony, but Kwame Nkrumah, Ghana's first post-independence president, was socialist and thus ultimately banned their import (Caldwell and Sai 2007). Nkrumah did, however, strongly support the modernization of Ghana, and so actively sought to participate in the United Nations' 1960 round of censuses, wanting Ghana to be the first African country to have a census (Caldwell and Sai 2007). The census showed that Ghana had a total fertility rate of seven children per woman and that the population was growing rapidly. The Population Council facilitated the training of Ghanaian demographers and the Planned Parenthood Association of Ghana, founded in 1967, focused its advocacy on the development of a national family planning program. These steps ultimately resulted in the 1969 *Population Planning for National Progress*, a policy document then implemented by the democratically elected government starting in 1970. Caldwell and Sai (2007) note that although the national family planning program received international acclaim, it was never supported by the highest levels of government, and was more a project of the Ministry of Finance and Economic Planning than the Ministry of Health. Furthermore, the government backed away from media campaigns soon after the family planning program was set up, as these campaigns provoked resistance from many Ghanaians who believed that they would promote immoral behavior.

The cases of Kenya and Ghana illustrate ambivalent government receipt of early international promotion of pregnancy prevention. In part to make up for less than enthusiastic, or nonexistent, government family planning programs, during the 1960s and 1970s private, family planning NGOs were founded in a number of countries, and by 1980, approximately half of sub-Saharan African countries had such an organization. During these early years, many non-US donors channeled funds for population activities through NGOs in order to avoid accusations of genocide, racism, and neo-imperialism (Schindlmayr 2004). Then, in the 1980s, donor support for family planning increased and many African governments began to view population growth as a burden that challenged their promises to educate and employ citizens, as well as keep them healthy, and so began to endorse pregnancy prevention as a means to achieve economic development and improve maternal mortality. In order to facilitate the distribution of contraception, former French colonies had to repeal a 1920 French law banning the sale of contraception, and doing so was the first proactive step related to pregnancy prevention taken by many countries (Economic Commission for Africa 1988).[2] Between the late 1980s and late 1990s, two thirds of countries in sub-Saharan Africa adopted national population policies designed to slow population growth by limiting fertility (Robinson 2015).

The experiences of Kenya and Ghana, as well as those in Senegal, Nigeria, and Malawi described in the following chapters, demonstrate that the process of population policy adoption in sub-Saharan Africa was the result of the intersection of local desires, international pressure backed by significant financial leverage, and, ultimately, the linkage of family planning to the globally sanctioned right to reproductive health (Robinson 2015). In particular, World Bank debt was a significant

---

[2] The law had been repealed in France in 1967, but remained on the books in most former French colonies as they had gained independence prior to that year.

predictor of population policy adoption, reflecting both the World Bank's belief that population growth inhibited socioeconomic development, but also the extent of the Bank's leverage in countries. Starting in the 1980s and continuing through the 1990s, the Bank promoted the adoption of population policies in sub-Saharan Africa in conjunction with structural adjustment programs and in general expanded support for family planning programs in the region (Conly and Epp 1997; Hartmann 1995; Sai and Chester 1990; World Bank 1992). Following the 1994 United Nations International Conference on Population and Development, even more countries adopted population policies as a way to demonstrate their commitment to the right to reproductive health (Robinson 2015). The countries today that remain without population policies have experienced greater levels of conflict, and are generally unstable, suggesting low capacity to adopt (population) policies, and low pressure from international donors to do so.

Whether family planning programs and population policies lower fertility remains an open question. The debate is primarily between those who passionately believe that providing contraceptive supplies the world over has helped reduce fertility (Bongaarts, Mauldin, and Philips 1990), and those who argue that because desired fertility drives actual fertility, family planning programs are much less important (Pritchett 1994). The truth probably lies somewhere in the middle. Sub-Saharan African countries that adopted population policies experienced a 21 percent decline in total fertility between 1987 and 2002, which is significantly greater than the 14 percent decline experienced by countries without policies during the same period.[3] But countries do not randomly adopt policies or programs, making assumptions of causality from such a comparison problematic. The best experimental evidence for the positive effect of family planning programs on fertility comes from a randomized control trial in Matlab, Bangladesh, where treatment villages received door-to-door family planning and maternal and child health services and experienced a 15 percent decline in fertility compared to villages that did not receive such services (Joshi and Schultz 2007; Miller and Babiarz 2014; Phillips et al. 1982). The Navrongo project implemented in Ghana in the 1990s drew inspiration from the Matlab experiment and while its effects were not

---

[3] Author's calculations, from World Development Indicators data (World Bank 2014).

as dramatic, it demonstrated that contextually appropriate family planning interventions could impact fertility, in particular child spacing (Phillips et al. 2012).

In sum, fertility remains high in sub-Saharan Africa, despite decades of primarily donor-motivated efforts to provide pregnancy prevention services. Part of the continued high fertility is explained by high desired fertility, but at least part of it is due to an unmet need for contraception. Generally speaking, governmental policies and programs have stemmed from the intersection of global and national interests, but such programs have not always been enthusiastically promoted by leaders, and insufficient capacity has inhibited their full implementation. While contraceptive prevalence rates in sub-Saharan Africa were uniformly low in all but parts of southern Africa during the period of focus for this book – the 1980s and 1990s – in more recent years, contraceptive use has increased dramatically in some countries, including Rwanda, Ethiopia, and Malawi, in part thanks to programs designed to ensure that people desiring contraception have been able to access it.

HIV Prevalence and Associated Prevention Interventions

As Figure 3.2 shows, HIV prevalence varies greatly across sub-Saharan Africa, from less than 1 percent in countries such as Madagascar and Somalia to over 20 percent in Botswana, Lesotho, and Swaziland. The causes of this variation are the source of heated debate, as are the implied interventions. The vast majority of HIV transmission in sub-Saharan Africa is through heterosexual sex, followed by vertical transmission from mothers to children through pregnancy, childbirth, or breastfeeding (Whiteside 2008). Homosexual sex and injection drug use, two common routes of transmission in other parts of the world, occur in sub-Saharan Africa, but are not the primary drivers of the epidemic. However, men who have sex with men and injection drug users constitute populations particularly at risk for HIV, even if both groups are relatively small. Along with sex workers, these three groups have the highest rates of HIV in Africa and the world over. A small, and difficult to measure, percentage of transmission occurs due to unsafe medical practices.

HIV transferred from primates to humans as humans butchered infected meat and probably emerged at numerous different points in

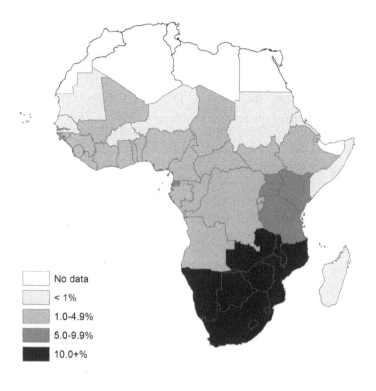

Figure 3.2. HIV Prevalence, Sub-Saharan Africa, 2013
Source: UNAIDS (2014).

sub-Saharan Africa during the twentieth century. The modern HIV epidemic truly began in the late 1970s in East Africa, in the Democratic Republic of the Congo and Uganda. A heterosexual epidemic in this region can be said to date from 1983 (Merson et al. 2008), and the first cases were diagnosed in most sub-Saharan African countries between then and 1986. The year of peak incidence, with the greatest number of new infections, occurred around 1990 in most countries and peak prevalence followed after a lag of five to seven years (Bongaarts et al. 2008). As of 2014, in ten countries the number of new HIV infections had declined by more than 75 percent, and in an additional twenty-seven countries it had declined by more than 50 percent (UNAIDS 2014).

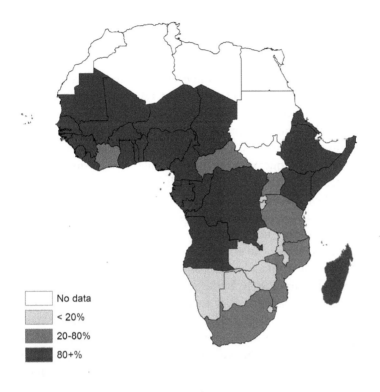

Figure 3.3. Prevalence of Male Circumcision, Sub-Saharan Africa, 2007
Source: World Health Organization and UNAIDS (2007).

The most frequently cited explanations for variation in HIV prevalence include male circumcision rates, sexual partnering patterns (including age at marriage), and virus type. Other drivers include wealth and unsafe injection practices. Circumcision helps protect men from contracting HIV because it removes parts of the foreskin that are highly permeable to HIV (Bongaarts et al. 2008; Cohen 2008; Hayes and Weiss 2006; Potts et al. 2008; Wilson and de Beyer 2008). Scholars had long noted the ecological correlation between circumcision rates and HIV prevalence (e.g., Bongaarts et al. 1989), as shown in Figure 3.3, which is close to the inverse of the map of HIV prevalence (Figure 3.2). But it was not until 2005 that randomized control trials were completed that showed that circumcision reduces sexual transmission from an HIV-positive woman to an uninfected man by up to 60 percent (Auvert et al. 2005; Williams et al. 2006). The results were so significant that the associated studies were stopped early on the grounds that it was unethical to continue without offering circumcision to all study participants. Many ethnic and religious groups in sub-Saharan Africa practice some form of male circumcision, and it is almost universal among Muslims, but its exact form and extent varies from group to group, so those advocating for male circumcision as an HIV prevention technique promote *medical* male circumcision, namely that performed by health care professionals in a clinical setting.

Because of the links between religion and circumcision, and because religion is so important in the lives of most Africans, many have looked to religion as a means for explaining variation in HIV prevalence. Scholars have confirmed the ecological relationship between the percentage of Muslims within a country and HIV prevalence (Gray 2004; McIntosh and Thomas 2004), but at least one summary of the literature (Gray 2004) concluded that there were no strong connection between Islamic codes, sexual behavior, and HIV outcomes. Most likely then, the ecological correspondence is via circumcision, while other observed connections between religion and HIV operate through religiosity, or the strength of religious belief. In their wide-reaching analysis of most sub-Saharan African countries, Trinitapoli and Weinreb (2012) find that no religious group is either more or less likely to be affected by AIDS, but that the religious climate influences both sexual behavior and HIV outcomes.

Many authors have attributed variation in HIV prevalence to differences in sexual partnership patterning, specifically what are referred to as multiple concurrent partnerships (Epstein and Morris 2011; Halperin and Epstein 2004; Morris and Kretzschmar 1997).[4] The logic behind this assertion is that when high percentages of a population have multiple sexual partners at the same time, as is presumed to more frequently be the case in southern and eastern Africa, it creates a dense sexual network through which HIV can

---

[4] There has been a debate in the literature regarding the extent to which multiple concurrent partnerships can explain the higher levels of HIV in sub-Saharan Africa. Those scholars who have argued most vehemently against multiple concurrent partnerships as determinants of variation in HIV prevalence point to other infectious diseases as well as poverty and inequality as the key drivers of HIV (Sawers and Stillwaggon 2010; Stillwaggon 2006)

rapidly spread. In particular, given the ease with which HIV is transmitted during the acute phase of infection (the month following initial infection), having a new partner during this period helps spread the virus quickly. The early work on the relationship between concurrent partnerships and HIV transmission was based exclusively on mathematical modeling, and it is only recently that more reliable estimates of concurrency at the population level have become available. Polygamy is another form of multiple concurrent partnership, but HIV prevalence is generally lower in places where polygamy is more common (Reniers and Watkins 2010). These lower rates result because women in polygamous unions tend to have sex with their husbands less frequently than women in non-polygamous unions, and because there are fewer extramarital partnerships in areas where polygamy is common, such that even if one of the partners in a polygamous family is HIV-positive, the number of people to whom the virus can be spread through sex is limited. Age at marriage is another factor that influences sexual partnering patterns and which can explain much of the variation in HIV prevalence across African countries (Bongaarts 2007; Garenne, Giami, and Perrey 2013). In contexts where people marry late, as in southern Africa, exposure to HIV is increased due to multiple partnerships during the premarital period that is longer than in places where people marry earlier, as in western Africa.

The relationship between wealth and HIV is somewhat counterintuitive. Although Africa is the poorest continent on earth and has the worst HIV epidemic, the richest countries in sub-Saharan Africa have the highest prevalence rates. In 2013, Botswana had the fourth highest GDP per capita in sub-Saharan Africa but the third highest adult HIV prevalence at 21.9 percent, while Namibia had the seventh highest GDP per capita and the sixth highest HIV prevalence of 14.3 percent (World Bank 2014). Prevalence in Zimbabwe actually declined as well-being *worsened* (Halperin et al. 2011). In part, these macro trends are the result of the aggregation of individual-level trends: greater income and education among individuals are frequently associated with a higher likelihood of being HIV-positive because of the opportunities that money provides for travel and purchasing sex (Fortson 2008).[5] But

---

[5] See Mojola (2014) for a nuanced discussion of the relationship between money and sex among young women in Kenya, and Haacker (2016) for a detailed treatment of the macroeconomic effects of AIDS.

the concentration of the HIV epidemic in southern Africa is also the result of the labor migration associated with natural resource extraction (part of what has driven GDP rates higher in the sub-region) and apartheid policies.

Finally, several other factors explain some of the variation in prevalence. HIV type 1 predominates in southern and eastern Africa, while HIV type 2 was initially more common in West Africa. Although both viruses lead to AIDS, HIV type 2 is less virulent (Gisselquist 2008; Marlink et al. 1994). The presence of other sexually transmitted infections greatly facilitates the transmission of HIV as such infections frequently create sores that serve as an easy point of entry for HIV and/or bring the very immune cells that HIV attacks to the genital area (Whiteside 2008). Sub-Saharan Africa has both high levels of sexually transmitted infections and relatively low levels of treatment for them, and the variation in sexually transmitted infections that cause the ulcers most likely to facilitate the transmission HIV maps well onto the variation in HIV levels (Caldwell and Caldwell 1996; Lewis 2011). Some small, but not insignificant, proportion of HIV transmission is due to unsafe injection practices and other poor hygiene in medical settings, but debate rages as to the extent that such transmission explains why HIV rates are higher in sub-Saharan Africa than elsewhere (Gisselquist et al. 2003; Hunsmann 2009; Sawers and Stillwaggon 2010). Lack of information on the differing extent of such iatrogenic transmission across countries makes it difficult to assess its impact.

Interpretation of the drivers of variation in prevalence has in turned shaped interventions to try to stop the spread of HIV, which can be classified as behavioral, structural, or biomedical. Behavioral interventions aim to change the ways in which individuals have sex, including condom use during sex, number and type of partners, and age at sexual debut. In short, the commonly used ABC approach to HIV prevention (abstain, be faithful, or use a condom) is a behavioral one. The goal of structural interventions is to alter the social, political, or economic context that puts people at risk for HIV but which people cannot easily change themselves, such as reducing gender inequality or improving economic opportunities. Biomedical interventions include medical male circumcision, treatment of sexually transmitted infections, antiretroviral therapy for HIV prevention, and vaginal microbicides. The vast majority of HIV interventions target individual behavior change, but the AIDS field has come to promote as most effective a "combination prevention" approach, which ideally includes all three categories of intervention. Below I discuss some of the common interventions from each category.

Condoms are approximately 90 percent effective in preventing HIV, with greater efficacy associated with correct usage (Hearst and Chen 2004). Even though condoms do a relatively good job protecting an individual from HIV, to have an effect as a population-level intervention requires almost universal usage, an outcome that is generally only achievable in situations where the epidemic is contained to a particular subgroup, such as sex workers (Caldwell 2000; Potts et al. 2008). Thailand is a good example of increased condom usage among sex workers and their clients helping to lower HIV prevalence dramatically (Phoolcharoen 1998). Such consistent usage is challenging among other groups at risk for HIV, particularly those who are in long-term relationships where condom usage would betray the appearance of trust, negatively define the relationship, or question the quality of its intimacy (Caldwell 2000; Potts et al. 2008; Tavory and Swidler 2009). For all these reasons, condom campaigns have not been a hugely effective response to the HIV epidemic in sub-Saharan Africa (Shelton 2007).

Maintaining one, monogamous sexual partner reduces individual level risk of HIV (Bongaarts et al. 2008; Gregson et al. 2006; Potts et al. 2008; UNAIDS 2008). While it is difficult to show definitively that partner reduction has led to changes in HIV outcomes, given measurement difficulties, reductions in the number of partners, and in particular the number of concurrent partners, is almost certainly at the root of the decline in HIV incidence that occurred in Uganda during the 1990s that I discuss in greater detail below.

Voluntary counseling and testing has been one of the main interventions in both rich and poor countries, motivated by the logic that knowing one's HIV status should lead to appropriate behavior change. Research shows that knowledge of HIV status generally does not reduce the risk of infection for those who test negative, but that it may reduce risk-taking among those who test positive, and in particular among those in serodiscordant couples, where one member is HIV-positive and the other is HIV-negative (Fonner et al. 2012; Potts et al. 2008; Shelton 2007).

Knowledge about how HIV is spread and how it can be prevented has increased to the point of saturation, achieved through explicit

interventions such as information, education, and communication programs as well as peer education, but there is little evidence that such
programs have reduced infection rates (Caldwell 2000; Medley et al.
2009; Oster 2012). Similarly, many interventions, particularly those
supported by the first round of PEPFAR, have promoted abstinence,
but have been relatively ineffective in achieving behavior change, in
particular because much HIV transmission occurs within marriage
(Dunkle et al. 2008; Lo, Lowe, and Bendavid 2016; Potts et al.
2008). We know that in some contexts, however, behavior change
has occurred, both from measuring it directly, as well as from declining
incidence rates. Such declines are likely the result of people talking with
each other and identifying meaningful ways to reduce the risks of HIV
transmission within the context of their particular epidemic (Ashforth
and Watkins 2015; Watkins 2004).

Biomedical interventions for HIV include long hoped-for, but as yet
unsuccessful, attempts at vaccines and microbicides, treatment of sexually transmitted infections, as well as more promising developments
with male circumcision and the use of antiretroviral therapy for prevention. Developing a vaccine to prevent HIV has proved difficult given
the number of different strains of HIV, its capacity to mutate, and its
strategy of attacking immune system cells. As of 2013, only 4 out of
more than 200 possible vaccines had been deemed safe enough to test in
humans (Tieu et al. 2013). While a vaccine remains years away at best,
the various trials conducted have provided valuable information on
how best to craft that future vaccine. Similarly, many have worked
towards the development of a topical vaginal microbicide as it would
be a woman-controlled means of HIV protection. As of 2013, there had
been eleven ineffective trials of six different products, with adherence
proving a fundamental challenge (Karim, Baxter and Karim 2013).

Treating other sexually transmitted infections, particularly through
simplified syndromic management techniques that rely on diagnosis
based on symptoms rather than laboratory tests, has long been used as
an HIV prevention intervention. While initial clinical trials indicated its
likely effectiveness as a population-level intervention, these large-scale
interventions have not decreased HIV incidence as hoped, although
there remains dispute about the quality of the trials to assess impact
(Grosskurth et al. 1995; Hayes et al. 2010; Potts et al. 2008; Shelton
2007; White et al. 2008). Male circumcision has become the closest
biomedical intervention to a vaccine, reducing HIV transmission from

an HIV-positive woman to an HIV-negative man through vaginal intercourse by up to 60 percent, far above those of the most promising vaccines. As a result, the World Health Organization, PEPFAR, and UNAIDS now all promote male circumcision as an intervention in highly impacted countries. As of 2011, fourteen such countries, all located in eastern and southern Africa, had male circumcision policies in development or in place (Wamai et al. 2011).

Finally, antiretroviral therapy has long been deployed as a mechanism to prevent mother-to-child transmission of HIV, and more recently has been shown to be effective at preventing transmission between adults. Antiretroviral therapy given to HIV-positive mothers during pregnancy and at the time of birth can reduce the risk of vertical transmission to the infant from 25 percent to less than 10 percent, and the elimination of vertical transmission of HIV by 2015 became a primary goal of UNAIDS in 2011 (UNAIDS 2011; Whiteside 2008). Also in 2011, the results of a randomized control trial were published showing a 96 percent reduction in the transmission of HIV between members of serodiscordant couples if the HIV-positive member began taking antiretroviral therapy before showing symptoms of AIDS (*The Lancet* 2011). Since then, much discussion has centered on so-called treatment as prevention, or TasP. The practicalities of such interventions in sub-Saharan Africa remain, however, challenging given that many countries still struggle to provide antiretroviral therapy to people who *are* showing symptoms of AIDS. As Figure 3.4 shows, countries differ in terms of the degree to which people in need receive drugs. Namibia and Botswana, countries with high HIV burden, decent roads, and small populations, have done the best, getting drugs to more than 90 percent of people who need them. But most of the worst-hit countries are still reaching less than half of those in need, despite treatment having been a major donor focus since the early 2000s with the emergence of the Global Fund and PEPFAR.

Structural interventions to prevent HIV are the least common, given their scope and cost, but have shown promising results. Most structural interventions related to HIV in southern and eastern Africa have sought to reduce gender inequality or increase financial security, and have had mixed success (Gibbs et al. 2012). In some cases, even though HIV incidence has not decreased, these programs have been effective in reducing factors associated with HIV transmission, such as intimate partner violence (Jewkes et al. 2008; Pronyk et al. 2006). Cash transfers

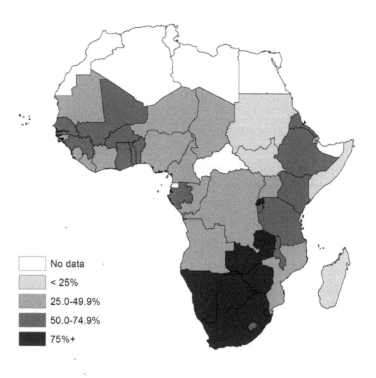

Figure 3.4. Antiretroviral Coverage Rates, Sub-Saharan Africa, 2012
Note: Shows percentage of HIV-positive individuals receiving antiretroviral therapy, relative to those eligible based on 2010 guidelines.
Source: World Health Organization (2014).

designed to change behaviors that put people at risk for HIV (as opposed to those that pay people to stay HIV or sexually transmitted infection free) have had largely positive effects, and reduced HIV risk even in cases where they were not intended to do so, such as when girls are compensated for staying in school (Baird et al. 2012).

As the debates about the drivers of variation in HIV and the relative effectiveness of various interventions indicate, the complexity of HIV makes it impossible to identify a single "best" way to respond to the epidemic. Just as the political, social, and economic context influences individual risk for HIV, the context also shapes the ways in which social organizations at all levels respond to the epidemic. In the following section, I thus turn to discussing African responses to HIV.

African Responses to HIV

Following the diagnosis of the first AIDS cases in the early- to mid-1980s in the majority of sub-Saharan African countries, most ministries of health folded HIV into the division that dealt with sexually transmitted infections, both because HIV *is* a sexually transmitted infection in sub-Saharan Africa, but also because many of the first populations severely impacted were sex workers, a focal population of those divisions. Most ministries of health developed some sort of AIDS committee early on to organize the national response (England 2006), and while some countries adopted HIV/AIDS policies, this type of response was not as popular as it had been with pregnancy prevention. By default, early interventions centered on prevention and care, given that there was no cure or even treatment at that point, and sought to increase knowledge among the population about HIV transmission routes as well as techniques for prevention.

In the early days of the HIV epidemic, many policymakers and large segments of the general African population expressed skepticism about the existence of AIDS. Sub-Saharan African governments claimed biased data explained high levels of prevalence in their countries, or that other health issues that affected more people should be prioritized (Piot 2012). Most governments also lacked the means to respond to HIV, making admission of the problem equivalent to admitting they were powerless (Dozon and Fassin 1989). Among those who believed AIDS to be real, many thought the disease came from the West, and closely associated it with gay men. Rumors spread widely that condoms actually contained HIV and were part of a plot by Westerners to decimate African populations. Many Africans questioned, and/or resented, that the HIV epidemic began in Africa, and with the transfer from primates to humans (Iliffe 2006). These origins suggested that Africans might have had sex with monkeys, and that Africans were to blame for a worldwide pandemic. Reflecting this perspective, Kenyan President Daniel Arap Moi said "African AIDS reports are a new form of hate campaign" (as quoted in Garrett 1994: 354). One African academic described the situation at the same time as: "Africa, already branded a dark and dying continent, once again was seen as the origin of bad things, the culprit in this deadly tragedy. African leaders were wary of this new finger pointing and justifiably scared that the world community might impose discriminatory regulations against Africans on the basis of this new menace" (Kalipeni 1997: 25). While AIDS denialism has lessened over time, even in the hardest-hit countries most Africans do not see AIDS as a pressing problem, but instead one among many, including poverty, unemployment, and overall insecurity (Fox 2014; Strand 2012).

Scholars and programmers alike have struggled to understand why some countries have put more effort than others towards HIV/AIDS, and why some interventions have been more effective than others. As described in Chapter 1, existing scholarship has identified political leadership and commitment, and government coordination with NGOs and other civil society organizations, as two main factors that explain country-level success in addressing HIV/AIDS. More generally speaking, though, the picture that emerges from research on this topic sometimes offers more contradictions than agreement. Counter-examples exist for every logical explanation for variation in countries' responses to HIV/AIDS. There are democracies with low HIV prevalence (Senegal) and with high HIV prevalence (Botswana), and autocracies that have experienced large declines in HIV prevalence (Uganda, Zimbabwe). There are rich countries that have struggled to combat the disease (Botswana, South Africa) and there are poor countries that have effectively lowered prevalence (Uganda). There are countries that have experienced war with low prevalence (Angola) and with high prevalence (Mozambique). And there are countries with high prevalence that at times have done very little (South Africa), while some with low prevalence have done a lot (Senegal). Overall, successful responses to HIV/AIDS have been few and far between (Merson et al. 2008).

The two most commonly cited instances of "success" in stopping the spread of HIV are Uganda and Senegal. These two countries (along with Thailand, and sometimes Brazil) feature as the highlighted boxes in United Nations reports and academic books alike,[6] and both indicate that political commitment and civil society participation facilitated

---

[6] Even a Nigerian government document has a side box describing "Governance Lessons from Uganda and Senegal" (National Agency for the Control of AIDS 2007: 22).

an effective response to HIV. I discuss Senegal at great length in Chapter 6 and provide a word about Uganda's response to HIV here.

HIV emerged in Uganda in the midst of a brutal civil war. Following the war's end in 1986 and Museveni's assumption of the presidency, Fidel Castro informed him of the extent of HIV in the military, apparently telephoning him personally after a large number of Ugandan officers sent to Cuba for training tested HIV-positive. Museveni then broadcast a message of "zero grazing," meaning that people should reduce their number of sexual partners, first to military personnel, whose support he needed in order to avoid the coups that had plagued previous governments, but then also more broadly (Ostergard and Barcelo 2005). He also linked HIV to what he perceived as declining morals, giving him powerful rhetoric and justification for intervention. Museveni thus demonstrated political commitment to slowing the spread of HIV, but not always for reasons associated with rights and other internationally sanctified perspectives, instead relying on surveillance and control of individual behavior to ensure his continued rule (de Waal 2006).

In Uganda, prevalence declined from approximately 20 percent to 10 percent in the 1990s (Low-Beer and Stoneburner 2004). Although debate exists about the relative role of increased condom usage in this outcome, a 60 percent reduction in the number of nonregular sex partners between 1989 and 1995 almost certainly deserves much credit (Green et al. 2006; Low-Beer and Stoneburner 2004). The key understandings for the drivers of this decline include political leadership on the part of President Museveni, a decentralized government which allowed for local experimentation and personalization of responses to HIV/AIDS, and active incorporation of different social groups into the response (Barnett and Whiteside 2006; Eboko 2005; Green et al. 2006; Parkhurst and Lush 2004; Patterson 2006). But even in this well-studied case, questions remain. Despite Museveni's political commitment, the behavior change that led to declines in HIV prevalence may have occurred before his interventions. Ugandans themselves, seeing many people sick with AIDS, most likely started talking about the disease and accordingly changed their behavior (Barnett and Whiteside 2006; Low-Beer and Stoneburner 2004). Decreased support for HIV interventions from Museveni in recent years has come in conjunction with flattening declines in HIV prevalence, and possible increases in HIV incidence among youth, suggesting the importance of *sustained* political commitment to reducing HIV (Green et al. 2013). More related to the themes of this book, it is also possible that a history of campaigns to "improve" public morality throughout the pre-AIDS era of the twentieth century in the Buganda and Buhaya regions of Uganda left people familiar with both discussing sexuality and external interventions targeting sexual behavior change (Doyle 2013).

As much as Uganda exemplifies the benefits of strong political commitment in responding to AIDS, political commitment can also come in counterproductive forms, as evidenced by President Mbeki of South Africa's persistent denial of the link between HIV and AIDS. The roots of South Africa's double-digit adult HIV prevalence rate lie in apartheid and the extensive labor migration associated with resource extraction, as well as low levels of male circumcision and a high incidence of sexually transmitted infections (Karim and Karim 2002). The HIV epidemic took off in the chaotic years preceding the transition to democracy in 1994, and during that time more closely resembled the epidemic in Europe and North America among gay men. As president, Nelson Mandela barely addressed the issue. Mbeki, however, railed against foreign governments' prioritization of AIDS and the drugs to treat it above other issues, such as poverty (Butler 2005; Decoteau 2013). His antagonistic stance on HIV, supported by and executed through Minister of Health Manto Tshabalala-Msimang, greatly slowed the spread of access to antiretroviral therapy and ultimately resulted in an estimated 330,000 additional deaths than would have otherwise occurred (Chigwedere et al. 2008). While interpretations for Mbeki's behavior vary, and are beyond the scope of the discussion here, South Africa's experience demonstrates the negative potential of political commitment.

While political commitment to HIV has varied across countries, so too has the magnitude of community and NGO responses to HIV (Merson et al. 2008). Although the sheer number of organizations working on HIV in a country does not necessarily translate into an effective response, Figure 3.5 shows the extent of variation in the distribution of local HIV/AIDS NGOs across sub-Saharan African countries in 2003 (United Nations 2003). Based on this one source, eighteen countries had fewer than ten domestic NGOs per ten million population dedicated to HIV. Countries with higher HIV prevalence, but also with more ties to international NGOs, had more local HIV/AIDS NGOs (Robinson 2010a).

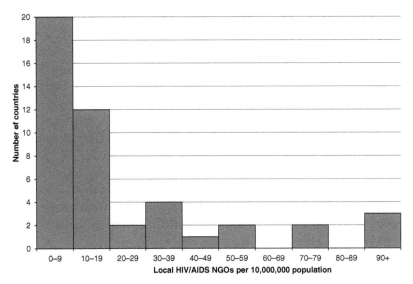

Figure 3.5. Distribution of Local HIV/AIDS NGOs, Sub-Saharan Africa, 2003
Source: United Nations (2003).

International organizations have particularly emphasized NGOs as a core component of the response to HIV. The primary, country-level grant-writing and managing entity for the Global Fund, the Country Coordinating Mechanism, is required to have local NGO representation. The first time the World Health Organization ever coordinated with NGOs was as part of its Global Programme on AIDS, and at least half of the World Bank's Multi-Country AIDS Program funds must target civil society (Harman 2010; Merson et al. 2008). PEPFAR has always worked with NGOs, with not insignificant proportions of its funding flowing through both international and African faith-based organizations (Burchardt, Patterson and Rasmussen 2013). More recently, its 2015 country guidance document emphasized the participation of NGOs to a far greater extent than at any previous point (PEPFAR 2015).

A number of noteworthy examples of local NGOs exist, many of which I discuss in the case study chapters that follow. Two examples in other countries include The AIDS Support Organisation, or TASO, in Uganda and the Treatment Action Campaign in South Africa. Noreen Kaleba, whose husband had died of HIV, founded TASO in 1987 as one of the earliest HIV organizations in sub-Saharan Africa. TASO initially sought to provide services to those living with HIV and to reduce stigma around the disease. Since then, it has grown into a major organization, with four centers throughout the country, and care provided to 100,000 people per year (The AIDS Support Organisation n. d.). Founded much later than TASO (in 1998), the Treatment Action Campaign started as a group of friends led by Zackie Achmat who knew each other from anti-apartheid activism (Grebe 2011). They modeled much of their response to HIV after Act Up, the New York-based organization founded during the peak of the AIDS crisis in the 1980s, but drew from their experiences, and networks, in the struggle against apartheid. The Treatment Action Campaign instigated the court case that ultimately led to the provision of antiretroviral therapy to pregnant women, and thus played a major role in Mbeki's decision in 2003 to finally implement a national antiretroviral program (Grebe 2011). Not all countries have such NGOs. The general lack of organized social movements in support of gay rights across sub-Saharan African countries left most without the organizations that had been crucial to AIDS activism in wealthy countries (Altman 1994). Among other reasons, family planning organizations thus became particularly important to the response to HIV.

Overall, research on responses to HIV in sub-Saharan Africa suggests the significance of political commitment and civil society engagement, both political factors in the model for explaining variation in country-level response to HIV developed in Chapter 1. I now turn to examining how transnational and political factors associated with family planning transferred to HIV prevention across sub-Saharan Africa.

From Pregnancy Prevention to HIV Prevention in Sub-Saharan Africa

As described in the previous chapter, resources in the form of funding, organizations, and human capital transferred between family planning and HIV prevention at the global level. To provide more evidence for that connection, this section presents findings from statistical analysis across all sub-Saharan African countries looking at the relationship between funding for pregnancy prevention and later funding for HIV, and between the existence of family planning organizations and population policies and HIV outcomes.

To measure global and local resources available for intimate interventions within countries, I consider USAID and the International

Planned Parenthood Federation[7] for pregnancy prevention and the Global Fund for HIV.[8] Countries with extensive USAID involvement were those targeted with RAPID presentations, or that were part of the OPTIONS program, both interventions designed to reduce fertility and explained briefly in the previous chapter. Information about which sub-Saharan African countries had a RAPID intervention comes from a WorldCat search for *The Effects of Population Factors on Social and Economic Development*, a series of reports that the Futures Group published prior to 1985 for the countries in which RAPID presentations were developed. Information about countries with OPTIONS interventions comes from Liagin (1996). Data on USAID funding for population activities in particular countries comes from Barrett and Tsui (1999).[9]

At the time of the emergence of AIDS and later, scholars and practitioners noted the capacity of local family planning organizations and programs in sub-Saharan African countries to support responses to HIV, citing their familiarity with communities and experience with facilitating behavior change (Greeley 1988; Green 1994; Sinding and Seims 2002; Williamson and Boohene 1990). Because so many family planning organizations are affiliates of the International Planned Parenthood Federation, the analysis below uses the existence of such an organization prior to the HIV epidemic as a marker for family planning resources. Founded in 1952 at the Third International Conference on Planned Parenthood in Bombay, the International Planned Parenthood Federation is a network of member associations with organizations in most countries around the world (International Planned Parenthood Federation n.d.-a). These organizations provide a broad array of reproductive health services, and in many cases serve as the focal point of nongovernmental organizing around reproductive health in a country. Much of the International Planned Parenthood Federation's support comes from bilateral aid agencies and at points in the past up to 90 percent of its annual budget of approximately US$125 million have come from governments (Crane 1993; International Planned Parenthood Federation n.d.-b; Kantner and

---

[7] It is unfortunately too difficult to disentangle UNFPA funding for family planning/population from that for HIV/AIDS to include UNFPA in this analysis.

[8] While PEPFAR is of course a major funder of HIV activities, it cannot be included in the analysis because its initial funding targeted only fifteen focus countries.

[9] My thanks to Deborah Barrett for sharing the raw data.

Table 3.1 *Results from Linear Regressions Predicting Log of Total Global Fund Disbursements for HIV/AIDS, Sub-Saharan African Countries, 2002–2010*

Variable	Model		
	(1)	(2)	(3)
IPPF Affiliate Founding Date	−†		
Country had Futures or OPTIONS Project in the 1980s		+†	
Funding from USAID for Population Activities 1976–85			+†
Average HIV Prevalence 2001–2009	+*	+*	+*
N	42	43	34
R^2	20.4%	19.0%	19.3%

† $p < 0.10$; * $p < 0.05$ (two-tailed tests).

Note: + indicates positive coefficient and − indicates negative coefficient. IPPF = International Planned Parenthood Federation.

Source: See text.

Kantner 2006). As described in Chapter 1, all but four countries in sub-Saharan Africa (Equatorial Guinea, Sao Tomé and Principe, Somalia, and Zimbabwe) had an affiliate by the end of 2009.

Comparing resources given to countries to prevent pregnancy in the 1980s with resources received to address HIV in the 2000s helps test for path dependence in funding streams across intimate interventions. Countries that had a USAID-funded population intervention in the 1980s (RAPID or OPTIONS) received, on average, almost US$57 million for HIV activities during the 2002–10 period from the Global Fund, while those without such USAID-funded programs received slightly less than US$24 million from the Global Fund during the same period, a statistically significant difference at the $p < 0.05$ level. Table 3.1 shows the results of linear regressions assessing the same relationships and reinforces these findings. Specifically, even after controlling for the HIV prevalence of a country, countries with an older family planning organization or that received more resources for pregnancy prevention received statistically more Global Fund HIV resources. These findings suggest that transnational ties to donors persisted from family planning to HIV, even after taking into account

Table 3.2 *Results from Linear Regressions Predicting Different HIV Outcomes, Sub-Saharan African Countries, 2001–09*

Variable	(1) Change in HIV prevalence 2001–09	(2) Change in HIV incidence 2001–09	(3) ARV coverage 2009	(4) PMTCT coverage 2009
Political factors related to history of population interventions				
Population policy indicator	–	–*	+*	+**
IPPF affiliate founded before 1986	–*	–	–	–
Sociocultural and economic factors				
Cultural fractionalization	–	+	–*	–
GDP per capita	–	–**	+*	+**
Former British colony	+	+*	–	+†
Transnational factors				
PEPFAR focus country	+†	–	+*	+**
Global Fund disbursements	+	–*	+***	+***
Controls				
Antiretroviral coverage	–	+†		
Epidemic peaked prior to 1999	–**	–*		
N	34	32	42	41
R^2	47.9%	46.4%	56.1%	72.9%

† $p < 0.10$; * $p < 0.05$; ** $p < 0.01$; *** $p < 0.001$ (two-tailed tests).

Note: + indicates positive coefficient and – indicates negative coefficient. IPPF = International Planned Parenthood Federation. ARV = antiretroviral. PMTCT = prevention of mother-to-child transmission.

Source: Adapted from Robinson (2011: 9).

that countries had different levels of HIV. As a result, some countries received disproportionately more funding for HIV than their level of HIV prevalence alone would suggest.

In addition to the link between pregnancy prevention and HIV prevention via donor funding, there is also a link between pregnancy prevention interventions and HIV outcomes, as summarized in Table 3.2 by a series of regressions. These regressions consider four

HIV outcomes: change in HIV prevalence (2001–2009), change in HIV incidence (2001–2009), the percentage of HIV-positive people in need of antiretroviral therapy receiving it (2009), and the percentage of pregnant, HIV-positive women receiving antiretroviral therapy to prevent transmission to their infants (2009). In addition to the political factors of interest (namely the existence of a family planning organization or a population policy), the analysis controls for sociocultural and economic factors – ethnic fractionalization, GDP per capita, and an indicator for former British colonies – as well as transnational factors – resources from PEPFAR and the Global Fund – likely to influence HIV outcomes and discussed in the model in Chapter 1. The first two regressions also include controls for the level of antiretroviral coverage and the age of the epidemic, which can independently influence changes in HIV prevalence and incidence.

The analysis in Table 3.2 shows that countries with an affiliate of the International Planned Parenthood Federation that predated the AIDS epidemic experienced greater declines in HIV prevalence between 2001 and 2009, even after controlling for a variety of other factors likely to influence such change (Robinson 2011). Although causality remains impossible to determine, this finding suggests that a preexisting, local organization familiar with providing services and information related to reproductive health and intimate behaviors allowed countries to better address HIV/AIDS when it first appeared. Table 3.2 also shows that countries that adopted a population policy provided more HIV-positive people with antiretroviral therapy. The beneficial impact of population policy adoption on HIV outcomes may reflect governmental willingness to address issues related to sex, good relationships with donors, or even government effectiveness (i.e., the ability to pass policies and implement programs).[10]

Although the statistical analyses provide support for positive transfers between family planning programs and responses to HIV, just as at the global level, certain factors inhibited such transfers within sub-Saharan African countries. I discuss some of these factors in greater

---

[10] Research at the individual-level from a study in Zambia shows a similar relationship: women who had ever used family planning were more likely to change their behavior in order to prevent HIV (Pillai, Sunil, and Gupta 2003). Similarly, an analysis of HIV prevalence across countries globally showed that contraceptive prevalence in 1990 was significantly associated with lower HIV prevalence in 2005 (Shircliff and Shandra 2011).

depth in the case study chapters that follow, but note several generalizations here. Interviews with population experts revealed that at the time of the emergence of HIV in sub-Saharan Africa, many family planning programs were still quite new, and in their quest to be successful, focused on marital sex.[11] As such, the contemporaneous HIV programs that targeted sex workers could not operate through the existing structures related to family planning. Donors also knew that African governments had been resistant to family planning, and so did not want to associate HIV with such a controversial topic.[12] Bureaucratic structuring also separated family planning from HIV: ministries of health initially placed HIV with sexually transmitted infections, rather than with maternal health and family planning. In addition, family planning programs generally did not promote condoms as a means of contraception (Zaba, Boerma, and Marchant 1998).[13]

Negative discursive links between family planning and HIV also existed across sub-Saharan African countries. In particular, a conspiracy theory developed in many different contexts that AIDS was actually a form of population control developed by the West, and specifically Americans, who infected donor-distributed condoms with HIV (Trinitapoli and Weinreb 2012). Such claims were made believable precisely because family planning organizations were the first to respond to HIV. The lack of a cure for AIDS, which became only more implausible as time went on and money poured into countries to fight AIDS, provided further support for the interpretation of AIDS as a man-made plague, whether for population control or other purposes (Trinitapoli and Weinreb 2012).

Despite these factors that separated family planning programs from HIV interventions, cross-national analysis supports the conclusion that resources in the form of funding and organizations associated with pregnancy prevention transferred to HIV prevention. Specifically, countries that received pregnancy prevention funding from USAID received more HIV funding from the Global Fund, and those that had an affiliate of the International Planned Parenthood Federation or that adopted a population policy experienced better HIV outcomes.

---

[11] E5. [12] E1.
[13] Zimbabwe's family planning program was an exception, however, and began to promote condoms following the emergence of the HIV epidemic there (Williamson and Boohene 1990).

Conclusion

As groundwork for the three case studies that follow, this chapter sketched the broad patterns in pregnancy prevention and HIV prevention across sub-Saharan Africa and examined how resources transferred from one intimate intervention to the other. Family planning programs began as early as the 1960s in Kenya and Ghana, but did not take off more broadly until the 1980s, when a combination of economic recession and World Bank interest prompted countries to begin adopting national population policies. Early HIV interventions focused on prevention and care as these were the only options available. Existing research suggests that the countries that have been most successful in addressing HIV had greater political commitment and strong civil societies.

Two key resources transferred between pregnancy prevention and HIV prevention across sub-Saharan African countries. The first was funding from external donors: countries that received above-average funds for pregnancy prevention also received above-average funds for HIV interventions. Although the causality of such a relationship cannot be determined – countries may have other characteristics that make them desirable funding recipients regardless of the program target – it is suggestive of the conclusion that strong path dependencies exist in foreign aid streams. The effect of prior funding for family planning on HIV funding persists even after controlling for HIV prevalence, indicating that country-donor relationships may supersede some level of "true" need for assistance.

A second resource-based transfer occurred through family planning NGOs and population policies. Countries with an affiliate of the International Planned Parenthood Federation that predated the AIDS epidemic, or with a population policy, experienced better HIV outcomes in terms of declines in HIV prevalence as well as provision of antiretroviral therapy. Again, although it is difficult to disentangle whether characteristics of the country led to both pregnancy prevention and the good HIV outcome, or if one caused the other, there are a number of reasons why having a family planning NGO on the ground prior to the emergence of the AIDS epidemic may have been beneficial. First, the importance ascribed to civil society organizations in effective responses to HIV. Their benefits include closeness to populations in need, as well as the capacity to channel donor funds, particularly in a period during which donors were suspicious of African states. Second, these NGOs had experience with sensitive issues related to sex that made them less likely to engage in denialism, as well as connections with key groups in society (religious and traditional leaders, other NGOs, the government, and even donors) that could then be employed to obtain and disseminate information about HIV.

The cross-country analysis thus supports the conclusion that the history of family planning positively influenced HIV prevention. These findings are in line with the path-dependent processes described in Chapter 1, as given investments in one field tend to lead to further investments in that same field. The analysis above demonstrates that such path dependence occurred through both transnational ties – countries that had received more donor attention for population also received above-average levels of funding for HIV – and local political factors, where organizational resources developed for family planning were likely deployed to address HIV. Finally, the positive association between population policy adoption and HIV outcomes may reflect an impact of policy feedback in that governments experienced with adopting policy in the realm of the intimate were more likely to engage in other intimate interventions. The following chapters address these relationships in detail for the cases of Malawi, Nigeria, and Senegal.

4 | Malawi: Negative Policy Feedback and Political Legacy

Of the three cases examined in this book, AIDS is most visible in Malawi. Malawi has, and has had, a more severe epidemic than either Nigeria or Senegal: adult prevalence was 9.1 percent in 2013, having declined from a peak of over 16 percent in the late 1990s (Government of Malawi 2012a; UNAIDS 2016a). But the people living with HIV are not readily recognizable given the widespread availability of affordable antiretroviral therapy. Instead, AIDS is visible because of the response to it. In 2009, the road from the airport to the capital of Lilongwe was flanked with billboards advertising Care brand female condoms as well as small signs for local organizations supporting those living with HIV. Larger signs for projects and offices doing HIV work and listing the supporting donors were liberally sprinkled throughout town. The daily newspapers published many articles that discussed AIDS as well as contained advertisements from local NGOs and donors for AIDS-related positions. The same pattern repeated itself throughout the country, driving down the M1 from Lilongwe to the biggest city of Blantyre. Shops in small towns were painted with ads for Chishango condoms – "shield" in Chichewa and the brand socially marketed by the in-country affiliate of Population Services International (see Figure 4.1) – and the signs for HIV-related organizations and projects, both large and small, were ubiquitous.

The "official" response to HIV is also more visible in Malawi than in either Nigeria or Senegal. Here, the National AIDS Commission is located in a large, fancy building, funded by donors specifically for this purpose, and referred to as "Glass House." In the restroom at the National AIDS Commission, as at the World Bank and many other AIDS-related organizations, boxes of free condoms rested on the backs of toilets. In parallel to the magnitude of the epidemic, AIDS researchers from numerous universities in the Global North implement projects in Malawi: some biomedical, randomized control trials of drugs and other interventions, and others more social science oriented, such as the

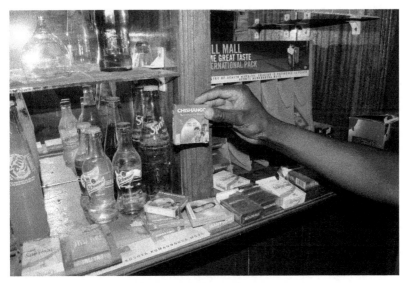

Figure 4.1. Malawi Condom Packaging
Source: Photo by Scott August, courtesy Population Services International.

University of Pennsylvania's long-running Malawi Diffusion and Ideational Change Project, now the Malawi Longitudinal Study of Families and Health (Kohler et al. 2014). While US-based institutions also have research projects in Nigeria and Senegal, Malawi's small cities and land area make the projects more noticeable. In Malawi, far more so than in Nigeria or Senegal, I joined a recognizable group of people "doing" research on AIDS.

Malawi would have had a difficult time avoiding a serious HIV epidemic, given the country's location in the hardest-hit area of sub-Saharan Africa and low male circumcision rates, but the government still responded late. It was not until the mid-2000s, when affordable antiretroviral treatment became available, that the government began to actively address HIV. This chapter explains that belated response with particular reference to the preceding history of intimate interventions. In particular, some of the roots of the delayed action on HIV can be found in Malawi's reticence to adopt family planning programs, demonstrating the potential for negative policy feedback loops.

The model developed in Chapter 1 identifies transnational, political, sociocultural, and economic factors as helpful in understanding responses to HIV across countries. Addressing transnational, political, and sociocultural, factors in particular, the chapter examines how the history of family planning in Malawi influenced the response to HIV. The country's relationship with the West – and with donors in particular – combined with the larger-than-life figure of President Banda are the most important transnational and political factors, respectively, that shaped intimate interventions. In particular, President Banda's rejection of contraception as anti-Malawian greatly influenced the course of pregnancy prevention in the country. Malawi's generally weak civil society and the absence of any family planning NGO until 1987, political factors, meant that the country had few organizational resources from pregnancy prevention campaigns to use in addressing HIV. Together, these forces led to damaging policy feedback processes, whereby the experiences of family planning limited options for responding to HIV. A sociocultural factor, higher rates of HIV in the region inhabited by an ethnic and religious minority, the Yao, has in particular complicated the development of medical male circumcision campaigns, a recent element of HIV prevention strategies. Finally, Malawi had the lowest gross national income per capita in sub-Saharan Africa in 2013, hovering at less than US$300 per person, leaving the population particularly dependent on government and donor-funded AIDS programs (World Bank 2014).

In this chapter, I first provide background on transnational and political factors in Malawi that were salient to both family planning and HIV prevention, which I then discuss in greater detail in the following section, describing the transfers that did and did not occur between family planning and HIV prevention. The evidence presented in this chapter comes from interviews I conducted in 2009 with Malawians working for donor organizations, federal ministries, and local NGOs.[1] It is supplemented by analysis of government and NGO documents, as well as the secondary literature. While Malawi's initial responses to family planning and HIV were somewhat underwhelming, today the country has gained a reputation as both a family planning and an HIV treatment success story, indicating that although history matters, it is but one factor in the complicated story of intimate interventions.

---

[1] References to interviews are denoted by "M" for Malawi, a number, and the type of organization for which the respondent worked.

Transnational and Political Factors in Malawi

The first and long-time president of Malawi, Hastings Kamuzu Banda, decisively influenced the adoption of intimate interventions in the country. An authoritarian leader, he opposed family planning and was reluctant to develop an official response to AIDS. His oppressive rule severely hampered the development of civil society organizations that might have filled the void in state-led service provision (Pact Malawi 2007; Venter 1995).

Banda became president of Malawi following Nyasaland's independence from Great Britain in 1964 and chose the name "Malawi" for the country, taking it from the Maravi people who had historically lived in the area. He spent much of his early adult life abroad, receiving medical training and then practicing medicine in the US and UK before returning to Nyasaland in 1958 to lead the Nyasaland African Congress (King and King 1992). He became the de facto prime minister after the 1961 elections gave his party a legislative majority, and then the actual prime minister in 1963. Following independence in 1964, Banda consolidated power in the newly created office of the presidency, and made his party, the Malawi Congress Party, the only legal party and one to which all Malawians had to belong. Then, in 1971, he declared himself "His Excellency the Life President of the Republic of Malawi." By the 1980s, Malawi was essentially a police state, where order was enforced by the Malawi Youth Pioneers, the paramilitary wing of the Youth League of the Malawi Congress Party that doubled as the secret police. Banda was useful to Western governments as he was very suspicious of socialism and maintained communication with apartheid South Africa; as a result, they did not question his authoritarian rule and even provided aid (Kerr and Mapanje 2002; Venter 1995; Wroe 2012). The situation continued largely unchanged for nearly thirty years, until pressure to democratize came from both external donors and an internal social movement led by religious organizations. Events came to a head in 1992 when a letter written by the country's Catholic bishops decrying the state of the country and calling for political change was read during Lent in every single Catholic church in the country (Meredith 2005; Mitchell 2002). By this point the Cold War was over, so donors no longer needed anti-Soviet allies and withdrew aid in response to Banda's treatment of dissidents, leaving him with fewer resources to maintain his power (Wroe 2012). Lack of resources as well as the bishops' Lenten letter and the protests it spurred led to a 1993 referendum, during which Malawians voted in favor of multi-party elections. In 1994, Malawi held its first multi-party election and voted Banda out of office; he died shortly thereafter, in 1997.

Banda was a dictator and could make things happen, or keep them from happening as was the case with both family planning and early HIV prevention. He was not only President for Life, but Father of the Nation, and cultivated cultural nationalism, particularly respect for hierarchy and authority with his image prominently displayed in all businesses and offices (Forster 1994). He heavily promoted Chichewa, the language of his region and ethnic group, as a national language even though he could not speak it well himself, and banned all other languages except for English (Kerr and Mapanje 2002). His companion and the official hostess, Cecilia Kadzamira, was referred to as "Mama," the mother of the nation (Meredith 2005). Among the matrilineal Chewa, women have a well-defined relationship with an older brother or maternal uncle, their *nkhoswe*, who serves as a source of support for the women in his family, his *mbumba*. Banda named himself "*Nkhoswe* No. 1," making all Malawian women his *mbumba* (Gilman 2009). Banda ensured that he was always met by "praise dancers" – dancing women wearing cloth with his image on it. Dancing had previously been a form of dissent against the British; Banda's control of such dancing simultaneously removed an opportunity for political expression and served to link women's bodies to the president, state, and nation (Gilman 2009). Although he acknowledged the need to improve women's status, and took concrete steps to promote education and employment for women, from Banda's perspective they remained subordinate to the male guardians of the family (Forster 1994; Forster 2001).

Banda's stance was not only paternalistic and authoritarian, but also deeply conservative. Despite, or perhaps because of, his Western education, Western "permissiveness" was particularly threatening to Banda (Forster 1994); his position as an elder of the Church of Scotland reflected and reinforced this conservatism. Women were not allowed to wear trousers or short skirts and men's hair was to be kept short and could be cut upon arrival at the airport if deemed of an inappropriate length (Gilman 2009; Lwanda 2002; Meredith 2005). Foreign movies and publications were censored, and in 1969, the Peace Corps was ejected from the country because of the Western values its volunteers promoted and symbolized, and perhaps even because of promoting family planning (Chimbwete, Watkins, and Zulu 2005). Intellectualism was threatening to Banda: all research had to be approved by the National Research Council, and permission was required for scientists to attend international conferences (Kerr and Mapanje 2002; Wangel 1995). Banda's regime used extensive surveillance techniques to monitor those working at the University of Malawi, and the Censorship Board heavily influenced syllabi for classes (Kerr and Mapanje 2002). Under these conditions, many intellectuals were exiled, deported, or fled Malawi, and among those who stayed, arrests without charge and imprisonment without trial were not uncommon (Kerr and Mapanje 2002).

Malawi's relationship with the international community improved upon the transition to democracy in 1994. While Banda had resisted pressure from other governments and international organizations to democratize and liberalize, in the post-Cold War era, the receipt of development aid depended on making strides towards democracy, and so Malawi followed suit (Englund 2006). After the multiparty elections, international aid organizations flooded into Malawi, among them ones that emphasized family planning and HIV prevention, as well as those that promoted democracy and the expansion of human rights.

Interactions with the international community since 1994 have been largely cordial, albeit interspersed with periods of conflict. When international financial institutions told President Bingu wa Mutharika in 2005 that he should no longer provide fertilizer subsidies to farmers, the largest occupational group in the country and an important electoral constituency, he rebuffed them and Malawi exported corn a mere five years after having suffered famine (Dorward, Chirwa and Jayne 2011; Dugger 2007; Sachs 2012). His second term in office was, however, marred by a turn towards authoritarianism, cronyism, and corruption. Government crackdowns on peaceful protests led to the withdrawal of British aid. Malawi also came under close international scrutiny in 2010 for jailing a transgender woman who married a cisgender man in a traditional wedding ceremony, for further government suppression of protests in 2011, and again in 2014 over a major corruption scandal. All of these incidents led to the threat, or actual suspension, of foreign aid. Finally, in 2015 the Global Fund took grants away from the country's national AIDS commission following claims of improper allocation (Banda 2015).

This brief background on Malawi illustrates transnational, political, and sociocultural elements important to understanding intimate interventions in the country. Specifically, Banda's conservative authoritarian rule through the mid-1990s led to the rejection of family planning as anti-Malawian, inhibited HIV prevention activities, likely reduced the volume of donor funding, and also limited the space for civil society. Banda used culture as a justification and rhetorical device for his rule. Although the provision of family planning and HIV prevention and treatment are much improved today, Banda's rule has had long-lasting negative effects.

Preventing Pregnancy in Malawi

Under Banda, the government of Malawi only reluctantly engaged in pregnancy prevention: starting from the early 1980s, reduction in family size was to occur by spacing births rather than preventing them. Until the late 1980s, there was no NGO providing services, and throughout the pre-1994 period, Malawians were suspicious of the motives behind contraception provision (Kaler 2004). As a result, the sum total of family planning services until 1994 consisted of the government child spacing program implemented in 1982 to which were added the clinics of the Christian Health Association of Malawi in 1984 and the local NGO, Banja la Mtsogolo, in 1989 (National Family Welfare Council of Malawi 1994). In 1994, following multiparty elections, the government adopted a national population policy, and family planning programs increased in reach and intensity as the global population field's access to the country grew.

As in many sub-Saharan African countries, in the decades following independence, the Malawian government viewed population growth relatively positively. For example, the government's report on the 1966 census acknowledged the rapid rate of population growth, but interpreted this growth as an opportunity for nation-building (Chimbwete, Watkins, and Zulu 2005). The uneven distribution of people between the south and north of the country was of greater concern to the government than population growth (Kalipeni 1992). Nonetheless, according to government documents as well as respondents, in the early 1960s family planning supplies were briefly available in Malawi. But soon after, likely in 1968, the government discontinued the program, and some say banned family

planning altogether, primarily because Banda viewed family planning as Western and the limitation of family size as un-Malawian
(Chimbiri 2007; Chimbwete, Watkins, and Zulu 2005; Government
of Malawi 1996). According to the 1994 population policy's
description of what happened, "The services' scope and objectives
were not clearly presented to the public so that many misconceptions led to the services being terminated" (Government of Malawi
1994: section 3.3.1.1). Similarly, the 1994 National Family
Planning Strategy explained the history: "Family planning services
were first introduced in Malawi in the early 1960s. However, the
approach, philosophy, and rationale of the programme were not
clearly articulated. This led to misconceptions concerning the intent
of the programme which, in turn, resulted in its abolition"
(National Family Welfare Council of Malawi 1994: 1). Another
source explicitly noted that those running the program were foreigners who did not understand the culture of Malawi (Government
of Malawi 1986). Perhaps not surprisingly, sex was not a topic of
public conversation in this atmosphere (Lwanda 2002).

Because Banda framed family planning as un-Malawian and because
donors were so enthusiastic about it, Malawians saw what little programming that existed as something from afar. Many Malawians also
interpreted the programs as an effort by donors and the government to
reduce the burden of a country that was constantly in need of aid and
emergency support (Kaler 2004). Those interviewed for the book
understood Banda's ban on family planning from this perspective,
stating that the ban was because the citizenry itself had reacted negatively to family planning, not because of Banda's personal views.
As a respondent explained: "Family planning in Malawi dates back
to the 1960s, when the first attempts to introduce the program failed,
because of misconceptions about population reduction. Like, the government didn't want us to be more people."[2] Another respondent
echoed this interpretation: "Family planning programs started well in
the late 1960s, but they were soon stopped, because people did not
understand the intent. People said that the government was trying to
control the population. So, Dr. Banda decided not to encourage the
Ministry of Health to provide family planning services."[3] The historical narrative is thus that Malawians believed the government tried to

---

[2] M35, bilateral organization.   [3] M32, local NGO.

limit the size of the population, and even though the government did not mean the program to be interpreted this way, because of this negative reception, stopped the provision of family planning services.

In the late 1970s elites from the medical field began to push for government provision of family planning. After attending a 1979 conference in Swaziland where family planning was discussed, Lucy Kadzamira, the director of nursing services in the Ministry of Health from 1977 to 1994, recommended family planning be introduced for the purposes of child spacing (Chimbwete, Watkins, and Zulu 2005). Her position in the Ministry as well as her connection to Banda through her sister Cecilia Kadzamira, his official hostess, gave her opinions weight. A "Workshop on Health and the Family" followed in 1981, funded by the UNFPA, hosted by the Ministry of Health, and attended by representatives from various other ministries and donor organizations (Chimbwete, Watkins, and Zulu 2005). After this meeting, a memo was sent to Banda that cautiously promoted family planning in the name of spacing, rather than limiting, births. As one respondent put it, "So the senior health professionals, I think really sat and said, 'We need to do something about this.' And so, eventually in the course of discussions, they convinced the president that we are not going to plan the family, that's not our business."[4] Instead, they would provide the technology to allow people to space their children.

Strategically written, the memo appealed to Banda's cultural nationalism in a variety of ways and several of its likely authors had close ties to the president (Chimbwete, Watkins, and Zulu 2005). First, it used the Chichewa term *kulera*, meaning child spacing (achieved through "traditional" means such as abstinence and breastfeeding), to refer to both child spacing and modern methods of pregnancy prevention. Second, it argued that a child spacing program would respond to existing demand by supplying modern family planning methods where traditional ones were currently being used, as opposed to converting non-users. And third, it urged Banda, as *Nkhoswe* No. 1 of the nation, to attend to his duties and reduce maternal mortality by providing contraception. The justification for the program echoed tactics that were successful in overcoming resistance to family planning in Zimbabwe and other African countries (Kaler 2003), and the Malawian National Child Spacing Programme was thus approved in 1982.

---

[4] M24, multilateral organization.

This program focused primarily on the timing of pregnancies and limited services to married women over the age of eighteen who had obtained their husbands' consent (Wangel 1995). It promoted family planning as a means to delay pregnancies that were too early, prevent pregnancies that came too late, increase the number of years between pregnancies, and reduce the number of women with "too many" pregnancies, all as a means to improve maternal and child health. Early materials produced by the program included *A Pictorial-Story Guide to Child Spacing* (Ministry of Health n.d.-b) as well as *Our Common Secret* (Ministry of Health n.d.-a), which were illustrated with large photos and produced in both English and Chichewa. The *Pictorial-Story Guide* followed Mr. and Mrs. Phiri,[5] who started with two children, had a third, and then sought assistance from the clinic to limit the size of their family, which later pictures depict as having better health care and more time to grow food. *Our Common Secret* presented different forms of contraception, including a picture of smiling women captioned, "We practice child spacing because We believe child spacing improves our health" and another of smiling men captioned, "Yes it is true we too have our own secret. We too have our own way of participating directly in child spacing. We use CONDOMS." In the 1990s, the term "child spacing" was pervasive, reflecting the framing that had helped bring the program into being in the first place. As one respondent explained: "We couldn't have used 'family planning,' because initially it wasn't accepted. So the name was changed. So in this child spacing was included permanent methods: even if you had your tubes tied, it was still 'child spacing!'"[6]

Following the adoption of the child spacing program, the global population field's interaction with Malawi intensified, and the World Bank, UNFPA, and USAID began to fund population activities (Kennedy 1984). With the support of international donors, the federal bureaucracy created new administrative units to manage population activities, Malawian demographers received training, and demographic data collection increased (Chimbwete, Watkins and Zulu 2005). The economic downturn of the 1980s provided donors with further justification for encouraging a more explicit population policy.

[5] "Phiri" is the Chewa equivalent of "Jones" or "Smith," so the authors intended the couple to be seen as average Malawians.
[6] M20, international NGO.

As in Nigeria and Senegal as well as in many sub-Saharan African countries, the World Bank promoted population activities, including a child spacing component in its first Malawi health project, identifying population growth as a priority issue for Malawi in the 1980s, and carrying out a population sector review in 1984 (Simmons and Maru 1988). The donor-funded RAPID model described in previous chapters was completed by 1990 (Newton 1990), and as one respondent explained: "This is the time when USAID broadened to focus on population projections, and impacts of population growth on the resources available in the country. The RAPID model was actually being developed around that time, and had an effect on what was going on in Malawi."[7]

In 1990, the Department of Economic Planning and Development created a Population and Human Resources Development Unit, and in 1992, the government established the National Family Welfare Council as a parastatal organization[8] under the Ministry of Women, Youth, and Community Affairs to manage the activities of the child spacing program. This same year, the government removed a number of barriers to family planning access, including the particularly steep criteria for use of the injectable contraceptive Depo-Provera: marriage and four children (Solo, Jacobstein, and Malema 2005). Finally, in 1993 the Principal Secretaries Symposium approved a draft population policy, one month before the referendum on multiparty elections (Chimbwete, Watkins, and Zulu 2005).

Malawi officially adopted the population policy in 1994, after Banda had left office, marking a change from an inward-looking preservation of culture to an active desire to engage the international community on population issues and more broadly (Chimbwete, Watkins, and Zulu 2005). As one respondent described the shift, "The family planning strategy started, and then the population policy followed. These were developed with the wind of political change."[9] In 1994, the Malawi National Child Spacing Programme was renamed the Malawi Family Planning Programme, but kept the term *kulera* to describe family planning (Chimbwete, Watkins, and Zulu 2005). In President

---

[7] M25, international NGO.
[8] A "parastatal organization" is a quasi-government organization. Such organizations cultivate the appearance of privatization for the benefit of neoliberal donors, without being completely free of governmental control.
[9] M35, bilateral organization.

Muluzi's first address to parliament, he mentioned the importance of family planning to development objectives, and in 1995, for the first time, the budget had a line item for family planning (Chimbwete, Watkins, and Zulu 2005).

Throughout the 1990s, institutional change promoted by the global population field drove an increasing emphasis on family planning. In 1997, the Family Health Unit evolved into the Reproductive Health Unit, reflecting the changes codified at the 1994 United Nations International Conference on Population and Development that shifted terminology for population activities away from population control towards the broader concept of reproductive health (Hodgson and Watkins 1997). The National Family Welfare Council moved to the Ministry of Health and was renamed the National Family Planning Council, and then in 1999 became the Family Planning Association of Malawi and the affiliate of the International Planned Parenthood Federation, making Malawi the last country in sub-Saharan Africa to affiliate (Hennink, Zulu, and Dodoo 2001; International Planned Parenthood Federation 2009). In 2001, the UNFPA formed a committee to revise the population policy to bring it in line with the concept of reproductive health (Chimbwete, Watkins, and Zulu 2005), and in 2002, the government adopted a reproductive health policy (Government of Malawi 2002). By 2012, Malawi had revised its population policy to better reflect the Millennium Development Goals, among other factors (Government of Malawi 2012b).

The donors most involved in family planning in Malawi have been USAID, the British development agency DFID, and the UNFPA. The World Bank has also funded population activities, including a 1999 project designed to increase the use of community-based distribution agents (Solo, Jacobstein, and Malema 2005), but neither family planning nor population policy was a condition of the Bank's 1981 structural adjustment policy (Chimbwete, Watkins, and Zulu 2005). International NGOs active in family planning in Malawi have included Jhpiego, EngenderHealth, Management Sciences for Health, Plan International, and Population Services International as well as the Adventist Development Relief Agency.

A local NGO, Banja la Mtsogolo, founded in 1987, has provided a major share of contraceptive supplies and services to Malawians. Banja la Mtsogolo, the "Family of the Future" in Chichewa, is the affiliate of the British NGO Marie Stopes International and receives funding from the Malawian government, as well as from multilateral and bilateral organizations and international NGOs. Since the late 1990s, Banja la Mtsogolo has provided half or more of the family planning in Malawi at heavily subsidized prices (Banja la Mtsogolo n.d.; Hennink, Zulu and Dodoo 2001). When Banja la Mtsogolo had to temporarily stop subsidizing services in 2000, client visits dropped by 46 percent (Opportunities and Choices Programme n.d.). In addition to services provided at clinics located throughout the country, Banja la Mtsogolo also sends mobile reproductive health assistants into rural areas (Banja la Mtsogolo 2009).

Concomitant with the government's shift towards greater support of family planning in the 1990s, the percentage of married women aged 15–49 using modern contraception increased dramatically from only 7 percent in 1992, to 26 percent in 2000, and to more than 40 percent by 2014 (National Statistical Office and ICF Macro 2011; Solo, Jacobstein, and Malema 2005). Although the magnitude of these figures may be somewhat overestimated given they come from self-reports potentially influenced by social desirability bias (Miller, Zulu, and Watkins 2001), the trend towards greater contraceptive use is certainly real. Contraceptive prevalence is higher among urban and wealthier women, but has also increased substantially in rural areas, and among women of all levels of wealth (Solo, Jacobstein, and Malema 2005). The most popular forms of contraception are hormonal, with the vast majority of women relying on injectables (National Statistical Office and ICF Macro 2011).

As a result of the increase in contraceptive prevalence, the total fertility rate declined from more than seven children per woman in 1970 to five in 2014 (Population Reference Bureau 2015). Malawi has thus gained somewhat of a reputation within the global population field as a family planning "success." When USAID began its Repositioning Family Planning program, it chose Malawi along with Ghana and Zambia as countries that had increased contraceptive use and reduced fertility (Malarcher 2005; Solo, Jacobstein, and Malema 2005). Malawi also received commendations for being one of the few countries to implement by 2010 many of the recommendations of the Maputo Plan of Action, the 2006 African Union design for ensuring universal access to sexual and reproductive health for all Africans (SAfAIDS and Ford Foundation n.d.). More recently, in 2012 USAID again used Malawi as an example of a "successful" sub-Saharan African family planning program, this time in conjunction with Ethiopia and Rwanda, with particular reference to achieving the Millennium Development Goals (Bureau for Africa 2012). While the drivers of these changes go beyond the scope of the book, they indicate that the nature of pregnancy prevention in a country can change over time.

In sum, family planning in Malawi followed a path similar to that in many other sub-Saharan African countries, but with particularly strong opposition to contraception from the government through 1994. Prior to that date, virtually all support for family planning came at the urging of medical professionals and international donors. Starting from the establishment of its first clinic in 1989, an NGO, Banja la Mtsogolo, also provided a significant share of contraceptive supplies and services (National Family Welfare Council of Malawi 1994). Thus transnational factors promoted family planning, while the effect of political factors was in two directions: leadership opposition, but some civil society support. The government's stance shifted with the election of President Muluzi in 1994 and his desire to broadcast widely that Malawi was ready to reconnect to the international community. One signal was the adoption of the 1994 population policy, and another was the expansion of contraceptive availability in health facilities. Since then, Malawi's contraceptive prevalence rate has increased steadily, a trend that may be partially attributed to government and organizational actions and also to other factors, but whose analysis falls outside the bounds of this book.

Preventing HIV in Malawi

HIV most likely entered Malawi in the late 1970s, and by 1985, when the first tests were completed, 2 percent of women in the antenatal ward at Queen Elizabeth Hospital in Blantyre were HIV positive (Lwanda 2002). Biometrics from a sample of sex workers the following year showed a prevalence rate of 46 percent, and in 1986, almost 4 percent of Malawian mineworkers in South Africa were HIV-positive (Chiphangwi et al. 1987; Iliffe 2006). HIV rates among antenatal patients rose steadily from that point forward: 8.2 percent in 1987, 18.6 percent in 1989, 21.9 percent in 1990, and 31.6 percent in 1993 (Taha et al. 1998). Prevalence among the adult population was approximately 10 percent in 1993 and by 2001 had reached 13.8 percent (Chirwa 1998; UNAIDS 2010). Factors that helped HIV rates climb so high include ubiquitous labor migration to tea and tobacco plantations in Malawi and mining opportunities further afield as well as low levels of male circumcision (Bryceson and Fonseca 2006). It is likely that South Africa's forced repatriation of 13,000 Malawian migrant workers between 1988 and 1992 facilitated the spread of HIV as some workers returned with HIV, and most came back with higher incomes that enabled behaviors associated with the spread of HIV, including alcohol consumption and transactional sex (Chirwa 1998).

At the time that AIDS was recognized in Malawi in the 1980s, the overall climate of the country was repressive both politically and socially as described earlier in the chapter (Forster 2001). Despite being a medical doctor, President Banda had minimal interest in HIV/ AIDS (Patterson 2006). Like poverty and malnutrition, AIDS was a "non-subject" and certainly not something to be discussed on the heavily censored radio, as admission of any of these problems would indicate governmental fault (Peters, Kambewa, and Walker 2010: 292; Wangel 1995). The government's general perception, as well as that of many Malawians, was that HIV came from the West, was the result of immorality and particularly homosexuality, and was spread by foreigners and those who had traveled abroad (Bryceson and Fonseca 2006; Lwanda 2002).

Although Banda did not himself acknowledge AIDS, an official response to the epidemic came relatively soon after the first estimates of HIV prevalence were available, and the global AIDS field also became involved in the country. In 1985, the government set up a committee to secure the blood supply and the Malawi Broadcast Corporation began to play traditional-sounding songs under the theme of *kwabwela edzi*, "AIDS has come" (Lwanda 2011). That same year, the German bilateral aid agency, GTZ, began providing HIV testing at Malawi's two major hospitals and the results led to funding from the World Health Organization (Wangel 1995). In 1986, the government created a Public Education Strategy on AIDS, and in 1987 the Ministry of Health started the National AIDS Control Programme as well as developed a short-term plan for addressing AIDS (Mkandawire, Luginaah, and Bezner-Kerr 2011; Putzel 2004; Wangel 1995). In 1988, the government and the World Health

Organization formulated the Medium Term Plan, a more comprehensive AIDS intervention program.

Many factors challenged an effective response to HIV. Given Banda's frequent cabinet shake-ups, there were six ministers of health between 1985 and 1991 (Wangel 1995). No national program for sexually transmitted infections existed when AIDS emerged, only the clinics from the colonial era that were run through the Christian Health Association of Malawi's hospitals, a situation that persisted through the early 1990s (Atkinson and Nkera 1993; Wangel 1995). Early on, the government allowed only one US-funded AIDS research project, refusing all other offers (Wangel 1995). As one respondent described the early period of AIDS, "The first five years, it was 'Shhhhh.'"[10]

Behind the silence, though, the government took advantage of funding from the global AIDS field and certainly had some sense of the extent of the epidemic. Although officially part of the Ministry of Health, the AIDS Secretariat reported directly to the president, allowing executive access to AIDS funds (Wangel 1995). The National AIDS Committee, flush with funds from donors, served as a source of patronage for Banda's Malawi Congress Party (Lwanda 2002). Rumors circulated that refrigerators and VCRs intended for HIV activities administered by the United Nations Children's Fund ended up with Malawi Congress Party officials and civil servants in 1988/89, and money designated for HIV work was diverted in order to alleviate shortages in foreign exchange (Lwanda 2002; Wangel 1995). At least one source suggests that the government agreed to the one US-funded AIDS project solely as a means to produce data on HIV in order to generate donor funding (Wangel 1995). Finally, and perhaps most egregiously, for a several-year period beginning in 1988, the government used donated HIV test kits for members of the president's staff, even after the blood donor program had run out of tests (Wangel 1995).

Starting from 1989, a series of events made HIV more visible. First, the military, which had a garrison in Mozambique from 1985 to 1993 protecting the Nacala railway, showed obviously increasing HIV prevalence (Lwanda 2002). A World Bank report about HIV in the Malawian military made it impossible to keep the high prevalence secret, and the widely-reported vandalization by army officers of the newspaper that published the report's findings only brought more

---

[10] M24, multilateral organization.

attention to the issue (Lwanda 2002). Second, South Africa repatriated approximately 13,000 Malawian migrant workers between 1988 and 1992 on the grounds that they were a high-risk group for HIV (Chirwa 1998). Although the explanation was somewhat of a smokescreen – unemployment rates in South Africa were increasing, causing a backlash against foreign workers, and the mining industry as a whole was performing increasingly poorly – the repatriation brought greater visibility to HIV in Malawi (Chirwa 1998). Third, prominent groups began to speak openly about AIDS. The Catholic bishops' 1992 Lenten letter justified its call for an end to Banda's regime in part based on health challenges facing the country, including AIDS, and new political parties added HIV to their platforms for the 1994 elections (Chiona et al. 1992; Lwanda 2002). Fourth, a review by the government and donors found the national response to HIV to be lacking on a number of dimensions and described a "pervasive culture of silence and persistent denial" around HIV/AIDS (as cited in Garbus 2003: 73).

Reflecting greater awareness of the severity of the epidemic, President Muluzi's first public appearance following his election in July 1994 was an AIDS awareness march associated with the August 1994 National AIDS Conference in Blantyre, and soon after, he launched an abstinence campaign called "Why Wait" (Probst 1999; Schoffeleers 1999). But the issue still remained on the backburner, overshadowed by the transition to democracy and other concerns. In 1994, the international NGO implementing USAID's AIDS program said there were "no counterparts to work with" at the National AIDS Committee, and by 1995, the head of the National AIDS Committee resigned in protest after not having been paid in months (John Snow 1998; Lwanda 2002).

The negative impacts of AIDS became yet more visible between 1994 and 1999. First, significant numbers of the president's party began to die. Between 1994 and 1998, twenty higher-level members of the United Democratic Front died, many likely from AIDS (Lwanda 2002). At the same time, South Africa began to disallow HIV treatment for foreigners, cutting off many HIV-positive Malawian elites (Lwanda 2002). President Muluzi's attendance at funerals, designed to demonstrate his connection to the people, began instead to showcase just how little the government was doing about AIDS (Lwanda 2002). Malawians themselves were constantly reminded of AIDS, as they attended funeral after funeral. As one respondent explained:

"Before the advent of antiretroviral therapy, people were dying like nobody's business. And, because of the rate at which people were dying, we didn't need statistics. Any professional would not have required the statistics to know we had an epidemic in our midst. In our culture, when there's a funeral associated with your neighbor, you can't just be in the house, you have to go and be part of it. It could be your relative, a friend, a relative of a friend, a friend's friend – we were in funerals almost every day. You really had to make a decision about which funeral am I going to go to, at least today I should stay at work. It was that bad."[11]

Increasing media coverage of AIDS demonstrated its mounting salience. Between 1985 and 87, very few articles in *The Daily Times* or *Malawi News* mentioned AIDS (Wangel 1995). Major coverage in *The Daily Times* was limited until it reported on a 1993 meeting regarding the government's medium term plan to address AIDS (Wangel 1995). Following the transition to democracy and the removal of censorship rules, however, media coverage of AIDS picked up (Peters, Kambewa, and Walker 2010). The number of articles in Malawi's main newspaper, *The Nation*, mentioning "AIDS" increased from eighty-one in 1999–2000 to 216 in 2005–06, paralleling the increase in availability of HIV testing (Angotti et al. 2014).

Alongside growing media attention, the number of local AIDS NGOs increased over time. The first local AIDS organization was founded in 1992, the Nkhotakota AIDS Support Organization (USAID 2004a). Other major organizations supporting those living with HIV formed during the 1990s and exist to this day: the National Association of People Living With HIV/AIDS in Malawi in 1993, the Malawi Network of AIDS Service Organizations in 1996, and the Malawi Network of People Living with HIV/AIDS in 1997. By 1997, there were approximately seventy-five local and international NGOs working on HIV in Malawi, and the number of AIDS/orphan care NGOs registered with the Council for NGOs in Malawi doubled between 1995 and 2002 (Lwanda 2002; Morfit 2011). By 2007, there were over 500 AIDS NGOs (Pact Malawi 2007). Many of these NGOs were and are small and heavily dependent on donor funding (Edström and MacGregor 2010; Pact Malawi 2007; Serieux et al. 2012). Indeed, a sample survey of local civil society organizations working in AIDS during the 2007–09 period found that half had

---

[11] M24, multilateral organization.

received funding from international organizations in all of the preceding years, and more than half had fewer than twenty-five employees (Serieux et al. 2012).

In the face of so much death, increasing media coverage, civil society pressure, and donor attention, President Muluzi declared AIDS a national emergency in 1999 (Garbus 2003), an election year, and made a public comment that "Men should learn to dim their (headlights) in the face of temptation" (quoted in Lwanda 2002: 163), meaning that men should reduce their number of sexual partners. Still, though, government HIV interventions focused primarily on disallowing sex work and imprisoning sex workers (Lwanda 2002). The removal of the National AIDS Control Programme from the Ministry of Health in 2001, in order to comply with World Bank guidelines, decimated the Ministry and further hampered HIV prevention and treatment, and the National AIDS Control Programme received harsh critiques of its effectiveness (Patterson 2006; Putzel 2004).

Notably absent from Malawi's response to HIV, particularly in the Banda years, were technocratic leaders. As in other countries, such policy entrepreneurs are crucial to setting government priorities, and evidence specifically from Malawi indicates that locally produced research can be particularly effective in influencing policy change (Hutchinson et al. 2011). The Banda regime had largely pushed out individuals capable of playing such roles, either directly through deportation or imprisonment, or indirectly through the destruction of intellectual freedom combined with low wages and poor working conditions (Kerr and Mapanje 2002). Malawi also had no particular intellectual reputation to uphold globally, unlike Senegal described in Chapter 6, thus limiting any need to take action. Indeed, at least part of the excitement about a supposed cure for AIDS found by a local healer in Malawi in 1994 was that it would help bring positive attention to Malawi. A middle-class professional noted at the time, "Wouldn't it be wonderful if [the cure] *did* work! It would put Malawi on the world map; it would show Westerners that Malawi had something to offer, that Malawian traditional medicine wasn't so stupid" (as quoted in Iliffe 2006: 95).

The energy of the response to the HIV epidemic in Malawi really only increased significantly with the availability of treatment. Before 2001, the cost of antiretroviral therapy had been 10,000–30,000 Kwacha per month, or about US$135–145, an impossibly expensive bill for the average Malawian when GDP per capita was approximately that much *per year* (Wilson 2013). The government launched a pilot program to provide antiretroviral therapy in Blantyre and Lilongwe in 2000, but it was not until 2004 after Malawi had received funding from the Global Fund that free antiretroviral treatment became more available (Garbus 2003; Jahn et al. 2008).[12] By June 2005, sixty government and mission facilities in the country were providing first-line antiretroviral therapy, and the number of people on treatment had increased to 46,000, up from just 4,000 in 2002 (Harries et al. 2007; Knight 2008). The government adopted a national AIDS policy in 2004, and that same year, HIV became a major issue for the first time in a presidential campaign (Iliffe 2006; Patterson 2006).

Much of the international funding for HIV received in the past ten years has gone towards antiretroviral therapy. As of 2013, an estimated half of HIV-positive Malawians and approximately 80 percent of HIV-positive pregnant women were receiving antiretroviral therapy (UNAIDS 2016a).[13] Unlike in Nigeria or Senegal, where lower prevalence rates reduce the odds of individuals knowing someone with HIV, such is not the case in Malawi, so when treatment became available, lots of people noticed. The availability of antiretroviral therapy created "[...] hope for treatment. When there was no access to treatment, people didn't want to know about HIV, but when the ARVs came, and especially when they came free, people were like, 'Well, now I need to know my status because I can get on ARVs.'"[14]

Recently, Malawi has gained a positive reputation within the global AIDS field for its implementation of Option B+ (e.g., Rosenberg 2014). The World Health Organization revised its guidelines for initiation of antiretroviral therapy in 2010, recommending that countries place HIV-positive women on one of two antiretroviral regimes (Option A or B) based on their CD4 count, a measure of the level of progression of HIV. Because of concerns about whether it would be feasible to test the CD4 count of positive women, Malawi instead decided to implement what is now called Option B+: all HIV-positive pregnant or breastfeeding women, regardless of their CD4 count, are put on

---

[12] Malawi was not an original PEPFAR focus country, and so did not receive significant funds from PEFPAR until 2008.

[13] When compared to all countries in sub-Saharan Africa, Malawi ranks in the top (best) third.

[14] M19, local NGO. "ARVs" refers to antiretroviral therapy.

antiretroviral drugs for life. The program began in 2011, and modeling indicates it is cost effective, particularly in terms of the years of life added for the HIV-positive mothers (Fasawe et al. 2013; WHO Regional Office for Africa 2014).

Malawi's HIV prevention efforts lagged in the early years of the epidemic, in large part because of President Banda. Not only was he unwilling to address HIV, but he pushed out the intellectuals and potential technocratic leaders and inhibited the creation of NGOs that could have helped counter his inaction. Ultimately, donor pressure and funding combined with the increasing severity of the epidemic led to government action. Thus transnational and political factors drove much of the country's response to HIV. In addition to these factors, as I discuss next, the experience of pregnancy prevention also left a lasting legacy.[15]

From Pregnancy Prevention to HIV Prevention

Transnational and political factors drove both Malawi's family planning programs and the response to HIV, and resources and strategies associated with family planning transferred to HIV, particularly within international and local organizations. A discursive transfer also occurred between family planning and HIV prevention, but one that was arguably less beneficial to the response to HIV. Finally, the HIV epidemic has itself influenced the ability to provide family planning.

Organizational Resources and Strategies

Family planning and HIV interventions in Malawi were linked through organizational resources, particularly Banja la Mtsogolo and USAID. USAID deployed a number of strategies, including community-based distribution and social marketing, that began with family planning but then easily evolved to include HIV interventions.

One of Malawi's primary pregnancy prevention resources was Banja la Mtsogolo, the family planning NGO founded in 1987, just as the

---

[15] For rich description and analysis of the on-the-ground experience of HIV in Malawi during particularly the past fifteen years, see Esacove (2016) and Swidler and Watkins (2017).

presence of AIDS in Malawi came to be recognized and five years before the founding of the first AIDS organizations in 1992 (USAID 2004a). Just as Banja la Mtsogolo made major contributions to pregnancy prevention, over time it has increasingly become active in HIV prevention. Since 2004, Banja has socially marketed condoms under the brand name Manyuchi (see Figure 4.1), which, like Chishango, target a young male audience with packaging showing an attractive young woman displaying a good deal of cleavage, but at a higher price (Banja la Mtsogolo 2009; Danart et al. 2004). During 2008, with funding from the Malawian National AIDS Commission, Banja la Mtsogolo expanded free HIV testing and counseling to all but one of its thirty-one clinics. Outreach, through reproductive health assistants who work directly in communities and mobile clinics, brings family planning, HIV, and sexually transmitted infection services to areas far from health centers (Banja la Mtsogolo 2009). Banja la Mtsogolo now provides male circumcision for HIV prevention, and in 2008, almost two thirds of Banja la Mtsogolo family planning clients received information about HIV (Banja la Mtsogolo 2009).

USAID also served as a major linking point between family planning and HIV prevention, and particularly emphasized integrating the two in Malawi from the earliest years of the HIV epidemic. USAID's priority objectives for the health and population sector in 1990 were to increase the use of family planning and control the spread of AIDS, as well as to reduce infant and child mortality/morbidity (Newton 1990). Early community-based distribution programs focused on both family planning and HIV. USAID's Support to AIDS and Family Health (STAFH) project funded Malawi's first program for community-based distribution of contraceptives starting in 1989, based at three Christian Health Association of Malawi facilities (National Family Planning Council 1998). The project expanded to other hospitals and regions, such that by 1995 there were eighteen different programs spread across the country (Kornfield 1996). In addition to contraception, community-based distribution agents were also expected to provide information on prevention of sexually transmitted infections and HIV, as well as to refer clients to other HIV-related services, such as testing and care (National Family Planning Council 1998).

Not long after community-based distribution began, so too did social marketing that connected family planning and HIV. Protector brand condoms were first socially marketed in 1991 with funding from USAID via the Futures Group and the SOMARC project (Brown 1994). While the SOMARC project was primarily a family planning program that socially marketed condoms, USAID explicitly saw it as contributing to AIDS control goals as well (Newton 1990; Nyanda and Mmanga 1990). At this time, Malawi was described as a place where "condoms previously had not been advertised, and in which open discussion about AIDS and condoms was very limited" (Brown 1994: 1). Following a reduction in price of more than a third to increase sales, SOMARC's condoms were offered at MK 0.50 (about ten US cents at the time) for a pack of three (Chirwa 1993). The initial advertising campaign was to "Be Responsible, Use Protector Condoms" but government restrictions limited the content of advertising and prevented promotion at either point of sale or through billboards (Atkinson and Nkera 1993). SOMARC's radio campaign did not explicitly mention AIDS, but instead talked about a dual message of "protection." An early evaluation concluded that, "Because of its 'soft-sell' approach to marketing condoms for AIDS prevention, the Protector campaign managed to escape negative publicity in a conservative country like Malawi, yet was able to effectively communicate an AIDS prevention strategy" (Tipping 1993: 4).

Population Services International took over marketing in 1994, and the Protector brand name was later changed to Chishango (Danart et al. 2004; Kaler 2004). Early on, Chishango advertising also included family planning as well as HIV prevention messages (Thompson 1995). Following a plateau in sales, Population Services International relaunched the condom in 2002 with new packaging designed to appeal to young men that shows a woman's bare thigh. The photographic image of the bare thigh caused controversy, and so Population Services International changed all billboards to the old logo, a shield, but for some time kept the image on the packaging (Danart et al. 2004). More recently, they have changed the picture on the packaging back to a shield (see Figure 4.1).

USAID included Malawi in its first two major AIDS programs, AIDSCOM and AIDSTECH, starting from 1989 (Newton 1990). Funded through AIDSCOM, the STAFH Project began in 1992 with a six-year, US$45 million budget that was then extended for an additional three years through 2001 (Solo, Jacobstein, and Malema 2005). Echoing USAID's overall objectives in Malawi, STAFH's goal was to reduce total fertility and the transmission of HIV and other sexually transmitted infections (USAID 1992c). One of STAFH's strategies was to integrate family planning (referred to as "child spacing" in project documents) and AIDS activities whenever possible (USAID 1992c). The proposal justified such integration as follows:

In many ways, these two activities will be implemented separately, but it is the intention of the Mission to integrate them in every way possible. *There is little precedent for this approach in terms of major project design elsewhere* [emphasis added], but it is an approach which displays specific advantages and which is gaining acceptance. To a large extent the target groups of the two activities are the same. Also, they both rely on significant participation by the Ministry of Health [MOH], require the allocation of substantial MOH resources, and utilize similar MOH services and facilities. This can make them competitors for scarce health resources, but if they are regarded in every way possible as complementary, then the resulting efficiencies should further enhance achievement of individual objectives. (USAID 1992c: xi)

Given USAID was the primary supplier of both contraception and condoms for HIV prevention in the country may have encouraged such an integration (Atkinson and Nkera 1993). The emphasis on both family planning and HIV prevention extended throughout the program's activities. Funding from STAFH supported the creation of *Tinkanena*, a Chichewa radio soap opera promoting family planning as well as prevention of sexually transmitted infections and HIV that ran through the 1990s and won three annual awards from the Malawi Broadcast Corporation for best-produced program (John Snow 1998). Grants to NGOs through the project focused on helping organizations provide both family planning and HIV services (John Snow 1998). A later NGO-focused project of USAID, the Umoyo Network, grew out the NGO component of STAFH and maintained the integration of family planning and HIV (Goyder 2003). Continuing earlier programs, STAFH focused considerable resources on the development of community-based distribution programs to provide contraceptive supplies as well as information about HIV.

The integration of family planning and HIV into the community-based distribution component of STAFH demonstrated some of the challenges to transferring strategies known from family planning to HIV. To integrate these two areas, community-based distribution agents were either to promote condoms for family planning *and* HIV prevention, or to provide information on HIV prevention and services. Doing so, however, was easier said than done. First, family planning clinics and staff had never promoted condoms for family planning, seeing them instead as a back-up method of contraception, a choice for preventing sexually transmitted infections for non-marital relationships, or for youth (Thompson 1995). Second, many of the agents were not comfortable talking about HIV at all and were confused about whether the Chishango condom was for family planning or HIV (Thompson 1995). One study found that only a quarter of clients received information about AIDS from a community-based distribution agent, and that the information tended to be superficial and vague (Kornfield 1996). Third, many clients felt that HIV should be addressed separately from family planning for one or more of several reasons: to prevent information overload, because one person could not be skilled enough to teach about both, or because HIV was related to promiscuity and family planning to family (Thompson 1995). As a result, the community-based distribution programs made little impact in addressing HIV.

Today, as in many sub-Saharan African countries, there is increased discussion of integration of family planning and HIV prevention (e.g., Government of Malawi 2011). For example, with USAID funding, the US NGO Management Sciences for Health implemented yet another major community-based distribution program from 2007 to 2011 that focused on the integration of family planning and HIV services (Barnes, Blumhagen, and Huber 2010). Pilot studies indicated that such integration is cost effective (Barnes, Blumhagen, and Huber 2010; Bollinger and Adesina 2013).

Organizational resources as well as strategies like social marketing and community-based distribution thus flowed from family planning to HIV in Malawi. As the discussion of transnational and political factors influencing intimate interventions demonstrated, the political climate did not engender widespread support for either family planning or HIV, and negative discourses about family planning also transferred directly to HIV in a policy feedback process unsupportive to the response to HIV. Condoms, although available in conjunction with family planning/child spacing programs, were never widely used to prevent pregnancy, and so did not serve as a point of technology transfer.

Discourses

A number of popularly-held suspicions about the motivations of family planning, the origins of AIDS, and the intentions of donors and the Malawian government mutually reinforced one another and complicated intimate interventions in Malawi. Like family planning, many Malawians viewed HIV as something dubious that came from abroad, and in the mid-1990s, there were still reports that some Malawians believed that AIDS was invented to frighten people into using condoms, or perhaps even to prevent them from having sex (Forster 2001; Lwanda 2002). Amy Kaler (2004) has described the suspicion about the relationship between condoms and AIDS as the result of the "long shadow of population control." Given this degree of suspicion about population control, when family planning organizations began talking about AIDS, many Malawians saw AIDS as an American family planning "plot" to reduce the size of Malawi's population (Lwanda 2004: 35). Concern about foreign interventions leading to sterility long predated the HIV epidemic in Malawi and elsewhere in sub-Saharan Africa (Kaler 2009). For example, during a smallpox outbreak in Nyasaland in 1960, rumors spread that the vaccine would cause sterility (Vaughan 1994). Even in the early 2000s, rumors circulated that because Malawians had not overwhelmingly adopted family planning, donors had developed alternative means to reduce the population size through hiding sterilizing agents and HIV within other products, such as condoms (Wilson 2012).

For all these reasons, some portion of Malawians viewed condoms as dangerous, ineffective, and possibly even the source of AIDS itself. They thus felt that the response to AIDS was too heavily based on condoms. Indeed, a nationally representative survey conducted in 2003 revealed that 44 percent of Malawians believed condoms were the top priority of the government's AIDS programs, but only 6 percent agreed that should be the case, instead preferring the government to focus on health education and medicines (Zogby International and Schneidman & Associates International 2003). Relatedly, condoms have been further removed from family planning in people's minds by their linkage with sexually transmitted infections – HIV in particular – and sexual relationships outside of marriage (Chimbiri 2007; Kaler 2004).

In addition to reservations about condoms, many Malawians were suspicious about the government's role in AIDS. The absence of a cure made the disease sound fantastical and perhaps invented. One of the Malawian names for AIDS, particularly in the earlier days of the epidemic, was *matenda a boma*, the government disease. AIDS was labeled such because the government talked about AIDS, and because people did not entirely trust the government, particularly because of the Banda regime's manipulation of the media, it became plausible that the government may have somehow caused AIDS (Forster 2001; Kaler 2004; Lwanda 2002; Wilson 2013). Even once antiretroviral drugs were available, people were concerned about their quality because a product that had previously been so expensive and inaccessible suddenly flooded the market (Wilson 2012). Suspicion was directed at both the government and donors. Some interpreted the government's unwillingness to support a traditional healer's 1994 claim that he had found a cure for AIDS as evidence that the government took the side of international donors, whose motives were also questionable (Schoffeleers 1999).

Indeed, some Malawians blamed donors directly for AIDS, noting that the donors' emphasis on free choice (referring to individualism and rights) led people to "freely" spread HIV (Lwanda 2002). The foreign connections with HIV were popularly expressed as alternative interpretations for the acronym for AIDS, such as an "American Invention Depriving Sex," "American Idea to Discourage Sex," or "American Initiative to Deny Sex" (Bonga 1999; Wangel 1995). The American connection arose because of the association between AIDS and gay men in the US, and also because primarily US NGOs promoted condoms and other HIV prevention techniques in Malawi (Lwanda 2002). Many among the Malawian elite took offense at the Western portrayal of African sex as different from Western sex, rejecting as racist narratives of particularly "African" sexual patterns used to explain the intensity of the HIV epidemic in southern Africa (Lwanda 2002).

In part because of these suspicions, but also because of the number of competing issues, AIDS has remained low on the list of pressing problems reported by Malawians. Results from a number of surveys across Malawi over time have indicated that food security and other poverty-related concerns have been of far greater importance to people than AIDS, even among those who were HIV-positive (Dionne 2012; Dionne, Gerland, and Watkins 2013). Such low prioritization of AIDS does not, however, imply that Malawians are ignorant of AIDS or unwilling to talk about it, just that they face a variety of problems that make daily life challenging (Lwanda 2003; Peters, Kambewa, and Walker 2010; Watkins 2004).

Where Transfers between Intimate Interventions Did Not Occur

A number of factors worked against a transfer from family planning experiences to the response to HIV. First, Malawi's Ministry of Health has long had the same bureaucratic structure as most other sub-Saharan African countries that separates the sexually transmitted infection division from the division focused on family planning, challenging integration between the two areas. Second, once AIDS emerged, there may have been some reticence to "taint" it with family planning, given the sensitive history of family planning in Malawi. As a respondent put it, "There was also fear that maybe government would come back and say, 'Hey, what are you talking about family planning?!' So it was actually important to compartmentalize family planning and HIV and take them as two different activities."[16] Third, discourse about pregnancy prevention in Malawi had been removed *so* far from sex – to child spacing – that it made it even harder to link pregnancy prevention to HIV prevention. As one respondent characterized it, "When you talk HIV, people think sex straightaway. When you talk family planning, the people think about children, and they're happier thoughts than the actual process of getting the children."[17] Another respondent described matters more bluntly: "It's very difficult to fight a sexually transmitted disease when no one will talk about sex."[18]

As this last quote suggests, Malawi may, however, have a deeper than average reticence to address intimate interventions that has made HIV prevention harder, and HIV treatment (including Option B+) easier. For example, Malawi's development in 1991 of an orphan task force – the first in the region (Garbus 2003) – suggests a capacity to address the effects of HIV, which are more distant from the moral culpability of HIV transmission. Malawi's experience with medical male circumcision for HIV prevention also reflects the particular challenges facing intimate interventions. Malawi was slower than other eastern and southern African countries with high HIV prevalence to

---

[16] M25, international NGO.   [17] M34, federal ministry.
[18] M23, local NGO.

implement male circumcision for HIV prevention (Dickson et al. 2011). Indeed, while conducting fieldwork in Malawi in 2009, I attended the annual AIDS research conference where a number of panels covered male circumcision. At this time, four years had passed since the publication of research results showing the significant effect of male circumcision in reducing HIV transmission, and Kenya was actively implementing a male circumcision program at the time. But the discussion at the conference included much laughter and discomfort. The Minister of Health had at that point publicly announced that there would never be a male circumcision program in Malawi. In addition, the association of male circumcision with a small minority ethnic group, the Yao, who are Muslim, linked negative discourses about an Islamization of the predominantly Christian country to male circumcision (Parkhurst, Chilongozi, and Hutchinson 2015). Furthermore, many Malawians doubted the scientific evidence supporting male circumcision as the Yao region had higher HIV prevalence. The observed counterintuitive relationship is due to non-Yao groups in the region having higher HIV prevalence as the Yao themselves, as well as women in the region with circumcised husbands, have lower rates of HIV (Dionne and Poulin 2013; Poulin and Muula 2011; Parkhurst et al. 2015). Simultaneously, the sense that donors were imposing an intervention as intimate as male circumcision reinforced broader discourses about the need for independence from donors (Parkhurst et al. 2015). Ultimately, however, the Minister of Health changed her stance and male circumcision was scaled up, with significant support from donor organizations.

Finally, the experience of AIDS has in turn influenced the provision of family planning in Malawi. Although some have attributed the increase in contraceptive prevalence that occurred during the 1990s to the AIDS-related condom promotion campaigns (Cohen 2000), the preponderance of evidence suggests that AIDS complicated the provision of family planning. As was the case globally, all the attention for HIV detracted attention from family planning, even as early as 1992, when a report noted that "district staff mentioned attendance at frequent AIDS seminars and workshops which has limited the time they have available for Child Spacing and other responsibilities. Concurrently, it seems that fewer workshops on Child Spacing are being held" (Atkinson 1992: 7). These trends continued into the present, particularly after 2000 (Government of Malawi 2011).

At a very basic level, it is difficult to implement a family planning program in the context of highly visible AIDS mortality, a factor of particular import in the 1990s when the government intensified the family planning program. The silences of government documents reflect this challenge: those from the 1990s focusing on population and family planning only rarely mentioned HIV, and those from the 2000s focusing on HIV had similarly infrequent mentions of family planning. As one respondent explained, "With HIV came the high mortality. And at the rate at which people were dying, it was just thought there was no room for family planning."[19] Another respondent echoed this sentiment: "Family planning's a sensitive topic in times of AIDS. I think there are even well-instructed people saying, 'Why should we care about family planning with our populations dying?'"[20] The difficulty talking about family planning in the context of AIDS mortality caused problems for people trying to promote contraception: "First, since they discovered HIV, it has been really something of a paradox for us. To still continue developing programs that will promote family planning, and then people are asking, 'But we are already dying?' And then we say, 'No, you can't leave HIV to space your children for you. You need to take responsibilities.'"[21] This belief that AIDS mortality countered high fertility persisted through the development of Malawi's 2010 RAPID report, which included a section demonstrating that although HIV had slowed population growth, high fertility still outweighed the excess mortality due to AIDS (Ministry of Development Planning and Cooperation 2010).

Furthermore, government, NGO, and donor programs alike have linked condoms so strongly to HIV, sexually transmitted infections, and nonmarital relationships, it has made it difficult to promote them for family planning (Chimbiri 2007; Kaler 2004). As one respondent described it, "I think the whole issue of promoting condoms, getting them used, has been greatly challenged by having them seen as an HIV prevention technique as opposed to family planning. I think if we had, and if we do, position condoms much more as a family planning method, even if a woman wants to use them for HIV prevention, you avoid all these dynamics about who's being unfaithful to whom, and she says, 'Look, I don't want to get pregnant.' It's an immediate

---

[19] M35, bilateral organization.   [20] M36, bilateral organization.
[21] M32, local NGO.

thing that everybody can appreciate. I think it's much easier to negotiate."[22]

Despite the indisputably negative "long shadow" family planning programs cast on HIV prevention and the associated policy feedback process (Kaler 2004), the response to HIV in Malawi bears resemblance to that which came before it. In particular, resources originally deployed for family planning were used for HIV, including those from donors like USAID, but also at the local level through organizations like Banja la Mtsogolo. Malawi's experience thus reflects the linkages and gaps between the global population and AIDS fields, mediated by political and sociocultural factors specific to Malawi.

Conclusion

Transnational as well as political factors have strongly dictated the story of intimate interventions in Malawi. Banda made it clear that he did not welcome Western advice or financial assistance that contradicted his social conservatism; thus the government did little to provide the scaffolding for preventing pregnancy or HIV until near the end of his regime. Banda was most interested in the maintenance of his own rule, and supporting women's access to contraception would have directly threatened his position as *Nkohswe* No. 1 by giving them control over their fertility. Even admitting that AIDS was a problem would have undermined his authority. The far-reaching extent of his power limited the possibility for technocratic leadership in federal ministries and forced many potential technocratic leaders out of the country. When technocrats did engage, it was on Banda's terms, such that a child spacing, rather than a family planning, program resulted.

The picture changed in the post-Banda era, when adopting a population policy allowed the newly democratic government to signal to outsiders that it was ready to engage with the international community on a number of issues, including population growth. International donors stood at the ready, but Banda's many years of authoritarian rule left a weak civil society that did not provide an alternate channel for advocacy, and a population that was skeptical, as Banda had been, that donor interest was benign. Malawi's recent

[22] M27, international NGO.

successes in increasing the contraceptive prevalence rate may indicate the waning impact of Banda's legacy on intimate interventions.

The story of intimate interventions in Malawi teaches us that histories of previous health interventions can have negative impacts through policy feedback processes as well as other mechanisms, but also that those negative impacts are not permanent. The long shadow cast by family planning programs helped minimalize claims that something needed to be done about HIV. Suspicions about family planning transferred directly to suspicions about HIV prevention, and factors related to Malawi's political history and perhaps even its sociocultural makeup enhanced mistrust of intimate interventions overall. While Banda practiced cultural nationalism, the higher HIV prevalence in the Yao region complicated male circumcision interventions and may have provided further fodder for anti-Islamist discourse, echoing some of the effects of ethnic fractionalization described by Lieberman (2009). But despite the long shadow of population control, Malawi has achieved some degree of success in treating HIV and contraceptive prevalence has soared in recent years to greater than 50 percent among married women, more than double that in Senegal and at least three times higher than in Nigeria (Population Reference Bureau 2015). The next chapters turn to discussing these two countries' experiences with intimate interventions.

5 | Nigeria: Transnational Pressure and Political Disruption

The response to AIDS is far less visible in Nigeria than in Malawi, in part because HIV prevalence in 2013 was a much lower 3.2 percent (UNAIDS 2014).[1] As the country in sub-Saharan Africa with the largest population and one of the largest economies, Nigeria's capital Abuja has much government and donor activity. While there are occasional billboards directing Nigerians to "Abstain, Be Faithful, or use a Condom" (ABC), visitors to Abuja are not constantly reminded of the AIDS epidemic. In 2009, the National Agency for the Control of AIDS was located in one repurposed office building. Even though the agency had spread into four neighboring buildings by 2014, its sign was tattered and the annexed office space was as recycled as the original building. Although HIV is certainly a problem, it competes for national attention with corruption, Boko Haram, and the ever-fluctuating price of oil.

As in Malawi, transnational and political factors best explain the extent and nature of intimate interventions in Nigeria. Pressure from donor organizations in the global population field led to a population policy while the priorities of the global AIDS field have driven much of the response to HIV, although Nigerian technocrats and organizations have certainly been deeply involved in the associated processes. A technocratic leader, Olikoye Ransome-Kuti, facilitated the adoption of the population policy, as did the strategic maneuvering of the country's then president, General Ibrahim Babangida. Another political factor, the country's long history of authoritarian rule, left civil society weak and unable to provide alternatives to the government for either family planning or HIV prevention. Sociocultural factors – specifically Nigeria's extreme ethnic and religious fractionalization – complicate all governance, and in particular have hampered the implementation of pregnancy prevention.

---

[1] UNAIDS' prevalence estimates for 2015 do not include data for Nigeria.

134

Economic factors – not Nigeria's poverty per se but the extensive interaction with international donors – have made the stakes higher for global actors both within, but also peripheral to, the population and AIDS fields. The political chaos Nigeria experienced during the 1990s inhibited the transfer of resources between pregnancy prevention and HIV prevention. During this time HIV rates also increased rapidly, to perhaps as high as 5 percent, and no technocratic leader emerged. The return to democracy in 1999 in Nigeria coincided with the global increase in availability of and funding for antiretroviral treatment, as well as a new government that wanted to reconnect with the international community. Simultaneously, the number of HIV-focused NGOs exploded. As such, Nigeria has more enthusiastically embraced HIV treatment than prevention, but challenges remain as more than 3 million people are HIV-positive, and the massive population of 170 million must be reached with HIV prevention messaging and technologies.

Following background on transnational, political, sociocultural, and economic factors in Nigeria that influence intimate interventions, this chapter presents the history of each intimate intervention and then discusses the transfers that occurred between family planning and HIV prevention. It draws from interviews I conducted with family planning and HIV programmers in Nigeria in 2006 and 2010, as well as from a variety of documents produced by donors, nongovernmental organizations, and the Nigerian government.[2] As in Malawi, transfers from family planning to HIV occurred primarily through resources and strategies associated with transnational and political factors.

Transnational, Political, Sociocultural, and Economic Background on Nigeria

Three key background factors help to understand intimate interventions in Nigeria. The first, a transnational and economic factor, is the intense involvement of international financial institutions, whose interest in the country stems from its massive economy and (at times) large debt. Second, alternating periods of military and civilian rule, a

---

[2] References to interviews are denoted by "N" for Nigeria, a number, and the type of organization that the respondent worked for. I conducted interviews 1–18 in 2006 and 19–52 in 2010.

political factor, led to an acute period of political crisis in the 1990s just as HIV took off, dampening civil society and reducing foreign aid. Third, Nigeria's unique politics of population with multiple competing subgroups, a sociocultural factor, has made population interventions politically risky.

Throughout recent decades, Nigeria has had intensive interactions with international financial institutions because of the size of its economy – the first or second-largest in sub-Saharan Africa depending on the year – and the extent of its economic struggles. These interactions have in turn made Nigeria more vulnerable to the desires of donors than would otherwise be the case given its potential for self-sustainability. Nigeria's economy as an independent nation has been based on oil, which in 2015 accounted for 92 percent of the value of exports and was also the primary source of foreign exchange (OPEC 2016). Despite this wealth, the majority of Nigerians are extraordinarily poor: in 2010, almost 85 percent lived on less than US$2 per day (World Bank 2014). While numerous factors drive this disparity, corruption and mismanagement of resources are at the top of the list. Nigeria's foreign debt reached approximately US$36 billion in 2005 before the country reached a deal with foreign creditors to pay off most of it at a steeply discounted rate (Polgreen 2005). Unlike many other African countries that made similar arrangements sooner, donors hesitated to strike a deal with Nigeria given its oil revenue and high levels of corruption.

For most of the 1980s and 1990s, Nigeria was under military rule. President from 1985 through 1993, General Babangida repeatedly delayed elections, and then annulled the results of the 1993 election of Moshood Abiola. As a result, there was ultimately a military coup which left Sani Abacha in power. Following the assassination of Ken Saro-Wiwa, the writer and environmental activist, and a long string of human rights abuses, including the imprisonment of Abiola, Nigeria was suspended from the Commonwealth of Nations[3] in 1995 and "decertified" from receiving USAID funds through any means other than American and Nigerian NGOs and for activities other than humanitarian assistance (USAID Africa Bureau 1998; Wright 1998).[4]

---

[3] The association consisting primarily of former members of the British Empire.
[4] The official grounds for US sanctions was Nigeria's tolerance for narcotics production/transit under the Foreign Assistance Act (Boss and Robinson 1994).

Following Abacha's death in 1998, the country began the transition to democracy that was finalized with the election of Olusegun Obasanjo in 1999. The 1990s were thus a period of great uncertainty, strife, and repression as various political factions jockeyed for power at the expense of actually governing (LeVan 2015). It was also the period in which the AIDS epidemic accelerated.

Population is political in Nigeria, increasing the stakes of those promoting any intimate intervention that might influence the relative sizes of different subgroups, defined by religion, ethnicity, or region. Not only does membership in a particular group serve as a source of identity, but it also influences access to central government resources, including those from oil. As a result, there is competition between regions, the more than 250 individual ethnic groups, and the 36 states that comprise the federal union. To help reduce such competition, in 1991 the government moved the capital from the largest city Lagos to Abuja, located in the more regionally, ethnically, and religiously neutral geographical center of the country (Falola and Heaton 2008). At the group level, the rough alignment between Muslims, the northern region, and military power has been pitted against the similarly rough alignment between Christians, the southern region, and oil (Gordon 2003; Yin 2007b). The central government algorithm for redistribution of resources to states depends in part on relative population size, motivating sub-regions and ethnic groups to (appear to) be as large as possible (Gordon 2003; Suberu 2001). As one respondent described the situation, "Population issues are highly contentious issues: it's about distribution of resources, it's about control of power and central authority, so people are always jockeying among themselves."[5] As a result, census taking has proved complicated in Nigeria, with double-counting, non-release of results, and ultimately a ban on the collection of data on ethnicity or religion (Falola and Heaton 2008; Suberu 2001; Yin 2007a).

Although Nigeria has experienced periods of relative abundance, generally speaking, in the absence of any government-backed social safety net, people must serve a variety of insurance purposes. The importance of "wealth in people" observed in Nigeria is common across African societies and alongside economic insecurity, high infant mortality, and the generally low status of women creates powerful

[5]　N15, international foundation.

incentives for high fertility (Dixon-Mueller and Germain 1994; Guyer 1995; Johnson-Hanks 2006; Pearce 1995; Renne 2003; Smith 2004a). As one respondent explained, linking the need for large group size as well as individual wealth in people, "Everybody wants to make sure that their base is large enough. The Muslims don't want to be less than the Christians and the Christians don't want to be less than the Muslims, so everybody kind of wants to have children. You can only have people when you have children."[6] To "have people" in Nigeria's patron-client-based political economy means to have the network and resource base necessary for survival.

Transnational/economic, political, and sociocultural aspects of Nigeria highlight several important characteristics of the context for intimate interventions. First, Nigeria is large as measured by the number of people, the size of the economy, the volume of debt, and the magnitude of donor projects, so donor organizations are deeply vested in the country with overall obligations far greater than countries like Malawi or Senegal. Second, the politics of Nigeria have led to periods of chaos, which have influenced the provision of foreign aid, as well as impacted the development of civil society. Third, the politics of population have made family planning programs and population policy particularly challenging, as the next section describes.

Preventing Pregnancy in Nigeria

Nigeria was one of the first countries in sub-Saharan Africa to adopt a population policy,[7] which it did in 1988. Political and transnational factors were paramount in the decision to create the policy, while sociocultural diversity complicated its implementation and associated programs. The Minister of Health provided the extensive technocratic leadership necessary to bring the policy into being. In addition, national leaders used the policy strategically to promote nationalism, deflect blame for economic woes, and represent commitment to political restructuring. At the same time, transnational actors such as the World Bank strongly advocated for a policy. Despite notable energy expended by the Ministry of Health and other Nigerian organizations

---

[6] N1, local NGO.
[7] Here I draw heavily from Robinson (2012), which includes greater detail on the process of population policy adoption in Nigeria.

in the late 1980s and early 1990s to implement the policy, as the 1990s continued, pregnancy prevention flagged with the loss of donor funding, political chaos, negative backlash to the policy driven by sociocultural factors, and continued high desired fertility among many segments of the population.

Government provision of family planning began in the early 1980s. Prior to this point Nigerians could, on a limited basis, obtain supplies and services through commercial outlets as well as from university-run clinics (De Sweemer and Lyons 1975). Another early source was the Planned Parenthood Federation of Nigeria, founded in 1958 as the Marriage Guidance Council and which affiliated with the International Planned Parenthood Federation in 1964 (Orubuloye 1983; UNFPA 1981). By the early 1980s, it was the only family planning agency with clinics throughout the nation, and promoted family planning with such slogans as, "When a family practices family planning, it is good for the nation" and "Plan your family for health, wealth, and happiness!" (Obetsebi-Lamptey and Thomas 1981). Two other important family planning NGOs were founded in the 1980s: the Society for Family Health, in 1985, and the Association for Reproductive and Family Health, in 1989. The Society for Family Health focused on social marketing of contraceptives (as described in greater detail below), while the Association for Reproductive and Family Health initially specialized in community-based distribution of contraception (USAID 1994). In addition to these organizations, approximately fifteen other NGOs founded prior to 1990 had some engagement with family planning or reproductive health, although not as their primary activity (Sullivan 2007).

From the 1970s onwards, a variety of multilateral, bilateral, and international NGOs from the global population field also worked on population and family planning projects in Nigeria. The World Health Organization funded rural health services, including family planning, starting in 1972, the same year that UNFPA began supporting a university-based family planning program in Ibadan (UNFPA 1981). The UNFPA also financed a variety of other family planning related projects starting in the 1970s and provided a particularly significant share of contraceptive supplies during the mid-1990s when USAID decertified the Nigerian government (Feyisetan 1998). USAID began population-related work in Nigeria in the early 1980s, supplied the majority of contraceptives to the country from 1985 to 1994, and by 1995 provided more than 85 percent of all family planning commodities (Feyisetan 1998; The Futures Group 1983; UNFPA 1986; USAID 1995). Despite these governmental, nongovernmental, and donor activities, contraceptive prevalence in Nigeria remained low in the early 1980s, largely because of people's continued desire for large families.

Two political factors drove Nigeria's population policy adoption. The first was the technocratic leadership of Olikoye Ransome-Kuti. Respondents described Ransome-Kuti, Minister of Health from 1985 to 1993, as "key" and "instrumental" to the population policy process, and as one put it, "The policy came from having the right minister, in the right place, at the right time."[8] A pediatrician trained in Ireland, Ransome-Kuti came from a prominent, activist, and Christian family: his mother a publicly outspoken promoter of women's rights and reportedly the first Nigerian woman to drive a car; his father a minister and teacher who formed the Nigerian Union of Teachers; his brother, Fela Anikulapo-Kuti, the politically-oriented founder of Afrobeat music; his brother Beko a human rights activist; and his cousin Wole Soyinka a Nobel Laureate (Ita 2006; Olukoya and Ferguson 2003; Raufu 2003). As Minister of Health he created the national health program, which focused on integrated, primary care. Ransome-Kuti framed the benefits of the population policy in similar terms, as a means to improve maternal and child health through increased reproductive health care and thus reduce both maternal and infant mortality and morbidity. As he explained in a 2000 interview, "That Policy was put there for the health of the woman. We told the woman, 'If you don't want to die, don't have more than four children.' That was what we were saying. Data shows that after the third child, maternal mortality goes up" (*Choices* 2000: 6). Following his retirement from the Ministry of Health in 1993, Ransome-Kuti went on to join and chair the executive board of the World Health Organization (Olukoya and Ferguson 2003; Raufu 2003). He died in 2003, garnering obituaries in both *The Lancet* and the *British Medical Journal* (Olukoya and Ferguson 2003; Raufu 2003).

The second political factor that helped bring the population policy into existence was its strategic benefit to national leaders as a means to promote nationalism, deflect blame for economic woes,

---

[8] N1, local NGO.

and demonstrate commitment to political restructuring. The Nigerian government was in a challenging position in the mid-1980s. Not only was the economy in terrible shape, but the public was clamoring for a return to civilian rule following successive military coups in 1983 and 1985. As a nation-building mechanism, the policy was published in pamphlet form, to aid dissemination of its ideas to citizens, with a green and white cover like Nigeria's flag. The policy emphasized Nigeria the nation-state, consisting of a government caring for and managing the population, and described the population as the "nation's most valuable asset" (Federal Republic of Nigeria 1988: 1). Supporting materials also emphasized nationalistic elements related to the policy. For example, after the policy was adopted the Population Information Communication Branch of the Ministry of Information published a pamphlet entitled, *A Nation's Population as an Asset, Not a Liability*. The pamphlet, also green and white like Nigeria's flag, had the national family planning logo on it: a couple and child superimposed on a map of Nigeria (see Figure 5.1). The pamphlet's subtitle conflated population management, government, and health: "A planned nation is a healthy nation," and under the heading "Population and Development," the pamphlet read:

A nation's population is its greatest asset. The quality of this asset depends on the quality of the population that constitutes it. Therefore, a nation's development is closely a function of its population. However, a nation starts with the individual family. The size and quality of the family determines the size and quality of the nation. If the family is managed properly at the individual family level, it will be easier to manage the country at large, through the judicious management of available resources to meet the demands of the population. (Population Information Communication Branch n.d.)

The population policy thus served as an opportunity for nation-building in the midst of a time when many Nigerians were highly skeptical about the nation as a whole.

The population policy, through its linkage of population growth and economic development, simultaneously presented population growth as a scapegoat for economic problems, as well as provided a solution to those problems. Specifically, the policy blamed population growth for the country's abysmal economic performance since the end of the oil boom in the 1970s, thus deflecting attention from

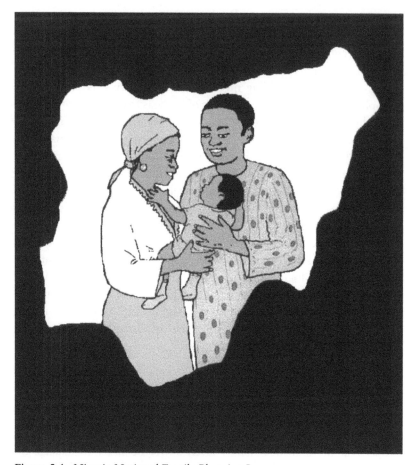

Figure 5.1. Nigeria National Family Planning Logo
Source: Kiragu et al. (1996: 6). Reprinted with permission of the Johns Hopkins University Center for Communication Programs.

government corruption and mismanagement, the real causes. It proposed lowered population growth as the solution, which would bring about socioeconomic development. In addition, the policy specifically attributed poor economic performance to factors outside the government's control, including the world economic recession of the 1980s, natural disasters, and immigrants. The television broadcast of a documentary entitled, *Our Destiny Is In Our Hands*, the day after the policy's inauguration reiterated these themes (Bankole 1994).

Against a backdrop of economic crisis, the policy also served as evidence that the government was preparing for a return to democracy. The 1987 report of the Political Bureau, a commission of academics created to propose a plan for political reform, recommended restructuring government institutions (Dibua 2004), which led to a flurry of policy activity. From 1985 to 1993, the government adopted at least thirteen different policies, including the population policy (Robinson 2012). The population policy was thus part of a larger process of policy adoption designed to demonstrate action on a number of social and economic fronts to both internal and external audiences.

Transnational factors were the third element that drove the population policy. International financial institutions, and particularly the World Bank, were active in Nigeria in the 1980s, as were other actors from the global population field. The World Bank's first population-related project was with Sokoto State in 1985 (World Bank n.d.). As described in Chapters 2 and 3, the World Bank promoted population policy across sub-Saharan Africa during this era, but because of negotiations over the structural adjustment program implemented in 1986 in Nigeria, the Bank was particularly involved in the country. Although some believe (e.g., Ebigbola 2000) the policy was a conditionality of the structural adjustment program, there is no evidence in World Bank documents for such a link between the two. In published documents the Bank has, however, described itself as influencing the policy change in Nigeria (World Bank 1989), and there is strong evidence in support of this claim. The Bank co-sponsored the group that drafted the policy and funded Nigerian consultants to carry out the research behind the RAPID presentations that showed a variety of negative outcomes associated with population growth (Hartmann 1995; Sai and Chester 1990; United Nations 1988). The president of the Bank, Barber Conable, met with President Babangida to discuss population issues (Hartmann 1995), and following the policy's adoption, in 1991 the World Bank gave Nigeria a credit of US$78.5 million for the National Population Project (Ehusani 1994; Odimegwu 1998).

To carry out the population policy, USAID also gave US$67 million for the Family Health Services Project,[9] making Nigeria the recipient of

---

[9] The Nigerian government was expected to contribute US$33 million.

the greatest amount of population aid from the agency at the time (Liagin 1996; Mazzocco 1988). The project employed a number of standard techniques to promote family planning, including the production of songs and radio dramas, traveling theater and mobile cinemas, the development of the family planning logo, and workshops to sensitize relevant organizations and their leaders. Major Nigerian recording artists produced two songs in 1989: "Choices" by Onyeka Onwenu and "Wait for Me" by King Sunny Ade. The songs promoted sexual responsibility, and the messages of, "Practicing family planning allows a couple to prepare for having children" and "Today there are ways of making love without making children" (Bankole 1994). Following their release, they were quickly top-ten hits, and associated public service announcements incorporated pieces of the songs and their videos (Babalola et al. 1992; Kiragu et al. 1996). Other public service announcements, with names like "The Compromise" and "Simple Solution," produced in Nigeria's major languages, advocated for the use of family planning to help manage family resources, instructed people to look for family planning services wherever they saw the national logo, and were so popular that many television and radio stations continued to air them after the program period had ended (Kiragu et al. 1996). The family planning logo (see Figure 5.1) resulted from a national competition followed by refinement by the Ministry of Health, USAID, and a marketing firm, and was launched nationally and at the state level starting in 1991 (Babalola et al. 1992). Finally, the Family Health Services Project ran workshops to promote family planning to traditional, religious, and political leaders.

Competition between subgroups as well as high desired fertility meant that the population policy's goal to *reduce* the number of people met resistance. Specifically, the negative reaction to the policy centered around the issue of four children per woman. One of the policy's goals was to reduce the average number of children per woman from six to four, General Babangida spoke of "four children is enough," and an early newspaper article described the policy as "limiting the number of children per woman to four," so the policy came to be known as a "four-child" policy (Abu 1988; Avong 2000; Caldwell, Orubuloye and Caldwell 1992; Renne 1996). One respondent summarized the negative response as, "We are Africans, and they are telling us we should have just maximum of four children. The layman was saying,

'What right has he got to tell me I should only have four children?'"[10] Particularly alert to the hypocrisy of political leaders, some Nigerians objected to the policy on the grounds that many leaders had more than four children (Orisasona, Akpan, and Adejoh 1996).

Women's groups supported some parts of the policy, such as its stated commitment to voluntary access to family planning as well as to improving infant and child mortality and the status of women. But women's groups also argued that the policy was discriminatory because fertility goals were expressed *per woman*, rather than per family, and because it enforced patriarchy (Dixon-Mueller 1993; Dixon-Mueller and Germain 1994; Osuide 1988). For example, section 5.3.1 read, "The patriarchal family system in the country shall be recognised for stability of the home." Maryam Abacha, the wife of future president and then-Chief of Army Staff Sani Abacha, denounced the policy as a threat to marital stability because it encouraged men to marry more wives in order to produce more children (Abu 1988). Christian religious leaders felt that the policy was unfair to Christians and non-polygynous families because it implied that a Muslim man, who could have up to four wives, could also have up to sixteen children, whereas a Christian man could only have four children total (Abu 1988; Faruq 1989). Others objected to the policy because it endorsed contraception and planned fertility in general, and Muslim groups in particular were disappointed that the policy proposed that population and family life education take place outside of the home, a responsibility they felt lay primarily within the family (Dixon-Mueller 1993; Dixon-Mueller and Germain 1994; Osuide 1988).

In addition to the issues related to the appropriate number of children, broader concerns existed about the population policy. The government's generally poor levels of performance at the time put into question the overall credibility of the policy (Renne 2003). Relatedly, minimal support existed at the subnational level for implementing the policy and other population-related programs (Sala-Diakanda 1996). More damning were the connections many Nigerians perceived between the West and the policy. Nigerians from the predominantly Muslim north of the country felt that the policy came from the West and was motivated by a desire to reduce the number of Nigerians, particularly Muslim ones (Renne 1996). One respondent

[10] N9, local NGO.

summarized this perspective: "There was a huge argument, particularly from the North. The policy's seen as Western population control – that was the major issue, Western population control. The northern Nigerian feels that because there's predominance of Muslims, now they want to reduce Muslim population, the African population."[11]

The negative backlash against the population policy combined with a loss of funding during the Abacha regime in the 1990s damaged pregnancy prevention efforts. As one respondent described that era, "Because we lost steam in the 90s, and we were short of commodities, so the family planning activities declined. And we lost steam, because the then-head of state was not acceptable to the US government, so we were decertified. And commodities did not come in except a few trickling in through UNFPA or International Planned Parenthood Federation."[12] Only US$10.5 million of the US$78.5 million designated by the World Bank for the National Population Project were ever disbursed, and the project was closed in 1998 (World Bank n.d.). In addition, when Ransome-Kuti stepped down as Minister of Health in 1993, the population policy and associated family planning program lost a major champion (Yaqub 1997).

The Nigerian government released a new population policy in 2004, which updated the 1988 policy to reflect the reproductive health agenda of the 1994 United Nations International Conference on Population and Development and included emergent issues, such as HIV, aging, and disability (Federal Republic of Nigeria 2004). Like the 1988 policy, the newer policy emphasized the interrelationship between population growth and socioeconomic development. The policy did not, however, produce the same sort of response as the 1988 policy. Nigerians had perhaps grown more used to intimate interventions, although continued low rates of contraceptive prevalence indicated little synergy between government interventions and population desires. Other factors also helped prevent backlash, including that the policy was not new, but a revision, and perhaps even that there was no technocratic leader like Ransome-Kuti championing the policy. The simultaneous rise in attention to HIV may have also detracted attention from the new population policy.

The 1988 population policy, as well as the family planning programs that preceded and followed it, came about largely because of

[11] N14, international foundation.   [12] N38, local NGO.

transnational and political factors. Support and pressure from donor organizations, a transnational factor, heavily impacted family planning outcomes until the political chaos of the mid-to-late 1990s. The World Bank's involvement with the population policy reflected trends across sub-Saharan Africa, but which were intensified in Nigeria because of the extent of the country's debt and the associated magnitude of the Bank's involvement there. Political factors, including the technocratic leadership provided by Minister of Health Ransome-Kuti and the strategic maneuvering of the Babangida regime, were crucial to the adoption of the population policy. More broadly, family planning NGOs founded mainly in the 1980s helped with the actual provision of services. Across the board, objections to the population policy and to family planning more generally resulted from sociocultural factors, and specifically the particular politics inherent to Nigeria's extraordinarily diverse population.

Preventing HIV in Nigeria

Nigeria has a generalized HIV epidemic with prevalence much higher among the most-at-risk groups: in 2010, approximately one quarter of female sex workers, and between 15 and 20 percent of men who have sex with men, were HIV positive (National Agency for the Control of AIDS 2014). HIV prevalence most likely rose from 1.8 percent in 1991 to over 5 percent in 2001, and then declined slightly from then onwards (Kanki and Adeyi 2006), plateauing around 2006 according to respondents. The epidemic varies greatly by state, with prevalence in some states less than 1 percent and in a handful of states over 8 percent (National Agency for the Control of AIDS 2014). A third or less of people who need antiretroviral therapy receive it, and similarly, only about a third of HIV-positive pregnant women take antiretroviral therapy at the time of birth to prevent transmission to their infants (National Agency for the Control of AIDS 2014). Because of the low coverage of pregnant HIV-positive women combined with high fertility, Nigeria accounts for one quarter of the new pediatric infections among the twenty-one countries targeted for elimination of mother-to-child transmission (UNAIDS 2014).

The first AIDS cases in Nigeria were diagnosed in the mid-1980s at the same time as most other sub-Saharan African countries, but HIV interventions were minimal until the early 2000s, after the country had returned to democracy and donors from the global AIDS field began to provide extensive financial support. Across all descriptions of the response to HIV in Nigeria, there is virtually no mention of the fifteen-year span between the discovery of the first cases and the return to democracy and arrival and expansion of treatment starting from the early 2000s. For example, as of 2011 USAID's AIDS web page for Nigeria stated:

"Nigeria's first case of AIDS was diagnosed in 1986, and the national prevalence soon rose rapidly, from 1.8 percent in 1991 to a peak of 5.1 percent in 2001... Nigeria has utilized numerous opportunities for collaboration and synergy across technical areas... A total of 1,043,000 HIV-positive individuals received care and support services, including HIV/TB services, in FY 2009."[13]

A publication from the Nigerian National Agency for the Control of AIDS has a similar gap in the narrative. After noting the founding dates of the government organizations created in the late 1980s, it then goes on to say that "Control efforts suffered [from a lack of] political will and poor funding over the years until the nation reached a turning point in 2000" (National Agency for the Control of AIDS 2008).

Like those from USAID and the National Agency for the Control of AIDS, the AIDS narrative as told by respondents started in 1986 with the discovery of the first AIDS case (a young, female "street hawker"), but then had few details prior to 2000 other than mentioning a minimal and medical response emanating solely from the Ministry of Health. Those who did comment on the late 1980s noted that at that point, there was a combination of doubt and denial. "Initially, in 1986 when the first case of HIV/AIDS in Nigeria was reported, even government doubted it,"[14] and "The health sector response in the 1990s was weak. Everyone thought HIV prevalence was low, so the AIDS unit was small."[15] With limited funding for testing and not enough people dying to *see* the problem as in countries like Malawi, many genuinely believed there was no AIDS "problem" in Nigeria. Indeed, a survey of 700 people in 1985 showed no one with HIV, leaving health experts in Nigeria and abroad skeptical. Apparently even Robert Gallo, the

---

[13] USAID (n.d.). None of the sentences removed refer to the 1985–2000 period, nor do they mention any other dates.
[14] N41, local NGO.   [15] N51, bilateral organization.

co-discoverer of the HIV virus, thought there might be a competing virus in Nigeria,[16] and a 1986 Nigerian expert panel concluded that AIDS was "not here yet" (*The Guardian* 1987). In 1990, *The New York Times* published an article on Nigeria stating, "Why infection rates in this West African country have lagged behind those of much of the rest of the continent is one of the great mysteries of Africa's AIDS epidemic," which referenced a hypothesis, although acknowledged to not be widely supported, that Nigerians might be immune to HIV (Noble 1990). In fact, low prevalence and a relatively concentrated epidemic made it difficult to identify anyone who was HIV-positive without purposively sampling at-risk groups.

Doubt was then compounded by denial, and a tendency to blame the epidemic on those outside the country. "At first there was denial – AIDS is not our own, it's not from us, it's from the West."[17] Even by 1989, most Nigerians did not believe AIDS existed in the country, as it was a disease associated with whites and gays, or at the very closest southern Africans (Bakare 1996; Behrman 2004; Smith 2014). As in other sub-Saharan African countries, many Nigerians interpreted global debates about the origins of AIDS as condemnations of Africa and resented that HIV's jump from primates to humans might imply that Africans had had sex with animals (Smith 2014). Such interpretations did not facilitate acceptance of the existence of HIV.

The military government did not take any sort of noticeable action. Unlike in Uganda, where Museveni's strong response to AIDS almost certainly flowed in part from his fear that he would lose his grip on power if the military succumbed to AIDS (Ostergard and Barcelo 2005), the Nigerian generals did little to nothing. They may have underprioritized HIV because of the relatively few cases, which they assumed soldiers contracted while on peacekeeping missions in Sierra Leone and Liberia, and they certainly were in a state of denial (Raufu 2001; Raufu 2002). Indeed, "the early cases of HIV were usually seen among military officers who were returning from duties outside the country, so government then was kind of making it a secret. They don't want people to know that we're dying from HIV, and they don't also want to popularize, to make issues of HIV public."[18] Similarly, "Denial

---

[16] Personal communication with former high-level Nigerian health official, 2011.
[17] N43, federal ministry. [18] N26, multilateral organization.

was the first response, the military government didn't care."[19] The military government had, however, "cared" enough to pass the population policy in 1988, suggesting that HIV interventions offered no political opportunity, whereas population policy had, and perhaps that the low number of cases and absence of active combat lessened the threat. Thus the response during the 1990s from the Nigerian government came solely from the Ministry of Health, and was not very subtle. "Once in a while, they would play 30 minutes or more documentary on HIV on national TV. And then what you could get from that documentary was that once you have HIV infection, you are finished. You are a dead man."[20] This film, *Dawn of Reality*, was produced by the Ministry of Health in 1992 and showed graphic images of Nigerians with full-blown AIDS (Fatusi and Jimoh 2006; Hellandendu 2012; Orisasona, Akpan and Adejoh 1996).

In the presence of such denial, the government built the scaffold of a response based on the blueprint promoted by the global AIDS field. The National Expert Advisory Committee on AIDS was founded in 1986 and the government set up the National AIDS and Sexually Transmitted Diseases Control Programme in 1988 with assistance from the World Health Organization Global Programme on AIDS (Federal Republic of Nigeria 2008; Folayan 2004). President Babangida mentioned a health education campaign on AIDS as part of his 1987 budget address and in 1991 launched a "War on AIDS" campaign, which included a promise of 20 million Naira for AIDS and a directive to all states and local governments to annually commit 1 million and 500,000 Naira, respectively (Folayan 2004; *The Guardian* 1987; USAID 1994). Early prevention programs included a small intervention for sex workers in the city of Calabar begun in 1987, and in the mid-1990s, there was a radio call-in show targeting youths (Bollinger, Stover, and Nwaorgu 1999). The Ministry of Health first collected HIV surveillance data in 1991 (Kanki and Adeyi 2006).

The state of the Nigerian response to HIV was, however, unremarkable in the mid-1990s. In 1996, the Nigerian government spent 5 percent of what the Ugandan government did on AIDS, for a population five times as large as Uganda's and with twice as many HIV-positive people (Iliffe 2006). The budget in 1997 for AIDS was just one million Naira, or US$10,000. In parallel, the national AIDS program had constant

---

[19] N32, bilateral organization.   [20] N22, local NGO.

turnover in directorship, with three between 1994 and 1997 alone (Alubo 2002; Iliffe 2006). Adopted in 1997, six years after the Federal Ministry of Health began work on it, the *National Policy on HIV/AIDS/ STIs Control* required that all condoms carry the statement that "The Federal Ministry of Health warns that abstinence and mutual fidelity remain the best protection against HIV/AIDS/STIs" (as quoted in Alubo 2002: 557; Falobi 1999; Federal Republic of Nigeria 2001; Iliffe 2006).[21] Media coverage of AIDS throughout this period (until 2001) was minimal, and more focused on the activities of NGOs than on educating the public about HIV and how to prevent it (Fatusi and Jimoh 2006; Odutolu et al. 2006).

But everything changed in Nigeria in the late 1990s, including politics and increasing awareness of AIDS. Sani Abacha died under mysterious circumstances in 1998, starting a chain of events that led to the 1999 election of Olusegun Obasanjo, a general who had briefly been head of state under military rule in the late 1970s. In 1997, Olikoye Ransome-Kuti announced at the public funeral of his brother Fela, the famous Afrobeat musician, that Fela had died of AIDS, thus putting a "face" on AIDS in Nigeria (Bollinger, Stover, and Nwaorgu 1999; *Choices* 2000; Raufu 2003).[22] More Nigerians observed others who were sick. In central Nigeria, near the capital, AIDS came to be known as the "Abuja disease," because of its association with women who had gone to the capital to engage in sex work and then returned home to neighboring states sick with HIV (Alubo 2002; Iliffe 2006).

Although the global AIDS field has not lauded Obasanjo as a transformational leader in the AIDS response (as it has Museveni), respondents credited Obasanjo with getting the ball rolling on Nigeria's response to HIV. After seeing the results of the 1999 seropre-valence survey, that same year Obasanjo formed the Presidential Commission on AIDS, and also mentioned AIDS in his speech to the United Nations General Assembly (Alubo 2002; Folayan 2004; TvT Associates 2002). At an AIDS-related event during President Clinton's 2000 visit to Nigeria, Obsanjo openly embraced an HIV-positive woman, a moment widely covered in the media (Henry 2000). He was publicly tested for HIV, and because of this, one respondent

---

[21] "STI" stands for sexually transmitted infection.
[22] The footage of this announcement is included in the documentary *Finding Fela!* (Gibney 2014).

went for a test the same day. As another respondent explained, "Obasanjo was a strong advocate – he didn't do what Mbeki [in South Africa] did, and acknowledged the issue."[23] The Harvard AIDS Prevention Initiative in Nigeria described Obasanjo as "a vocal advocate for addressing the HIV epidemic both in Nigeria and throughout Africa" (AIDS Prevention Initiative Nigeria n.d.-b).

In addition, during the early days of Obasanjo's presidency, new data became available that indicated there was a more serious epidemic than previously thought. "The turning point was when there was a quantum leap of HIV prevalence among pregnant mothers, to above the 4 percent level. And it was a good thing, of course, that we now got into civilian governance, in the sense that the then-head of state, General Obasanjo, felt that this was a threat really to the nation."[24] A 2000 report from the Nigerian Institute of Medical Research projected a doubling in the number of Nigerians who were HIV-positive between 1999 and 2003 and suggested that the 5.4 percent prevalence calculated from the 1999 sentinel surveillance survey might be an underestimate (National HIV/AIDS Database Project 2000). The 2001 *HIV/AIDS Emergency Action Plan* stated that "We are now in the explosive phase of the epidemic with potentially grave consequences" (National Action Committee on AIDS 2001: 2).

In 2001 Obasanjo hosted the first African Heads of State Summit on AIDS and Malaria on behalf of the Organization of African Unity, at which he urged African countries to commit more resources to AIDS (Kanki, Kakkattil, and Simao 2012). This summit produced the Abuja 2001 Declaration, one of the key steps in the creation of the Global Fund. At the summit, Obasanjo also announced the first antiretroviral program in Nigeria, which launched in 2002 and whose aim was to serve 10,000 adults and 5,000 children (out of 500,000 in need) with generic drugs purchased from the Indian firm Cipla (Idoko 2012; Iliffe 2006). Nigeria took great pride in both the summit and the antiretroviral program. A government publication described the government as "convening" the summit,[25] which "paved the way" for the Global Fund, while the initial announcement of the antiretroviral program referred to it as "Africa's largest" (as cited in Falobi and Akanni

---

[23] N37, international foundation.   [24] N38, local NGO.
[25] Piot's (2012) description of the same events differs slightly: the Organization for African Unity called the meeting, and Piot asked Obasanjo to host.

2004: 34) and noted that the government began the antiretroviral program "at a time [when] no government in Africa was doing that and that many others were afraid to do the same" (National Action Committee on AIDS 2005: 3).[26] Shortly after the summit, Obasanjo made a state visit to Washington, during which President Bush pledged US$200 million for what would become the Global Fund. It was then during Obsanjo's campaign for, and election to, a second term in 2003 that massive donor resources via the Global Fund and PEPFAR became available for purchasing antiretroviral drugs in Nigeria.

Like most sub-Saharan African countries, a national AIDS commission leads Nigeria's response to HIV. This commission grew out of the 1999 Presidential Commission on AIDS and transitioned to the National Action Committee on AIDS in 2000. In 2001, the government adopted the three-year HIV/AIDS Emergency Action Plan, and the amount in the budget for AIDS reached US$40 million (TvT Associates/The Synergy Project 2002). Revised HIV/AIDS policies were adopted in 2003 and 2009 (Federal Republic of Nigeria 2008; National Agency for the Control of AIDS 2009b). The National Action Committee on AIDS became the National Agency for the Control of AIDS in 2007, gaining a line in the federal budget, and benefitted greatly from the technocratic leadership of Dr. Babatunde Osotimehin from 2002 through 2008, who staffed it with energetic people and created an open environment. According to one respondent, President Obasanjo came to refer to Osotimehin as "Mr. AIDS." Osotimehin went on to be the Minister of Health in 2008, and then in 2011 became the Executive Director of the UNFPA.

Access to antiretroviral therapy in Nigeria grew steadily during the 2000s. Prior to the existence of the Nigerian National Antiretroviral Program, antiretroviral therapy had cost 30–50,000 Naira per month (US$300–500) (Kanki and Adeyi 2006). The program reduced the price to 1,000 Naira per month, or approximately ten US dollars (NEPWHAM, 2010) but suffered from a number of implementation challenges and failed to put many people on drugs quickly (Umeh and Ejike 2004). Nigeria's prevention of mother-to-child transmission program began in 2002 and soon received support from the Global Fund and PEPFAR, which after several years greatly increased the

[26] As described in the next chapter, Senegal, Côte d'Ivoire, and Uganda had actually all begun antiretroviral programs by this point, in 1998.

availability and reduced the cost of antiretroviral therapy (Idoko 2012; Odutolu et al. 2006). Nigeria received funding from Rounds 1, 5, 9, and 10 of the Global Fund, and PEPFAR made Nigeria one of the original focus countries. As a result of donor support, in 2005, Obasanjo announced that antiretroviral drugs would be free to all who needed them, which became the case in 2006 (National Agency for the Control of AIDS 2009c; Smith 2014).

The global AIDS field's commitment to Nigeria stemmed in no small part from a widespread concern that the HIV epidemic was going to become very, very severe there. Not only was it the most populous country in Africa, but a US National Intelligence Council report in 2002 identified Nigeria as one of five countries (along with Russia, China, Ethiopia, and India) anticipated to bear the greatest burden of HIV (Gordon 2002). The projections for the HIV epidemic in Nigeria included in that report were exceedingly grim – 10–15 million people HIV-positive, and a prevalence rate of 18–26 percent by 2010 – and accompanied by dire predictions of the impact on the economy, society, and government stability (Gordon 2002). This report was widely publicized in Nigeria, and led more Nigerians to believe that AIDS was a crisis in need of attention (Smith 2014). Capturing the widespread concern about AIDS at the time, a brochure describing the work of the AIDS Prevention Initiative in Nigeria was titled, *An Endangered Nation: Nigeria confronts an Escalating Epidemic* (AIDS Prevention Initiative Nigeria n.d.-b).

Along with ample donor funding, numerous HIV NGOs sprang up, building the local AIDS field and continuing a trend that had begun immediately prior to the transition to democracy when donors had circumvented the military government by passing funds through NGOs. They joined a handful of organizations that had begun working on AIDS much earlier, including STOPAIDS as early as 1987 and the Nigerian chapter of the Society for Women and AIDS in Africa starting in 1989 (Odutolu et al. 2006; Society for Women and AIDS in Africa Nigeria Chapter n.d.). Some of the new NGOs were highly opportunistic, taking advantage of the availability of funds with no real plan or capacity to address HIV, but many were real (Ogbogu and Idogho 2006; Smith 2007; Smith 2010). With donor urging, a support organization for people living with HIV/AIDS, the Network of People Living with HIV and AIDS in Nigeria, formed in 1998 but did not establish a permanent office until 2003, so the AIDS Alliance in Nigeria, founded in 1999 is credited for being the "first" support group (Ogbogu and Idogho 2006). The AIDS NGO umbrella organization, Civil Society for HIV and AIDS in Nigeria, was established in 2000 with donor support.[27] In order to achieve representation of constituencies deemed important by the global AIDS field, particularly UNAIDS, a handful of other umbrella NGOs emerged around 2005 – Association of Positive Youths Living with HIV in Nigeria, Association of Women Living with HIV/AIDS in Nigeria, and National Youth Network on HIV/AIDS – all of which are headquartered in the same building in Abuja, along with Civil Society for HIV and AIDS in Nigeria, called Civil Society House. The National Agency for the Control of AIDS also created the National Faith Based Coalition against AIDS and the National Business Coalition against AIDS (National Agency for the Control of AIDS 2009a). As one respondent described it, "the National Agency for the Control of AIDS is supposed to be the voices of the constituencies, but the constituencies had to be created,"[28] which was partially achieved through starting a separate NGO for each subpopulation. Despite their perhaps less-than-organic creation, some of these organizations have gone on to receive major funding: Civil Society for HIV and AIDS in Nigeria received a large World Bank credit, and has been a principal recipient for the Global Fund (National Agency for the Control of AIDS 2007). While there are examples of NGOs doing important HIV prevention, treatment, and care work, many Nigerians remain suspicious of AIDS NGOs more broadly, seeing the donor money that flows through them as yet one more example of the rich getting richer while the poor suffer. As late as 2012, narratives still circulated about AIDS as a conspiracy designed to fill the pockets of the already wealthy with donor funds (Smith 2014).

Overall, HIV prevention in Nigeria has never been strong, which can be explained by transnational and political factors. The return to democracy in 1999 immediately preceded the global AIDS field's shift towards funding antiretroviral treatment, and Nigeria's position as a PEPFAR focus country and major recipient from other donor organizations has strongly reflected these organizations' bias towards treatment. For example, through 2012, the Global Fund and PEPFAR had put only 1 percent and 16 percent, respectively, of their Nigeria budgets towards prevention (Fan et al. 2013). The chaos and military rule in

---

[27] N41, local NGO.   [28] N32, bilateral organization.

1990s, political factors, were a distraction that led to the loss of donor funds and severely damaged civil society, thus impeding HIV interventions. Finally, although Nigeria's diversity complicates governance overall, and challenges the implementation of all social programs, HIV has never been associated with one particular ethnic, religious, or regional group, indicating that the effects of ethnic fractionalization, a sociocultural factor, on HIV interventions have been more indirect than in some other countries.

From Pregnancy Prevention to HIV Prevention

Transnational and political factors drove intimate interventions in Nigeria, and are where resources, strategies, and discourses transferred from pregnancy prevention to HIV prevention. Both governmental and nongovernmental donor organizations deployed similar intervention strategies for family planning and HIV, and security concerns in particular prompted US involvement in both areas. The specific resources that transferred from pregnancy prevention to HIV prevention in Nigeria included three local NGOs that became important players in the response to HIV/AIDS as well as human capital, including a technocratic leader. As in Malawi, other factors prevented transfers from family planning to HIV prevention, including sanctions by donors against Nigeria during the 1990s, the structure of the Ministry of Health, and negative discourses associated with family planning.

Organizational Resources

USAID was a primary link between family planning and HIV prevention programs in Nigeria. It first funded major family planning programs in the country starting in 1985. Although the USAID documents about the Family Health Services project (1988–1994) do not reference AIDS, USAID brought AIDS under its programmatic umbrella as time passed, first funding HIV/AIDS activities in 1987 through AIDSTECH, and then from 1992–1997 through AIDSCAP (Fatusi and Jimoh 2006; TvT Associates/The Synergy Project 2002). By 1992, USAID's Nigeria Country Strategic Plan focused primarily on family planning, child survival, and HIV prevention (USAID 1994). Between 1992 and 1998 USAID provided just US$5.5 million for AIDS, all of it going to NGOs because of decertification, and was one of few donors with

HIV programs in Nigeria (Family Health International 2007a; USAID 1999a). With the funding going to just NGOs, USAID merged its HIV activities into other programs, including family planning (Family Health International 1997). "Without inflow and distribution of condoms through the USAID Family Planning program, Nigeria's war to stop the epidemic of HIV/AIDS will falter," a USAID report stated bluntly in 1995 (USAID 1995). USAID then ultimately became the largest HIV donor to Nigeria from 2003 onwards with the creation of PEPFAR (Family Health International 2007a).

International NGOs that had worked on family planning in Nigeria also increasingly incorporated HIV over time, particularly those funded by USAID. Family Health International, the major USAID implementing partner described in earlier chapters, started work in Nigeria in 1988, and from around 2007 onwards has promoted and piloted the integration of family planning and HIV services, particularly through the Global Health HIV/AIDS Initiative Nigeria (Chabikuli et al. 2009; Family Health International n.d.; Federal Ministry of Health 2007). Other USAID-funded organizations that had worked in family planning in Nigeria but then incorporated HIV into their activities included EngenderHealth, which had operated in Nigeria since 1985 (EngenderHealth n.d.), the Johns Hopkins University Center for Communication Programs, and the Center for Development and Population Activities (TvT Associates/The Synergy Project 2002).

Foundations committed to family planning in Nigeria also built HIV/ AIDS into their work. In particular, the Ford Foundation's Lagos office, established in 1960 and initially engaged in family planning, funded HIV activities very early on, motivated in particular by a staff member working there (Brier 2009). The Ford Foundation thus funded the earliest extant AIDS organizations in Nigeria, such as STOPAIDS and the Nigeria chapter of the Society for Women and AIDS in Africa. The latter received US$1 million from Ford between 1993 and 2002 (Brier 2009). As described in Chapter 2, the connections between family planning and HIV that Ford made in their Lagos office went on to influence the organization overall. Although the MacArthur Foundation did not open their Nigeria office until after the AIDS epidemic began, in 1994, from that point on they included many HIV activities under the umbrella of reproductive health (TvT Associates/ The Synergy Project 2002).

Three local family planning NGOs in Nigeria predated the AIDS epidemic or formed just as it began: the Planned Parenthood Federation of Nigeria (the International Planned Parenthood Federation affiliate); the Association for Reproductive and Family Health; and the Society for Family Health (the Population Services International affiliate). All three started as pregnancy prevention organizations and then became engaged in HIV prevention and treatment, although with a delay that paralleled the lack of government action in the 1990s. As stated on the Planned Parenthood Federation of Nigeria web site,

"The original core mission of Planned Parenthood Federation of Nigeria, a private, not-for-profit organization founded in the late 1950s, was to promote adoption of child spacing and contraceptive practices among individuals and couples. Over the years, Planned Parenthood Federation of Nigeria has evolved from this initial narrow emphasis to a broader, more comprehensive mission which takes on board the implications and needs arising from [the International Conference on Population and Development], the Beijing International Women's Conference, the concern with adolescent [reproductive health], and the HIV/AIDS pandemic."[29]

The Planned Parenthood Federation of Nigeria is primarily a service provider, with clinics in almost all of Nigeria's thirty-six states, and community-based distributors in the remaining areas (International Planned Parenthood Federation Africa Region n.d.). Since 1999, HIV has become a more prominent part of their portfolio, and they served as a sub-recipient for the Global Fund Round 5 (2007) to scale up AIDS treatment and care, and as a prime recipient for Round 9 (2010) on strengthening health systems. They have thus become a major player in the response to AIDS in Nigeria.

The Association for Reproductive and Family Health is a nonprofit organization "committed to improving the quality of life of under-served and vulnerable communities" whose mission is to "initiate promote and implement in partnership with other organizations, developmental, HIV & AIDS, [sexual and reproductive health] and family planning program" (Association for Reproductive and Family Health n.d.). That they list HIV before reproductive health shows how deeply they have become involved in the response to AIDS. The organization began by focusing almost exclusively on family planning, but by 2002

---

[29] Planned Parenthood Federation of Nigeria (n.d.).

was working to integrate HIV and sexually transmitted infection prevention into their family planning services (Adeokun et al. 2002). In 2007, they became a principal recipient for a grant from the Global Fund Round 5 to scale up AIDS treatment and care, for which more than US$18 million was ultimately disbursed (The Global Fund n.d.-c). They have one main clinic in Ibadan, and two satellite clinics in Ibadan and Ogbomosho (an hour and a half north of Ibadan). In addition to providing services, they are a major grant recipient for interventions and trainings of service providers and educators, receiving funds at one point or another from all the major population funders (the MacArthur Foundation, UNFPA, Population Council, the Packard Foundation, and the Ford Foundation, among others) as well as from the government of Nigeria.

The Society for Family Health is the Nigerian affiliate of Population Services International. Founded in 1985 as a "one-man show" working in only three states, today it has offices in seventeen of Nigeria's states and franchises in twenty-one (Boss and Robinson 1994; Population Services International n.d.-a). The organization initially focused on family planning and received support from the Population Crisis Committee, and began socially marketing condoms in 1990 (Boss and Robinson 1994). When their surveys in the mid-to-late 1990s showed that many Nigerians were unaware that an HIV-positive person might not necessarily look ill, they created the "AIDS no dey show for face" campaign (AIDS does not show on faces). One of the posters featured Femi Kuti, the son of Fela Kuti, and nephew of Minister of Health Ransome-Kuti.[30] The organization's HIV-related work grew exponentially starting in 2002, when they received a large grant from the British bilateral aid agency DFID, and then in 2005, when they became the first Nigerian NGO certified to receive funding from USAID (Population Services International n.d.-a). The shift to AIDS-related work has been beneficial to the organization. When I first talked with employees in 2006, they were in a somewhat rundown building, but when I returned in 2010, they had been upgraded to a brand-new, multistory facility, funded by donors in association with their AIDS-related work. By 2013, they were one of the top-five non-US NGOs receiving USAID funding for global health (Moss 2015).

---

[30] Image can be seen at http://assets.irinnews.org/s3fs-public/images/20038296.jpg.

Despite these three pregnancy prevention organizations ultimately migrating to HIV prevention work, both the Planned Parenthood Federation of Nigeria and the Association for Reproduction and Family Health came to HIV work relatively late. The Planned Parenthood Federation of Nigeria did not really expand their work beyond family planning until 1999. As someone from that organization explained:

RSR: So, before the shift to the broader view of reproductive health in 1999, if a woman had come in for family planning, would she have been told about HIV?

PPFN: That would have been very, very unlikely.

RSR: And would she have heard about any sexually transmitted infections?

PPFN: Yeah, we were really involved in sexually transmitted infection management, using the syndromic management approach. So, if you came for family planning, you definitely would have been counseled on sexually transmitted infections.

RSR: So that means that HIV was not being treated as a sexually transmitted infection?

PPFN: That's the point – it was just an emerging disease area.[31]

So the perception of HIV as a disease not even linked to other sexually transmitted infections limited the organization from early prevention activities.

Similarly, although the Association for Reproduction and Family Health engaged in some activities related to sexually transmitted infections (including HIV) prior to 2000, it was not until after that date that they became heavily involved with AIDS activities, first with support from the AIDS Prevention Initiative in Nigeria, a major Gates-funded, Harvard-run project, and then from the Global Fund. As someone from the Association for Reproduction and Family Health explained:

Because we felt we had low HIV prevalence, of 1.8 about 1990, people were still not very keen to invest a lot of resources in that area. Even the reproductive health and family planning community, that should have seized the opportunity of integration, didn't see the wisdom in doing so, until there were more cases discovered, across the nation. There were some at

---

[31] N47, local NGO.

that time who felt that integrating family planning and HIV will reduce the patronage, because HIV is an infection, thought to be sexually acquired. It was a subject not to be discussed. And anybody with sexually transmitted infection, has a stigma to it.[32]

So although both the Planned Parenthood Federation of Nigeria and the Association for Reproductive and Family Health were assets to Nigeria's response to HIV as established and well-functioning organizations that could collaborate with major funders, their contribution to HIV came relatively late, delayed in part because of broader conceptions of HIV as a disease, and its associated stigma. The Society for Family Health, with its condom campaigns in the 1990s, is likely the earliest family planning organization to have begun work on HIV prevention in Nigeria.

Other resources within Nigeria transferred from pregnancy prevention to HIV prevention. The 1997 National Policy on AIDS suggested equipping family planning clinics with HIV counseling facilities (Strachan et al. 2004). Many people who had worked in family planning and reproductive health moved to HIV/AIDS, including the head of the National Agency for the Control of AIDS, Babatunde Osotimehin (Goldenberg 2011). Ransome-Kuti, the Minister of Health and driving technocratic leader behind the population policy, also threw his energy behind HIV prevention. While still Minister, he developed the federal program to respond to HIV and built the initial architecture of a national response to HIV (Falobi 1999; Fatusi and Jimoh 2006; Iliffe 2006). At least one source reports that he was involved in the creation of the Society for Family Health (Odutolu et al. 2006). His public announcement that his brother the Afrobeat musician Fela had died of AIDS was crucial to greater Nigerian acceptance of the epidemic. He also served as Chairman of the National Committee on AIDS (Oluwaseun 2003).

Thus a variety of organizational resources transferred from family planning to HIV, both globally and within Nigeria. Nigerian family planning NGOs became major players in the response to HIV, albeit primarily only after the global AIDS field became deeply interested in Nigeria, and human capital originally supporting family planning came to work on HIV interventions.

---

[32] N38, local NGO.

Strategies

As in Malawi, the social marketing of condoms was a major crossover point between techniques for family planning and HIV prevention supported by international organizations. Even though condoms had not widely been used as a family planning technique in Nigeria, contraceptive social marketing programs readily incorporated condom promotion for HIV. Even before the AIDS epidemic, USAID was very enthusiastic about the possibility of contraceptive social marketing in Nigeria. A 1981 study characterized the situation as, "No country in which a [contraceptive social marketing] project has been undertaken is more commercially-oriented than Nigeria" (Obetsebi-Lamptey and Thomas 1981: 8). Gold Circle condoms for the purpose of family planning and HIV prevention were ultimately built into the exact same social marketing program, operated through Population Services International and the Society for Family Health starting on a small scale in three states in 1990 but expanding nationally by 1992 (Boss and Robinson 1994). Despite the ultimate integration, a 1988 USAID study had worried that a dual message about condoms would confuse consumers or detract from the condom as a contraceptive: "The issue arises from the new focus on the condom as a prophylactic against AIDS, and the question is whether this use will tarnish the image of the condom as a family planning method that is appropriate within a marital relationship" (Population Technical Assistance Project 1988: iv).

But the emphasis on social marketing remained, particularly once Nigeria was decertified and USAID had to find alternate pathways for funding family planning and HIV activities. During this period, USAID program documents again spoke of the benefits to integrating family planning and HIV strategies to maximize efficiency (Williams et al. 1995). USAID funded condom social marketing through AIDSCAP in the early to mid-1990s, and then the AIDSMARK program from 1999–2001 (Family Health International 1997). Then in 2002, the Promoting Sexual and Reproductive Health for HIV/AIDS Reduction program – funded by USAID and DFID, managed by Population Services International, and implemented by the Society for Family Health – merged the social marketing of contraception and condoms, and stated that it built "on lessons learned... in the development and management of a national contraceptive social marketing program" (TvT Associates/The Synergy Project 2002: 10).

Strategies beyond those associated with condoms also transferred, including edutainment. USAID sponsored the creation of a film about HIV, *Awakening*, which was made by the northern city of Kano's Kannywood film industry (USAID 2003a). The Society for Family Health produced in-person dramas, radio dramas, and billboards around the country on the topic of HIV and family planning (Odutolu et al. 2006). As in Malawi and as in the global AIDS field, a number of strategies initially used for family planning in Nigeria were repurposed or expanded to include HIV activities, with condom social marketing a point of particular transfer.

Discourses

USAID's involvement with both family planning and HIV was at least partially driven by US security concerns. A 1974 memo from Henry Kissinger entitled, "Implications of Worldwide Population Growth for US Security and Overseas Interests" identified Nigeria, and twelve other rapidly growing nations, as countries of "special US political and strategic interest" (Information Project for Africa 1991). Again, in 1989, a US defense-related publication identified Nigeria as of strategic interest given its projected population size (Foster, Sabrosky and Taylor 1989). And as described above, the 2002 National Intelligence Council report on HIV and security singled Nigeria out along with only a handful of other countries (Gordon 2002).

As in Malawi, suspicion about the motives behind pregnancy prevention interventions may have spilled over to HIV prevention. Much, but not all, of the negative discourse about family planning has occurred in the Muslim north of the country, where some have perceived pregnancy prevention interventions as a Western plot to reduce the number of Muslims (Renne 1996). For example, a 1989 publication on Islam and family planning noted how strange it was that Nigerians had to pay for all drugs except for those for family planning, and argued that current superpowers were implementing family planning programs in Nigeria in response to secret reports that Nigeria was poised to take over Africa because of its population size, natural resources, and foreign-educated population (Faruq 1989). Although this author's interpretation was perhaps creative, it corroborated a 1989 article in *The Washington Quarterly* that warned that Nigeria would "surpass" the US and Soviet Union to be the third largest country in the world by 2035 (Foster, Sabrosky, and Taylor 1989). Similarly, some Nigerians worried that they were being used as guinea pigs and dumping grounds by foreign companies and governments to test new contraceptives and dispose of expired ones (Orisasona, Akpan, and Adejoh 1996). More broadly, the vast sums of donor funding associated with the population policy only confirmed suspicions that it was not Nigerian and did not serve Nigerian interests (USAID 1994). As in Malawi, rumors have circulated that the US Central Intelligence Agency created HIV to reduce population growth, and that condoms might spread HIV (Smith 2014). Mistrust of the government and external actors has extended beyond family planning and HIV to include vaccines, which severely hampered polio eradication campaigns (Renne 2010).

The response to HIV in Nigeria has also at times reflected the politics of population, in particular the intense competition between states and subgroups. A 2002 USAID report noted that "Some states and local government authorities are fearful of being tagged as 'AIDS epicenters' due to stigma and attitudes of denial" (TvT Associates/The Synergy Project 2002: 7). As one respondent explained, there are no political benefits to addressing HIV/AIDS at the state level, and so governors are more likely to build a specialist hospital, which does bring them benefits, than to become a champion for HIV.[33] More recently, the release of state-level estimates of HIV prevalence led the Minister of Health for Rivers State, which had been ranked among the states with the highest prevalence, to question the accuracy of the data (Zaggi 2013). Thus there are examples of negative discourses associated with family planning spilling over to HIV.

Where Transfers between Intimate Interventions Did Not Occur

As in Malawi and Senegal, the reproductive health division of the Ministry of Health in Nigeria is separate from the division that focuses on sexually transmitted infections, and which first responded to HIV. The reproductive health division is under family health, while the sexually transmitted infection division is under public health (and across the street from the National AIDS Control Agency). A respondent explained this separation as a result of HIV not being

[33] N26, multilateral organization.

seen as a reproductive health issue when it first emerged, but instead as a disease.[34] Another respondent pointed out that all "donor diseases" (tuberculosis, AIDS, malaria) have their own buildings, and so are not even incorporated into the Ministry of Health. These administrative distinctions, although common across countries, complicated any transfer of resources from pregnancy prevention to HIV prevention.

Sanctions against Nigeria in the mid-1990s reduced aid flows to the country and made it more difficult for family planning organizations to apply their knowledge, skills, and resources towards HIV. More broadly, the military dictatorship neglected the health sector overall, including both family planning and HIV (Performance Needs Assessment Team 2001). In addition, soon after activities picked back up again with the transition to democracy in 1999, President Bush reinstated the Mexico City Policy, and US funding for family planning diminished. As one respondent explained: "I think the US government also added to the shift in focus from reproductive health to HIV. You had a Republican government that was not friendly to reproductive health. And then there was the gag rule [Mexico City Policy], and then there was all the reproductive health organizations starved of funds for eight years."[35]

Today, foreign and local organizations involved in the reproductive health area are focusing more on the integration of family planning and reproductive health services with HIV-related activities. As many respondents noted, however, such integration is easier said than done. Nurses and doctors at understaffed health facilities do not necessarily have the time to address yet one more issue, and all parties involved, from patients to policymakers, are used to separate, vertical programs.[36] In addition, as in Malawi, the AIDS epidemic made it difficult to talk about limiting family. Babatunde Osotimehin, former head of the National Agency for the Control of AIDS, said in a 2011 interview that "It was going to be impossible for me to stand up in a country where young men and women are dying and to say 'Excuse me I think you need to cut down on birth rates'. It was just not kosher... You couldn't begin to tell people 'You know, you are still

[34] N47, local NGO. [35] N47, local NGO.
[36] Immediately before my fieldwork in 2010, however, the former head of the reproductive health unit in the Ministry of Health had recently become the head of the sexually transmitted infection unit, suggesting a possible moment for synergy.

having too many children,' when they had just lost their kids" (as quoted in Goldenberg 2011).

Transfers from family planning to HIV prevention in Nigeria occurred primarily through transnational and political factors. International organizations that had supported family planning in Nigeria incorporated HIV into their portfolios and deployed similar strategies of intervention. Nigerian NGOs that had formed first to provide family planning became the lynchpin in the local response to HIV, and technocratic leaders involved with family planning participated in HIV prevention. Not all of the transfer was positive however, as the history of population interventions made some suspicious of the motives around HIV interventions, and bureaucratic structures as well as the political chaos of the 1990s proved to be forceful impediments.

Conclusion

Transnational, political, sociocultural, and economic factors each determined to some extent the nature and degree of intimate interventions in Nigeria. Resources associated with both transnational and political factors were particularly important relative to the transfers that occurred between family planning and HIV interventions. Political upheaval in the 1990s and weak civil society did, however, limit the family planning resources that transferred to HIV prevention. During most of the 1990s, Nigeria also largely lacked technocratic leadership to promote HIV, as Ransome-Kuti had resigned his post in the Ministry of Health in protest of the Babangida regime's manipulation of the 1993 elections (Renne 2016). Babatunde Osotimehin, who led the National Agency for the Control of AIDS from 2002 until he became Minister of Health in 2008, provided technocratic leadership, but at a later point in time, when donor funding and focus was on treatment. In addition, there is some evidence that suspicions around family planning may have cast a "long shadow" on HIV prevention, as in Malawi. The timing of Nigeria's return to democracy coincided with both the increase in the availability of HIV treatment and funding for it, and a transition away from US support for pregnancy prevention. As in other countries, the bureaucratic structure of the Ministry of Health inhibited a transfer between pregnancy prevention and HIV prevention.

Sociocultural factors make the implementation of social programs in Nigeria difficult, regardless of topic or target, as states compete for

central resources and strive to avoid being shamed for high HIV prevalence. Economic factors in Nigeria particularly intersected with
transnational factors, making the World Bank extremely interested in
population policy and keeping Nigeria at the forefront of the global
AIDS field's agenda. Nigeria's larger strategic importance to the US, as
well as the size of its population, has led to high levels of funding for
intimate interventions via USAID and PEPFAR.

Family planning NGOs – in particular, the Planned Parenthood
Federation of Nigeria, the Association for Reproductive and Family
Health, and the Society for Family Health – did become prominent in
the response to HIV. But only the Society for Family Health was active
in HIV prevention before the transition to democracy. A sense that the
epidemic was not extensive, that HIV was a disease different than the
other areas in which they worked, and that engaging with a stigmatized
disease like HIV might hamper pregnancy prevention-related work
appears to have kept the other two organizations from becoming
more deeply involved at the outset of the epidemic.

In Nigeria, as in Malawi, transnational and political factors had the
greatest influence on the scope of intimate interventions, and primarily
in similar ways. Effective technocratic leadership and political considerations led to a synergy between global promotion of, and national action
on, population and family planning. This situation did not, however,
reproduce with HIV prevention during the 1990s, when a variety of
domestic political factors limited donor involvement and hindered the
creation and action of civil society. Once the country returned to democracy, and donor funding became available for generic antiretroviral
therapy, Nigeria's HIV response shifted sharply towards treatment.
Lingering governance problems related to the competing sources of
authority in Nigeria, corruption, and weak democracy remain
a challenge for all forms of health interventions, whether intimate or not.

6 | Senegal: Transnational Ties and Technocratic Leadership

Similar to Nigeria, to "see" AIDS in Senegal requires seeking out the relevant local and foreign organizations. With less than 1 percent HIV prevalence, and a population of 14 million, there are only about 40,000 people in the entire country who are HIV positive. Billboards with AIDS messages are relatively infrequent, and the newspapers do not feature much discussion of HIV, instead covering health problems that affect more people, such as malaria. Dakar is the political and economic capital of the country, with the region home to a quarter of the country's population and located on a peninsula jutting out into the Atlantic Ocean. More cosmopolitan than either Abuja or Lilongwe, it is both a vibrant city in its own right as well as the seat of numerous donor activities and (West) African regional headquarters. Most donor organizations, including those working on AIDS, are now located in the Ngor area, close to the fancy hotels catering to European package vacation tourists. The Conseil National de Lutte Contre le Sida, Senegal's national AIDS commission, was actually hard to find, located down a dusty road from a beachfront hotel in Ngor (see Figure 6.1).[1] While here for an interview with someone else, I was casually introduced to the head of the commission himself, Dr. Ibrahim Ndoye, one of the key figures in Senegal's HIV success story whose contributions I detail below. The ease with which I was able to access the national AIDS commission, and its humble building, contrasted sharply with Malawi, where my repeated efforts to contact its members inside the commission's gleaming glass building were unsuccessful.

Senegal is the HIV success story in the book: a country where the government, civil society, and other actors have enthusiastically responded to HIV, and HIV prevalence has remained near 1 percent. The roots of Senegal's strong HIV prevention efforts lie in its

---

[1] It has since moved to a more central location at the main hospital, the Centre Hospitalier Universitaire de Fann.

168

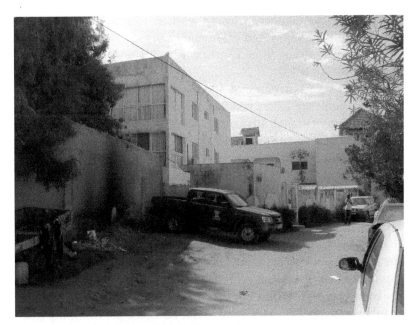

Figure 6.1. National AIDS Commission, Dakar
Source: Author's personal photo, 2010.

longstanding positive relationship with the international community and
a robust and active civil society. These transnational and political factors
have been bolstered by the sociocultural setting. Relative ethnic homogeneity, and low fractionalization, has resulted in stability and other
positive outcomes. Senegal's religious leaders form a core component of
civil society, and have shown a greater willingness to constructively
address HIV than those in Malawi or Nigeria. As in Nigeria, technocratic leadership enabled intimate interventions, but has had an even
greater impact because these leaders constitute, reflect, and reify the
strong bond between Senegal and the international community.

While Senegal is an HIV success story, contraceptive prevalence
remains low. Although fertility has declined from 6.7 children per
woman in 1970, women still have five children on average
(Population Reference Bureau 2015). A participant at a 2011 conference on family planning in Africa held in Dakar even described
Senegal as the "wild, wild west of family planning" (Boseley 2011).
However, a recent push to improve the availability of contraception

and increase the number of health workers to provide it, combined with continuing social and economic changes, raised modern contraceptive prevalence from 12 percent in 2010–11 to 20 percent in 2014 (Stratton 2015).

Although the outcomes of intimate interventions are different, a strong similarity exists between them in that Senegal has readily followed international advice regarding both family planning and HIV. That Senegal has long been an HIV, but not a family planning, success results from differences in how the template for intimate interventions from the global field matches the reality on the ground. With family planning, the population field promoted discourse about family planning increasing socioeconomic development that appealed to technocrats. Technocrats and programmers translated these frames down to the micro level to encourage family planning as a means to improve the health and living standards of the family. As in many places, this rationale alone was not, however, sufficiently compelling to overcome the benefits to high fertility nor the challenges associated with accessing family planning. With HIV prevention, Senegal's government participated willingly in a number of activities – targeting sex workers, involving civil society, speaking openly about HIV – in large part because it was relatively straightforward to do so because of the transnational and political factors described below. As a result, the global AIDS field labeled Senegal a success once HIV prevalence did not increase.

The chapter begins by presenting background on the relevant transnational, political, sociocultural, and economic factors that influence intimate interventions. It then provides the history of each intimate intervention, and concludes with discussion of the transfers that occurred between family planning and HIV prevention. As in Malawi and Nigeria, transnational and political factors best explain the contours of intimate interventions in Senegal. The most important transnational factor was Senegal's strong and positive connections with the international community. These connections were forged through colonial history, more recent economic dependence, and persistent outreach by both global and Senegalese actors. Key political factors in family planning as well as the response to HIV include technocratic leadership and the strength of civil society. More so than in either Malawi or Nigeria, religious leaders have been particularly supportive of HIV prevention, which relates partially to their connections to civil society (a political factor), but also to their position in society more broadly (a sociocultural factor). The analysis is based on interviews I conducted with family planning and HIV programmers in Senegal in 2006 and 2010, as well as from a variety of documents produced by donors, nongovernmental organizations, and the Senegalese government.[2]

Background on Senegal

Senegal's history of transnational ties as well as characteristics of its politics, sociocultural makeup, and economy help in understanding intimate interventions. Senegal's connections to France, and to the West more broadly, have existed since the seventeenth century. The capital of France's West African colonial holdings was always located in present-day Senegal: first in Saint Louis, at the mouth of the Senegal River on Senegal's northern border with Mauritania, and then from 1902 onwards in Dakar, which became the seat of Afrique Occidentale Française (French West Africa), formed officially in 1904.

Compared to Great Britain, France had relatively inclusive relationships with its colonies, stressing assimilation, and this was particularly so with Senegal. France's connection with Senegal began in 1659 when the Compagnie du Cap Vert – a French company that traded slaves and commodities – founded what would become the town of Saint Louis (Chafer 2012; Foley 2009). Long before the Scramble for Africa in 1885, France had a small colony in present-day Senegal that consisted of the towns of Dakar, Saint Louis, Rufisque, and Gorée, the so-called Four Communes of Senegal. When the French established equal political rights for all citizens in 1848, Senegal was granted a seat in the Chamber of Deputies in Paris, and those who could prove residence in the Four Communes for five years became eligible to vote in French parliamentary elections (Diouf 1998; Gellar 2005). By 1887, the Four Communes had the status of French municipalities, including the right to elect a deputy to the French National Assembly (Foley 2009). The ability to elect representatives was a unique right among French colonies – residents of all other colonies were subjects, rather than citizens – and ultimately Blaise Diagne of Senegal became the first African elected to the French National Assembly in 1914.

---

[2] References to interviews are denoted by "S" for Senegal, a number, and the type of organization that the respondent worked for. I conducted interviews 1–12 in 2006 and 13–44 in 2010.

Shared political goals and values led to a relatively exclusive and strong relationship between France and Senegal's elites, both traditional elites like chiefs and particularly modern elites like those in business and government (Chafer 2012). Senegal's first political leaders were trained in French schools, had experience in the French National Assembly, and were as committed to the ideals of republicanism as the French (Chafer 2012). Following World War II, France allotted ten seats to French West Africa in the constituent assembly that would write France's new constitution. Six Africans were elected, with Senegal disproportionately well-represented by Léopold Sedar Senghor and Lamine Gueye (Chafer 2002).[3] Both men became key political figures in Senegal's transition from colony to independent nation-state, and Senghor went on to be Senegal's first president. Senegal did not attempt any sort of radical break from France upon independence as neither Senghor nor de Gaulle saw decolonization as the exit of France from Senegal, and Senegalese post-independence political leaders were committed to ideals of modernization and development that depended on the transfer of financial and technical assistance from France to Senegal (Chafer 2012). Although technically a socialist, Senghor remained aloof from the Marxist streams of socialism more common in other parts of the continent, and emphasized the importance of connections to the West. This openness paralleled the Négritude movement, developed by Senghor with Aimé Césaire and Léon Damas, which was grounded in the idea of a distinct African culture that did not completely reject European culture. A poet and a writer, Senghor was the first African to be elected a member of the French Academy (Foley 2009).

The secondary literature on Senegal is full of references to the West's positive image of Senegal, and the ways in which Senegal benefits from its "brand" and "stellar international reputation" as a stable democracy (Foley 2009; IRIN 2012). Gellar (1995: 83) called Senegal "One of the most active and influential Black African countries on the international scene" and he noted further that "Senegal's diplomatic efforts have been remarkably successful in giving the nation a place of honor in

---

[3] Others elected included Felix Houphouet-Boigny (Ivory Coast/Upper Volta), Sourou Migan Apithy (Dahomey/Togo), Fily Dabo Sissoko (Soudan-Niger), and Yacine Diallo (Guinea). All would go on to make important contributions to the transition to independence in their respective countries, and Sissoko, Diallo, and Senghor were also prominent intellectuals.

various regional and international organizations." Bayart (1993) viewed such actions as strategic, with countries like Senegal purpose-fully inserting educated elites into international organizations in order to obtain various benefits and capitalize on their reputation: "It is no exaggeration to say that the export of [Senegal's] institutional image... has replaced the export of groundnuts," Senegal's long-time agricul-tural commodity (Bayart 2000: 226). Coulon and Cruise O'Brien noted Senegal's appeal to the West as a moderate, stable, democracy but also to Arab states as a strongly Muslim country, and concluded that "Senegal looks after its international image... [that] no doubt permits it to get the support indispensable to its survival" (Coulon and O'Brien 1989: 163–64). Much of this reputation is due to Senegal's first pre-sident, as "Senghor's mastery of international diplomacy and reputa-tion as Senegal's poet-president ensured a legacy of political and cultural prominence for Senegal" (Foley 2009: 32). In short, Senegal's international reputation forms a major part of its identity, which government and other representative actors strive to preserve.

A variety of other factors have helped maintain, and reflect, Senegal's connections with France and the West. Dakar is one of the most cosmopolitan cities in Africa, has long had direct air connections to Europe, and has consistently been one of the few places in sub-Saharan Africa with direct flights to the US. Unlike Nigeria or Malawi, Senegal is a major tourist destination for Europeans, with package tours from France and Germany, and a Club Med. The first three of Senegal's post-independence presidents (in office through 2012) were Catholic and married to white, French women. As a respondent described the situation,

"There has been lots of exposure to Western culture: Senegal was the capital of French West Africa, Senghor stressed respect and openness. Senegal was also well supported by donors, due to Senegalese diplomacy. It's a little country in terms of land and population size but it has a bigger image internationally than its size would suggest. Bigger than Mali or Nigeria, even though those are 'bigger' countries. Everyone international has some presence in Senegal."[4]

The government has also gone to great lengths to cultivate these rela-tionships, and prizes its global reputation as a stable democracy within

[4] S17, international NGO.

Africa. Respondents shared this pride in Senegal, with one noting, "Senegal is the door to Africa. It has been a leader in Africa for a long time."[5]

Political continuity combined with sociocultural factors, including a high degree of linguistic and particularly religious homogeneity, has produced relative stability in Senegal and also facilitated good relationships with the international community. Senegal has remained one of the most stable, relatively democratic countries in sub-Saharan Africa since independence from France in 1960. In particular, Senegal has never had a coup d'état, is known internationally for its positive civil-military relations, and in 1980 was the first country in sub-Saharan Africa where the executive branch voluntarily turned over (Diop 2013). The main driver of what political insecurity exists is the activities of separatist groups in the Casamance, the region to the south of The Gambia, which is ethnically and physically separated from the rest of Senegal. The Wolof account for approximately 40 percent of the population, followed by the Pulaar (~25 percent) and the Serers (~15 percent) (Central Intelligence Agency 2014). Wolof serves as the de facto national language, facilitating communication between different groups. Both ordinary Senegalese and scholars attribute ethnic harmony in part to the "joking" relationships that exist between different groups that ascribe particular roles and responsibilities by both ethnic group and patronym, which in turn allow gentle teasing (de Jong 2005; Villalón 1995). The population is predominantly (94 percent) Muslim, with the remaining 6 percent almost exclusively Catholic (Central Intelligence Agency 2014). Relations between Muslims and Christians are overwhelmingly positive, a fact that many Senegalese explained to me as the result of numerous families having members of both faiths.[6] Small gestures exemplify this conviviality, such as the tradition of Catholics bringing peanut and millet porridge to their Muslim neighbors at Easter, and Muslims sharing meat with Catholics following Tabaski, the major Muslim festival commemorating Ibrahim's willingness to sacrifice his son. Positive relations between ethnic groups may also result from the country's near total lack of

---

[5] S37, local NGO.
[6] Given how relatively few Senegalese are Catholic, however, good relations between religions cannot be explained by intermarriage alone as there simply are not enough Catholics to go around.

valuable natural resources, leaving fewer spoils for any one group to monopolize or covet (Collier and Hoeffler 2004).

Senegal's economic situation, while a reflection of inequality in the world system, also provides it with connections to the international community, in similar ways as in Malawi and Nigeria. Overall the population is poor, as more than half of people live on less than US$2 per day (World Bank 2014). In 1980, Senegal was the first country in sub-Saharan Africa to receive a structural adjustment loan from the World Bank and International Monetary Fund, and qualified as a highly indebted poor country in 1996, eligible for full relief from the same lenders (Dembele 2003). Senegal's currency, the CFA Franc, is guaranteed by the French treasury, was originally pegged to the French Franc, and is now tied to the Euro. Senegal is also a financial seat in West Africa. The CFA Franc is used by eight countries in West Africa which make up the West African Economic and Monetary Union and is issued by the Union's central bank in Dakar.

Transnational, political, sociocultural, and economic elements of Senegal's history and current position in the world are thus important for understanding intimate interventions, including the continuous and strong connection with France, Europe, and the West; democratic space for civil society (described in greater detail below); relative stability and harmony within the population; and economic dependence that has invited the involvement of foreign actors.

Preventing Pregnancy in Senegal

Senegal adopted a national population policy in 1988, the first population policy in a Francophone African country (Robinson 2015). As in Nigeria, transnational, political, and economic factors explain the early policy adoption, while sociocultural factors prevented the policy from having any real effect on fertility. Donor organizations and technocratic leadership in particular helped bring the policy into existence.

Senegal firmly supported "development as the best contraceptive" at the United Nations 1974 international population conference in Bucharest, rejecting the global population field's desire to implement family planning programs to slow population growth and improve development prospects (Locoh and Makdessi 1996). In 1976, however, President Senghor recommended the creation of a family planning program to lower population growth rates and the 1976 census ultimately showed the population growing rapidly at 2.2–2.5 percent annually (Mbodj, Mané, and Badiane 1992; Nortman and Hofstatter 1980). By 1978–79, the government had integrated family planning into all maternal and child health facilities, had solicited support and technical assistance for population from USAID, the international NGO Pathfinder, and UNFPA, and had established a National Population Commission (Nortman and Hofstatter 1980; World Bank 1992). One of the purposes of the population commission was to develop a framework for a population policy as part of long-term development planning (Sène 2005). To facilitate these goals, in 1980 Senegal repealed the 1920 French anti-contraceptive law that had up until that point made illegal even the distribution of information about contraception (Economic Commission for Africa 1988; Locoh and Makdessi 1996). Even with these changes, by 1983 there were only three sources of family planning in Dakar: ASBEF, an NGO whose clinic had opened in 1981 and whose work I describe later in the chapter; a Ministry of Health clinic (Protection Maternelle et Infantille) founded in 1976 and supported primarily by USAID and UNFPA; and a private clinic (Clinique de la Croix Bleue) founded in 1964 and funded by Pathfinder (Nichols et al. 1985). During the 1980s, USAID and UNFPA were the two primary donors supporting family planning in Senegal, and with their support, the number of public sector family planning service delivery points increased from twenty in 1984 to 150 in 1991 (UNFPA Ministry of Health and Social Action, National Family Planning Program of Senegal and Population Council 1995; Sanogo et al. 2003; UNFPA 2009; USAID 1992b). By 1989, population issues were included in the national primary and secondary school curricula (Devres, Inc. 1991).

Senegal adopted a population policy because of pressure from the global population field and technocratic leaders who saw various health and economic benefits to slowing population growth. As in other countries, USAID in particular emphasized fertility reduction and among other activities, sent consultants to the Ministry of Planning and Cooperation to facilitate drafting of the policy and organized a study tour to Zaire for Senegalese officials to learn about its family planning program (Hartmann 1995). USAID also funded the RAPID presentations, described in greater detail in Chapter 3, which were first used in Senegal in 1982 and ultimately shown to leaders in all the countries' regions, as well as to the president himself (Devres, Inc. 1991; Hartmann 1995; Mbodj, Mané, and Badiane 1992). Later, USAID attributed the government's adoption of the population policy in part to these presentations (USAID 1992b). In addition, the World Bank, which had scaled up population lending only recently, tied the creation of a population policy to the release of part of its third structural adjustment loan to Senegal, and took credit for the creation of the population policy (Sai and Chester 1990; World Bank 1989; World Bank 1992).

As in other countries, significant donor lending for population followed the adoption of the population policy, specifically from USAID and UNFPA, but also through the World Bank's Integrated Health Sector Development Project (Conly and Epp 1997; World Bank 1996). 1988 included an intensive mass media campaign promoting family planning (Devres, Inc. 1991). In 1991, with major support from USAID, the government initiated the National Family Planning Program, a vertical family planning program attached to the cabinet, separate from the Ministry of Health, that became operational in 1992 (Wickstrom, Diagne, and Smith 2006; Wilson 1998). Also in 1991, as part of the broader decentralization process, the Ministry of Health defined a minimum package of health services that was to be offered at every level of the health system, which included family planning (Hardee et al. 1998). The family planning program, however, changed departments eleven times in nineteen years, and the Minister of Health changed seven times in seven years, leading to major discontinuities in program implementation (Wickstrom, Diagne, and Smith 2006).

Economic factors also helped bring the population policy into existence, namely the sluggish economy and unfavorable balance of payments that initiated the structural adjustment program. Senegal's 1985–89 development plan noted that population growth would have a negative impact on existing and future resources (Sène 2005). As in most other sub-Saharan African countries, the Ministry of Planning, rather than the Ministry of Health, developed and managed the population policy (Robinson 2015). And almost all respondents described the creation of the population policy as a necessary response to the imbalance between population growth and socioeconomic development. As someone from the Ministry of Planning explained, "It was necessary to make a policy that could permit the harmonization of the rhythm of demographic growth with the rhythm of resource creation."[7]

In addition to donor interest and the economic situation, technocratic leaders helped the population policy come into being. In particular, among respondents who spoke specifically about the population policy, a quarter noted the participation of technocratic leaders in its production. One such technocrat was Landing Savané, a long-time politician as well as a demographer who published *Population: Un Point de Vue Africain* (*Population: An African Point of View*) in 1988. A respondent captured the contributions of such experts:

"What's important to me is that the position of the government is prepared by the professoriate. These professionals are demographers, men of science. Demographers, like Landing Savané, played a very important role in the formulation and documentation of the position of the Senegalese government."[8]

In his 1988 book, Savané strongly critiqued the dominant perspective of the global population field that rapid population growth hindered development, and instead argued that large populations could be a resource to African countries. While such a perspective might be viewed as contrary to a population policy, it actually reflected a compromise with what the Senegalese perceived as the Anglo/neo-Malthusian tendencies of donors, and as a result, Senegal's population policy contained no specific fertility targets. Respondents explained that the policy was a *population* policy, not a family planning policy, which thus encompassed much more than contraception or the limitation of births, and that Senegal's policy was not "demographic," like that of China or Anglophone African countries, whose primary goal was to limit births. Instead, it was about child spacing and protecting the health of mother and child (as was also the case in Malawi and Nigeria). As one respondent described this strategy, "It's only with a *global* policy that family planning could succeed," as opposed to one that focused solely on family planning.[9] Respondents also noted two other academics in particular, Abdoulaye Bara Diop, a professor of sociology at Senegal's main university, the Université Cheikh Anta Diop, and economist Malick Sow. Along with Savané, they served as

---

[7] S1, federal ministry.   [8] S9, local NGO.   [9] S8, university.

consultants for the population policy. While it is not surprising that the Ministry of Planning hired consultants to help formulate the population policy, that respondents remembered the exact names of consultants twenty years later, as well as explicitly noted the relevance of science to policy, reflects the import of technocratic leadership to intimate interventions in Senegal.

A variety of family planning NGOs were founded starting in the 1970s and particularly 1980s. By 1985, there were at least 30 local NGOs doing some work in the area of reproductive health in Senegal and this figure grew to over 50 by 1989 (Sullivan 2007). The most important, the Association Sénégalaise pour le Bien-être Familial (ASBEF, the Senegalese Association for Family Wellbeing), was founded in 1968 and affiliated with the International Planned Parenthood Federation in 1975 (Association Sénégalaise pour le Bien-être Familial n.d). One of its first activities was to lobby the government to repeal the 1920 anti-contraceptive law (Wickstrom, Diagne, and Smith 2006). It provides sexual and reproductive health services, particularly contraception, to adolescents as well as women through clinics located in half of Senegal's fourteen regions. By 1997, ASBEF provided almost a fifth of all contraceptive needs in Senegal, but this figure flagged in the 2000s when the organization lost funding from USAID with the reinstatement of the Mexico City Policy (Wickstrom, Diagne, and Smith 2006).

NGO and government interaction with religious leaders to reduce opposition to family planning started in the 1980s and was fully institutionalized by the mid-1990s. Many Islamic leaders and laypeople have viewed family planning as against Islam if used to limit fertility. To counter this view, ASBEF and the National Population Commission hosted a seminar on Islam and family planning in Dakar in 1982. The seminar, attended by more than 200 people, including Islamic leaders and members of the Senegalese government, concluded that Senegal should adopt a family planning system that took Islamic teachings into account (Omran 1992; Wickstrom, Diagne, and Smith 2006). ASBEF again hosted a roundtable on Islam and family planning in 1989 (Wickstrom, Diagne, and Smith 2006). In addition to ASBEF's activities, UNFPA supported the creation of a document authored by the Association National des Imams et Ulemas du Sénégal (National Association of Imams and Ulemas of Senegal)[10] that outlined how

---

[10] Imams are Islamic leaders of worship; ulemas are Muslim scholars.

family planning was not contradictory to Islam (Gueye 1995). Following the 1994 United Nations International Conference on Population and Development, the Ministry of Finance and Planning and the UNFPA facilitated the creation of the Réseau Islam et Population (Islam and Population Network), which had representatives from all of Senegal's Muslim brotherhoods and facilitated workshops for the general population led by religious leaders to provide education on family planning and sexually transmitted infections (Hardee et al. 1998; Renders 2002). The Réseau also published a document in 1996 explaining the population policy from an Islamic perspective (Réseau Islam et Population 1996). All of these meetings and publications were designed to demonstrate that the Koran is not against family planning, in particular if family planning is used to space, rather than limit, births. These efforts met with some success, as one respondent explained: "Even though some Muslims were against family planning, there were imams who collaborated and helped the population understand that Islam does not oppose contraception."[11] Although my respondents felt this outreach helped reduce religious opposition to family planning, a 2006 evaluation found that many Islamic religious leaders remained uninterested in family planning and that many Senegalese, including lower-level imams, still believed that family planning was against Islam (Wickstrom, Diagne, and Smith 2006).

Senegal's population policy received a muted response. Relatively minimal publicity around the policy likely contributed to this outcome: the bureaucracy responsible for the policy, the Directorate of Human Resources Planning within the Ministry of Economy, Finance, and Planning, had a relatively low position following ministerial reorganization in 1990 and was separated from the Ministry of Health and the National Family Planning Program (Wilson 1998). In addition, the several years following the policy's adoption were characterized by a short period of political and economic crisis (Wilson 1998). More broadly, despite increased acceptance for family planning through the 1980s and 1990s among programmers as well as individuals, the topic remained politically sensitive. For example, the Ministry of Health cancelled the rollout of a community-based distribution program for

---

[11] S8, university.

family planning in the 1990s when the opposition party, prior to an election, attacked it (Wilson 1998).

Very few women took up family planning, in large part because of continuing limited demand and barriers to access, but also because of a disjuncture between the population's desires and those of programmers. Sociocultural and economic factors drove this disjuncture. The template adopted from the global population field by the Senegalese technocrats simply did not mesh with the day-to-day experiences of Senegalese people, and particularly Senegalese women. Respondents noted that high fertility was itself the result of high mortality and the need for the social protection and labor provided by large families, cultural values that gave women status as a result of fertility, and religious dictates for people to go forth and multiply. As one respondent described it, "Family planning isn't the key issue to people – you can't start with it. Women are preoccupied with things other than family planning."[12] As another respondent noted, "When people are dying and you say you have to limit population, it doesn't make sense. The discourse used by programs has not been so good: 'You need to have fewer kids so that you can pay for school.' It's much better to tell people that not using family planning will lead to death. The socioeconomic motivation for family planning didn't work."[13] So while technocrats largely accepted the socioeconomic "motivation" promoted by the global population field, that frame failed to match local realities and thus did not increase contraceptive prevalence.

Senegal's experience with pregnancy prevention nevertheless still laid the groundwork for HIV prevention along several different dimensions. The country developed good relationships with donors, a transnational factor, that would come to be important in the response to HIV: USAID, the World Bank, and UNFPA. Family planning NGOs, most notably ASBEF, came into being and joined Senegal's already strong civil society, a political factor. Finally, the government and donors gained experience in dialoguing with religious leaders on the sensitive topics of contraception and sexuality, demonstrating a positive synergy between political and sociocultural factors. In the next section, I move to discussing HIV prevention in Senegal, with particular attention to these same factors.

[12] S22, local NGO.   [13] S24, federal ministry.

Preventing HIV in Senegal

The global AIDS field has labeled Senegal an HIV success story for keeping HIV prevalence near 1 percent and engaging in a number of best practices. Across the literature, the primary factors identified as driving this success include political commitment and active engagement with civil society, particularly its religious elements, mediated through effective management of sexually transmitted infections among sex workers, made possible by historical, transnational relationships (Barnett and Whiteside 2006; Eboko 2005; Iliffe 2006; Meda et al. 1999; Patterson 2005; Pisani 2000; Putzel 2004; Putzel 2006). Other key factors that have prevented a more extreme HIV epidemic and are unrelated to active government or organizational intervention include almost universal male circumcision, a less virulent form of the virus (HIV type 2),[14] and a geographic location far from more heavily impacted countries (cf. Engelberg 2005; Meda et al. 1999; Moran 2004; Putzel 2006). Others have identified the truly multidisciplinary nature of the response to the epidemic, distinguishing it from more surface-level multilateral responses that evolved much later in other countries (Niang 2001; Putzel 2003). Mapping these factors onto the model for country-level responses to HIV developed in Chapter 1, the literature has clearly emphasized political factors, with some attention to transnational ones. Relative to the predominant understanding presented by the literature, I stress the importance of transnational relationships and technocratic leadership.

The first AIDS case in Senegal was identified in 1986, and a number of official actions quickly followed. The government's first response came that same year: the commitment of federal budget for HIV and the creation of the National AIDS Committee (Comité National de Lutte contre le SIDA), which was part of the Ministry of Health and drew members from federal ministries, NGOs, and academe (Conseil National de Lutte contre le Sida 2002; Putzel 2003). The National AIDS Committee then created the National AIDS Program (Programme National de Lutte contre le SIDA). The government implemented HIV screening procedures for the blood supply in 1986, an action that came on the heels of a long history of good management:

---

[14] HIV type 2 predominated at the beginning of the epidemic in Senegal, but existed in equal proportion with HIV type 1 by the late 1990s (Meda et al. 1999).

Senegal had a blood bank as early as 1943, has had a transfusion center since 1951, a blood transfusion policy since 1970, and has screened the blood supply for hepatitis and syphilis since the 1970s (Conseil National de Lutte contre le Sida 2002; Meda et al. 1999; Niang 2001; Schneider 2013; USAID 2003b). In 1987 the government instituted an emergency plan of action for HIV, and with the assistance of the World Health Organization, developed Medium Term Plans for 1988–92 and 1994–98 (USAID 1999b). In 1989 sentinel surveillance, the measurement of HIV among specific populations, such as women attending antenatal clinics, began producing relatively constant and reliable data on HIV (Conseil National de Lutte contre le Sida 2002; Meda et al. 1999), and changes in syringe regulations in 1990 led to disposable syringes for vaccines and better means for disposal of used needles.

Senegal implemented a number of additional HIV interventions much earlier than in other countries. HIV has been included in teacher training as well as the national curriculum since the early 1990s (Pisani 1999; Quist-Arcton 2001). Behavioral surveillance – surveys of populations at particular risk for HIV – began in 1997 (USAID 2002). The government introduced a pilot program for prevention of mother-to-child transmission in 2000, described as one of sub-Saharan Africa's first (Family Health International 2007b; USAID 2002). In the early 2000s, Senegal became one of the few sub-Saharan African countries to have an HIV program targeting men who have sex with men (Awondo, Geschiere, and Reid 2012; Niang et al. 2004). And the Senegalese army has been described as using more condoms than any army in Africa (Singhal and Rogers 2003).

A number of organizations from the global AIDS field were involved in HIV prevention. USAID's first major HIV-related program in Senegal was AIDSCAP, described in Chapter 2 and implemented by Family Health International in Senegal beginning in 1992. The project authorization for the grant described the HIV epidemic in Senegal as being at an "early but potentially explosive phase" (USAID 1992a: 1). USAID funds constituted slightly more than half of all foreign aid for HIV given to Senegal between 1994 and 2001, and by 2003, USAID had provided Senegal with more than 10 million condoms (Seck 2001; USAID 2003b). In addition to supporting conferences for religious and political leaders on appropriate responses to HIV, described in greater detail below, AIDSCAP also funded training for journalists on HIV in the 1990s, enabled increased participation of civil society in the response to HIV, and developed the *Emma Dit (Emma Says)* comic series to teach about HIV and other sexually transmitted infections (Badge, Engelberg, and Sarr 1997; Barnett 2004; Family Health International 1997).

In addition to USAID, other donors from the global AIDS field funded HIV interventions in Senegal. Reflecting its favored status with donors, in 1996 Senegal received many times more aid per HIV-positive person than did worse-affected countries, including Malawi and Nigeria but also Kenya, Zambia, and Zimbabwe, such that the government contributed less than 8 percent of the total funding available for HIV (Putzel 2003; UNAIDS and Harvard School of Public Health 1999). The World Health Organization facilitated the creation of the National AIDS Program in 1986 as well as the development of Medium Term Plans for 1988–92 and 1994–98 (USAID 1999b). The World Bank, through the Multi-Country AIDS Program, also provided significant financing of HIV-related activities, one of the requirements of which was the creation of the National AIDS Commission in 2001 (Putzel 2003). PEPFAR was notably absent from the HIV response in Senegal until 2009, in part because the legality of sex work prevented the country from agreeing to PEPFAR's "anti-prostitution pledge"[15] (Reaves 2007).

It is of course impossible to definitively identify any particular element of HIV interventions as *causing* the positive outcomes observed in Senegal, but there are several pieces of evidence presented in a key 1999 UNAIDS report that Senegalese, and particularly those in Dakar, changed their behavior during the 1990s in ways likely to lower HIV incidence (Pisani 1999). First and most convincingly, the levels of sexually transmitted infections among sex workers and pregnant women in Dakar declined between 1991 and 1996. In addition, rates also declined among workers at the Port of Dakar (Simmons 2001). Second, in a 1997 household survey in Dakar, among men who reported casual sex, 67 percent used a condom, which was almost certainly a significant increase from prior to the AIDS epidemic, although comparable figures are not available. Third, condom sales increased from 800,000 in 1988 to 7,000,000 in 1997. The extent to

---

[15] This element of PEPFAR required organizations receiving money from the US government to have a policy in place opposing sex work.

which these apparent behavioral changes were due to the actions of government, donors, or civil society cannot be determined, but they suggest that people did actually change their behavior in ways that helped prevent the spread of HIV and thus may have contributed to Senegal's continued low HIV prevalence.

Transnational Factors Influencing HIV Prevention

A number of transnational factors facilitated HIV prevention interventions in Senegal, including the management of sex work and a general openness to the international community. Legal, managed sex work in Senegal is largely the result of historical factors, but is also something the government has maintained and which has benefitted the response to HIV. Positive relationships with the international community are also the result of history, but Senegal has worked hard to preserve them, and they have helped prevent AIDS denialism like that which occurred in South Africa under Thabo Mbeki.

The management of sex work, and the management of sexually transmitted infections, both predated HIV in Senegal. Surveillance and treatment of sexually transmitted infections among sex workers and the military in Senegal began in the late nineteenth century, and stemmed from a general French interest in hygiene (Becker and Collignon 1999). French concerns about depopulation bolstered colonial administrators' support for the health of colonial subjects, heightened first by the need for troops during World War I, and later by the belief that the productive labor of the colonies could help build the might of France (Becker and Collignon 1999). When antibiotic injections became available in the 1950s, the French began using them vigorously to treat sexually transmitted infections in Senegal (Echenberg 2006).

Sex work was legalized in France and some colonies in 1946, and even though France repealed the law in 1960, it remained on the books in Senegal, which became independent the same year (Poleykett 2012). Details of the law in Senegal were codified in 1969, and little has changed since then (Poleykett 2012). The legality of sex work is unusual among African countries, is not justified on the basis of rights, and stems in likely part from unique aspects of Senegal's colonial history relative to other French protectorates (Ngalamulume 2011; ProCon.

org 2015).[16] Women are not allowed to solicit clients on the street, but can work in clubs or discos, and those over the age of 21 may register as sex workers, which entails the issuance of health cards, regular check-ups that include annual HIV tests, semi-annual syphilis tests, access to free condoms, and prescriptions for treatment of sexually transmitted infections (Homaifar and Wasik 2005). If a woman is found to have a sexually transmitted infection, her card will not be stamped until the infection has been cured. A site for check-ups since 1970 has been the Social Hygiene Institute (Institut d'Hygiene Social) in Dakar, which facilitated early scientific access to one of the populations at greatest risk for HIV (Do Espirito Santo and Etheredge 2004; Poleykett 2015).

Other governmental and nongovernmental support structures integrated HIV into their work or emerged anew. The government created the National Office for Controlling Sexually Transmitted Infections (Bureau National de Lutte contre les MST) in 1978 as part of the Hygiene and Health Protection division of the Ministry of Health (Conseil National de Lutte contre le Sida 2002; Meda et al. 1999). When HIV appeared, it was straightforward to include it as part of extant programs, particularly since it shared the primary means of prevention – condoms – with other sexually transmitted infections. The Ministry of Health, starting in 1989, began integration of HIV and sexually transmitted infection prevention strategies (USAID 2003b). A local NGO, Association Awa, since 1993 has carried out extensive peer-to-peer HIV prevention outreach to sex workers (Ebin 2000).

Senegal's capacity to manage sexually transmitted infections and sex workers most likely helped stem the spread of HIV among sex workers, and from sex workers to the general population. The provision of services to sex workers also exemplifies global best practices for responding to HIV. Nonetheless, after growing to first 10 percent in 1994 and then 19 percent in 1997, HIV prevalence among sex workers in Dakar remained relatively constant at around 20 percent through

---

[16] Because the first French settlements in Africa were in Senegal, there was greater mixing of the African and European populations than in areas colonized later. This mixing led to concern about the transmission of sexually transmitted infections from the single, "free," African women to the European male population, particularly soldiers, and in turn to regulation of the African women. By the time the French empire expanded, however, cities were more segregated, decreasing the motivation to manage sexual relations (including sex work) in other locations.

2009 and a large number of unregistered, or "clandestine," sex workers exist (Diouf 2007; Foley and Nguer 2010; Homaifar 2006;
UNAIDS 2010). These women do not register because of shame, or
because they do not anticipate that they will engage in sex work for
a long period of time (Renaud 1997). As a result, programs cannot
reach them, leaving them at high risk for HIV.

In addition to the history that led to Senegal's capacity to manage sex
work, a number of other transnational factors have facilitated HIV
prevention. By virtue of having been the capital of French West Africa,
Dakar has excellent medical facilities, and came to have two world-
class HIV labs, the French Pasteur Institute and the Laboratory of
Bacteriology and Virology at Le Dantec Hospital (Eboko 2005;
Iliffe 2006; Putzel 2006). Senegal has hosted a number of conferences
related to HIV, which have provided ample opportunities to present its
success story to an international audience (Green 2003). Senegal has
also hosted a number of other conferences, including the 1992
Organization of African Unity summit, which produced the Dakar
Declaration on the HIV Epidemic in Africa, behind which Senegal
has been described as the driving force (Pisani 1999). According to
a respondent, "We accepted the reality of AIDS at the beginning, there
was no denial. Why? *Openness of spirit.*"[17]

Senegal benefits from its ties to international organizations, but so
too do international organizations. These organizations have fostered
and enforced the idea of Senegal as an HIV success story, and once
Senegal gained this status, it has worked hard to keep it (Eboko 2005;
Iliffe 2006). For many years, the global AIDS field was without
a success story, and most of the news related to AIDS was very, very
bad. As Peter Piot, the executive director of UNAIDS, described the
situation in the mid-to-late 1990s, "For UNAIDS to get its message
across, we needed success stories, because to mobilize money and
convince policy makers, it's not enough to demonstrate that something
is a really bad problem. If you can't do something about it, and it's
a hopeless case, then what's the point?... [Uganda and Thailand]
became our beacons of hope in a grim landscape. A little later we
added Senegal" (Piot 2012: 235). It was indeed in the late 1990s that
Senegal was first referred to as a "success," by the head of the National
AIDS Program, Ibrahim Ndoye, but also by the United Nations, which

---

[17] S36, bilateral organization.

recognized Uganda, Thailand, and the Philippines along with Senegal as successes at the official opening of the 1998 International AIDS Conference (Masebu 1997; Masebu 1998; Wone 1996). Also in 1998, the Society for Women and AIDS in Africa presented President Diouf of Senegal and President Museveni of Uganda with awards recognizing their support of the response to HIV in their countries (Mwaura 1999). Then, in 1999, UNAIDS published *Acting Early to Prevent AIDS: The Case of Senegal* (Pisani 1999), formally bestowing "success" status on Senegal, and creating the list of factors and facts that almost all subsequent discussions of the response to HIV in Senegal cite. That same year, Meda et al. (1999) published in *AIDS*, the official journal of the International AIDS Society, their key scientific article on the same topic, "Low and Stable HIV Infection Rates in Senegal: Natural Course of the Epidemic or Evidence for Success of Prevention?" Senegal's reputation as a success story was quickly cemented, and by 2001, the World Bank justified its proposed second round Multi-Sectoral AIDS grant for Senegal on the basis that it would "assist Senegal in maintaining its all-important 'success story' – a powerful force for emulation by other countries in the sub-region struggling with significantly higher levels of prevalence" (World Bank 2001: 3).[18]

Senegalese who work for the government, donor organizations, and NGOs are proud of their country's response to HIV, including prevention programs as well as the antiretroviral initiative described below. This pride confirms and reinforces Senegal's self-image as a leader in Africa on HIV as well as more broadly. For example, at the opening ceremony for the National AIDS Commission in 2002 President Wade stated: "More than a national responsibility, it is before the international community that we will respond to the hope that the continent has placed in us" (Conseil National de Lutte contre le Sida 2007: 3). Similarly, the country's 2002 Strategic Plan for responding to HIV noted that, "Senegal's AIDS program has played a leading and influential role in the African Region" (Conseil National de Lutte contre le Sida 2002: 25). Such confidence and pride have helped maintain

[18] Even before Senegal's international reputation as an AIDS success story solidified, USAID justified the country's inclusion in the AIDSCAP program on the grounds of its "status in the region [and] the opportunity to provide an example, or model program for the region" (USAID 1992a: 119).

government support for the response to HIV, creating a virtuous policy feedback loop.

Political Factors Influencing HIV Prevention in Senegal

A number of political factors influenced HIV prevention in Senegal, including an active civil society and strong technocratic leadership, which this section describes in detail. Civil society organizations helped link the government to religious leaders as well as everyday people, while technocratic leaders legitimized HIV to political leaders as well as constituted and reified Senegal's positive relationship with the international community. Other political factors, such as the centralized nature of the Parti Socialist that led Senegal through 2000, enabled the actions taken by government (Putzel 2003).

Senegal has a thriving civil society, with religion serving as a key point of social organization, but also many *groupements de promotion féminins*, or women's support groups. These groups and others like them are connected into the political apparatus of the country, which some have argued facilitated their involvement in the response to HIV (Putzel 2003). One estimate indicates that there were 6,000 such groups around 2000, comprising more than one million women (Conseil National de Lutte contre le Sida 2002). In addition, relative to other countries in sub-Saharan Africa, Senegal has an above-average number of NGOs: in 2003, Senegal had more NGOs per capita than 60 percent of sub-Saharan African countries (Robinson 2010a). Although accounts of actual numbers of NGOs vary greatly by source, most suggest significantly more of such organizations operating in Senegal than in other countries: perhaps 200 AIDS NGOs by 1995, with many of them formed in the immediately preceding years (International HIV/AIDS Alliance 1999; Niang 2008).

As a testament to the strength of HIV-related civil society in Senegal, five local NGOs banded together in 2003 to form the Observatoire, a watchdog group for the government's AIDS response. The Observatoire put forth an influential press release in 2005 to demand that the National AIDS Commission better incorporate NGOs into its activities, and simultaneously criticized the Commission for other lapses (International HIV/AIDS Alliance and Global Fund to Fight AIDS Tuberculosis and Malaria 2008; Jurgens and Dia 2006). Simultaneously, both the Global Fund and World

Bank insisted on change in Senegal's HIV response, with the Global Fund threatening withdrawal of funding. As a result, a local NGO, the Alliance Nationale Contre le SIDA (National Alliance against AIDS), founded in 1994 to organize civil society activities around HIV/AIDS, became a principal recipient of the Global Fund in 2006 (Mbodj and Taverne 2004). Senegal thus became one of the first countries with an NGO as a principal recipient, setting a trend for future Global Fund grants the world over. The existence and success of the Observatoire reflects the strength of civil society in Senegal, primarily its willingness and ability to express dissent, but also its diversity of opinions, because although the Observatoire represented the views of many NGOs, others publicly disagreed with its actions (Jurgens and Dia 2006).

Several religious NGOs became actively involved in the early response to HIV/AIDS, particularly Jamra (Arabic for "embers") and SIDA Service (AIDS Service). These NGOs helped pave the way for religious leaders to discuss HIV with their followers by providing legitimacy to acknowledging and addressing AIDS. Jamra, an Islamic NGO founded in 1982, has a primary mission to reduce substance abuse and sex work, and has targeted urban youth in particular. After signing an agreement with the National AIDS Committee in 1989, Jamra traveled all over the country and was instrumental in convincing the khalifs that lead each of Senegal's Islamic brotherhoods to discuss HIV with their followers (Delaunay and Quinio 1999; Gomez-Perez 2011; Lom 2001; Sayagues 2004). Jamra ultimately became the key link between donors, the government, and Muslim authorities. In reference to Jamra, a respondent noted that, "It was hard to talk about sex and HIV, but because a religious NGO did it, people believed."[19] Jamra's approach was based on promoting a *préservatif moral*, or a moral condom, to help prevent the spread of HIV (Delaunay and Quinio 1999). Then, in 1995, Jamra published the *Guide Islam et SIDA* (*Guide to Islam and AIDS*), a compendium that stressed the ways in which Islam could be used to help prevent HIV (Ministere de la Santé Publique et de l'Action Social et al. 1995; Sayagues 2004). In 1997, Jamra helped organize the first International Colloquium on AIDS and Religion, held in Senegal (Green 2003; Thioye 1998). Jamra was also involved in the 1999 creation of the Alliance des Religieux et des Experts Médicaux contre

[19] S43, local NGO.

l'épidémie du Sida au Sénégal (Religious and Medical Alliance against the AIDS Epidemic in Senegal), which brought together religious NGOs that focused on AIDS, such as SIDA Service (described in the following paragraph), as well as those that did not, the National Association of Imams and Ulemas of Senegal, and the National AIDS Program (Gomez-Perez 2011).

SIDA Service, a Catholic NGO founded in 1992, provides care and support to those who are HIV-positive, and was the first organization in Senegal to offer free voluntary HIV testing and counseling services. Although founded specifically in response to HIV, SIDA Service emerged out of Senegal's pre-existent Catholic health care infrastructure. During its first two years, SIDA Service visited all archbishops and bishops in Senegal to discuss HIV (Sayagues 2004). SIDA Service also organized the 1996 conference on Christianity and AIDS (Putzel 2003). There was widespread agreement among respondents that the cooperation of religious leaders was crucial to Senegal's effective response to HIV. As one respondent put it, "We carried out awareness-raising activities with religious leaders, and as a result, there were no burnt-down condom billboards like in Niger."[20] SIDA Service has grown to have 23 centers across Senegal, and has expanded to Guinea-Bissau and The Gambia (UNAIDS 2009).

Environnement et Développement du Tiers Monde (ENDA, Environment and Development in the Third World), founded in 1972 and one of the oldest NGOs in Senegal, set up a team exclusively devoted to HIV in 1986, the year that the first HIV case was diagnosed in Senegal (Mbodj and Taverne 2004). ENDA has a health program, ENDA-Santé (ENDA-Health), has supported organizations for people living with HIV/AIDS, and has also been particularly active in outreach to men who have sex with men (Niang et al. 2004). In addition, ENDA's Director of Health and Development Programs from 1988–1997, El Hadj As Sy, was well connected globally and as a result, even though the organization had relatively limited experience working with HIV, ENDA was selected to be one of the handful of NGOs on the task force that helped create UNAIDS (Gordenker et al. 1995).[21] ENDA also helped form the regional branch of the

---

[20] S26, international NGO.
[21] Sy himself went on to become regional director for Africa for UNAIDS (Piot 2012).

International Council of AIDS Service Organizations, an outcome again due in part to global connections (Delaunay, Blibolo, and Cissé-Wone 1999; Putzel 2003).

Respondents emphasized the importance of civil society to Senegal's HIV activities, noting that Senegal has a rich history of social organization that predated HIV and could be drawn upon to address HIV. As one respondent described the situation, "We were able to build on something that already existed: civil society structures and *groupements des femmes* have always been involved with vaccination and primary health care issues."[22] Similarly, another respondent said that "Senegal was lucky – it has a long history of associations, which are in the Senegalese tradition. We used the force of associations to develop a community response to HIV. Every region and sector had associations engaged in the fight, and organizations really started structuring around 1990–91."[23]

In addition to NGOs, technocratic leadership is another political factor particularly important to Senegal's HIV prevention interventions. Respondents attributed much of Senegal's early and effective response to HIV to three technocrats: Soulemayne Mboup, Ibrahim Ndoye, and Awa Marie Coll-Seck. While technocrats were crucial to intimate interventions in Nigeria, and their absence influenced outcomes in Malawi, they predominate in both the external and internal narrative of the understanding of Senegal's successful response to HIV. Piot (2012: 162) referred to all three as "stars of AIDS, public health, and medical research." Not only did technocratic leadership directly facilitate the response to HIV, but it reflects Senegalese openness and has deepened links between Senegal and the international community through scientific networks (Eboko 2005).

Mboup, a virologist, co-discovered the HIV type 2 virus in 1985, and directs the Laboratory of Bacteriology and Virology at Le Dantec Hospital in Dakar, one of the best virology labs in Africa. Mboup has more than 200 peer-reviewed articles listed in Web of Science, of which 20 have been cited over a hundred times.[24] The most frequently cited (more than 350 times) is the *Science* article from 1994 describing the longer incubation period of HIV type 2 relative to HIV type 1 (Marlink et al. 1994). He was also an editor on a major publication, *AIDS in*

---

[22] S36, bilateral organization.
[23] S39, local NGO.   [24] As of September 2014.

Africa (Essex et al. 2002), and has served as the point person for Harvard's AIDS research in Senegal, a collaboration that has helped train Senegalese researchers as well as develop laboratory infrastructure in Dakar (AIDS Prevention Initiative Nigeria n.d.-a; Poleykett 2015). Academic sources, the popular press, and the media all attribute much of Senegal's successful response to HIV to Mboup (e.g., Garrett 1994; Piot 2012; Putzel 2006; Quist-Arcton 2001). His reputation and stature have made him a global spokesperson for Senegal, and in particular, the response to HIV. For example, in 2007 he led a group of African scientists to write a letter denouncing President Jammeh of The Gambia's claim to have found a cure for AIDS (Cassidy and Leach 2009; Piot 2012).

Ndoye ran the government's sexually transmitted infection program prior to the advent of AIDS as the head of the Social Hygiene Institute, was the director of the National AIDS Program from its founding in 1987, and then was the executive secretary of the National AIDS Commission from when it was founded in 2001 until 2014 when he retired.[25] Ndoye's position as the head of the executive committee of the Commission essentially placed him above the cabinet ministers that lead federal ministries. Even those organizations and individuals most critical of him and the Commission have cited the importance of his continued and long leadership to the fight against HIV in Senegal. Much like Mboup, official narratives describing HIV prevention in Senegal frequently mention Ndoye. Importantly, he never joined a political party, facilitating continuity in (his) leadership of the national response to HIV (Putzel 2003).

Seck's activities have in particular connected Senegal to a variety of international organizations. In Senegal, she worked with the National AIDS Program after it was first created, then started an NGO, then moved to Geneva where she directed two departments at UNAIDS from 1996 to 2001, was the Minster of Health of Senegal from 2001–2003, and then the executive director of the World Health Organization's Roll Back Malaria Partnership in Geneva from 2004 to 2012, after which she again became Senegal's Minister of Health.

Respondents regularly mentioned all three technocrats, and identified various ways in which they led the country's response to HIV. As one

---

[25] Safitou Thiam, a former Minister of Health, has since become the executive secretary.

respondent described, "There were university doctors, respected specialists who legitimized HIV/AIDS, made it easier for politicians to follow suit – Mboup, Seck, Ndoye."[26] By legitimizing HIV, these experts helped Senegal's response start early. "Why the early response? Well-advised men. Dr. Ndoye – very engaged. Prof. Mboup – all were on point with the fight."[27] The presence and notoriety of people like Mboup helped provide scientific legitimacy to HIV, making it something about health, and not just about morals. Following the discovery of HIV type 2, Mboup, Ndoye, and Seck called on President Diouf, who immediately provided support for a response to HIV because "work on HIV/AIDS was seen as something that added value to, rather than detracting from, Senegal's reputation" (Putzel 2003: 22). According to Mboup himself, "The pride the country felt in discovering HIV type 2 helped slow the course of the virus. People wanted to talk about Senegal's role; AIDS was not shunned as a topic. 'It meant you could talk about AIDS in a positive way here in Senegal!... That made things easier than perhaps any other country. We were the scientists in front of the problem. And that gave us legitimacy'" (as cited in Donnelly 2003). The existence of such technocratic leaders, who strongly promoted HIV prevention, was particularly crucial at the beginning of the epidemic when the relative invisibility of HIV in Senegal made the media and general public doubt it was a problem (Becker and Collignon 1999; Hardee et al. 1998; USAID 1992a; Wone 1996). These technocratic leaders also helped shape the contours of HIV research collaboration in other countries, including Nigeria. Promotional material for the Harvard-supported AIDS Prevention Initiative in Nigeria states, "In supporting Nigeria's efforts... researchers are modeling their approach on a long-term collaboration with another West African nation, Senegal" (AIDS Prevention Initiative Nigeria n.d.-b).

Technocratic leadership in conjunction with a desire to be a trailblazer helped spur Senegal's 1998 antiretroviral program, the Initiative Sénégalaise d'Accès aux Antirétroviraux (Senegalese Antiretroviral Access Initiative), which the government funded in part from its own coffers. This program was one of the first public antiretroviral distribution systems in sub-Saharan Africa (Ndoye et al. 2004).[28] It was only

---

[26] S36, bilateral organization.   [27] S33, local NGO.
[28] Uganda and Côte d'Ivoire also began distributing antiretroviral drugs in 1998 with support from UNAIDS.

two years earlier, in 1996 at the biannual International AIDS Conference in Vancouver, that researchers had announced the discovery of effective combination antiretroviral therapy. When Senegal launched its program, the cost of such therapy was still extraordinarily high (on the order of US$7,000–10,000 per patient per year), and international opinion generally held that adherence to antiretroviral regimens was not feasible in the African context (Ndoye et al. 2004). But Senegal forged ahead, and after having treated approximately 400 people in a handful of sites, programmers both within and outside the country viewed the program favorably, and other West African countries were encouraged to replicate it (Desclaux 2004; Ndoye et al. 2004). As part of the antiretroviral program, the Senegalese government was also the first African government to negotiate a massive reduction in the cost of antiretroviral drugs from international pharmaceutical companies, reducing the cost by approximately 40 percent to US$600 per month (Bollinger, Stover, and Diop 1999; Family Health International 2002).

Political factors were thus very important to the response to HIV in Senegal. In particular, the strength and religious connections of civil society as well as the depth and international renown of technocratic leaders facilitated conversations about HIV with everyday Senegalese as well as political leaders. These factors set Senegal apart from Malawi and Nigeria, but also from all other African countries.

Sociocultural Factors Influencing the Prevention of HIV

Religious leaders were involved in HIV prevention from an early point, mainly through the facilitation of local NGOs such as Jamra and SIDA Service, but also through interaction with the government and donors. In 1994, the primary US-funded AIDS program in Senegal, AIDSCAP, and the National AIDS Program published a survey of religious and political leaders carried out by the NGO Africa Consultants International regarding the leaders' attitudes towards AIDS (Badge, Engelberg, and Sarr 1997). One of the resulting recommendations was a national colloquium on religion and HIV, as religious leaders had indicated that they wanted to be involved in the response to AIDS (Badge, Engelberg, and Sarr 1997). A conference in 1995, "AIDS and Religion: The Response of Islam," provided an important opportunity for interchange and produced the key statement that condom use was acceptable within serodiscordant couples, where one member was HIV-positive (Badge, Engelberg, and Sarr 1997). A second conference in 1996, "AIDS and Religion: Responses of Christian Churches," served as a further point of dialogue and was also attended by Islamic leaders (Badge, Engelberg, and Sarr 1997). As a result of these interactions, respondents noted religious leaders and the rest of the AIDS field struck a tacit bargain that religious leaders would discuss abstinence and fidelity with their followers, but would neither condone nor condemn condoms. A respondent described the benefits to such outreach: "People listen to *marabouts* more than to the president. This is sometimes good, and sometimes bad. With HIV, it was good."[29]

Governments and organizations have reached out to religious leaders and organizations in many countries, but rarely with as much success as in Senegal. Respondents acknowledged that something was different about religion in Senegal, but could not explain what. The overall positive relationships between Muslims and Christians in the context of a stable country presumably facilitated such open dialogue, as did the interrelationship between religion and civil society.

That Senegal stands out for supportive religious involvement in HIV activities does not, however, imply that all such involvement has been positive. In 1997, for example, some religious leaders attacked the Réseau Islam et Population for its promotion of condoms (Wilson 1998). Furthermore, a 2008 survey of religious leaders in major cities of Senegal showed that many Muslim leaders in particular held beliefs about HIV that facilitated stigma and discrimination, and that religious leaders in general were relatively unsupportive of condom use outside of marriage (Ansari and Gaestel 2010). Finally, and as described in greater detail below, although the NGO Jamra was instrumental in building initial bridges between the government and Islamic organizations to promote a constructive response to HIV, Jamra's more recent stand against homosexuality is hindering HIV prevention and treatment among men who have sex with men, one of Senegal's most-at-risk populations.

Senegal addressed the HIV epidemic early and in ways that the global AIDS field has recognized as effective. Transnational factors, including the historical legacy of legal sex work and long-cultivated and positive

---

[29] *Marabouts* are religious leaders from Senegal's Sufi brotherhoods. S17, international NGO.

relationships with the international community, were particularly important. But political factors were also highly relevant, including a strong and deep civil society and domestically and globally recognized technocratic leaders. Senegal's actively involved religious leaders and organizations as well as the country's relative lack of ethnic and religious fractionalization were sociocultural factors that also contributed positively to HIV interventions. Across the board, transnational, political, and sociocultural factors interacted in highly productive ways to support the country's HIV interventions.

From Pregnancy Prevention to HIV Prevention

As in Malawi and Nigeria, most of the transfers from family planning to HIV prevention in Senegal occurred through resources and strategies associated with transnational and political factors. As one respondent explained, "Although the techniques and tools of HIV are new, the questions are not. Experience with reproductive health allowed discussion of sex, of male-female relations."[30] And the seminal 1999 UNAIDS report that first identified Senegal as an HIV success story, stated among the reasons for that success that "Reproductive health and child health are well established priorities... family planning services are expanding: modern contraceptive use doubled in the five years to 1997" (Pisani 1999: 7–8). Donors involved in the provision of family planning quickly engaged with HIV, deploying similar strategies, such as condom social marketing, but also clearly piggybacking their HIV programs on the earlier family planning activities. Local NGOs that worked in family planning also came to include HIV prevention in their portfolios, and NGO communication with government regarding religion and family planning repeated in discussions about religion and HIV. As in Malawi and Nigeria, however, the structure of health bureaucracies may have prevented expertise associated with pregnancy prevention from transferring to HIV prevention.

Organizational Resources and Strategies

As in Malawi and Nigeria, the footprint that donors laid for family planning in Senegal structured the response to HIV/AIDS. USAID was

[30] S31, university.

a major link, first funding family planning in 1981, and HIV work in 1987 (USAID 2004b). But so too were other international organizations, as well as local NGOs.

One element of that footprint was the explicit division of the country's regions among donors funding family planning activities, apparently an arrangement that originated with a request from the Senegalese government (Conly and Epp 1997; Wickstrom, Diagne, and Smith 2006). Through the 1990s, USAID worked in six of Senegal's then-ten regions (USAID 1998), while UNFPA covered the others. This divide then carried over to HIV, indicating how funding patterns like those observed cross-nationally in the analysis in Chapter 3 may come into being. Similarly, when USAID set up the AIDSCAP project in 1992, it maintained the same urban focus of the Family Planning/Child Survival project that preceded it, and limited its work to four of the same six regions, justifying its geographic choices in part because of the "possibility of liaisons with the Mission's proposed family planning project" (USAID 1992a: 16). In short, the funding structure developed for family planning flowed directly into that for HIV.

Other elements of AIDSCAP resembled those of earlier family planning programs, including study tours to neighboring countries with successful HIV programs and the use of RAPID-style computer simulations and presentations to stress the economic, social, and other impacts of AIDS to policymakers and leaders. USAID also described the AIDSCAP-Senegal project design as having "addressed many of the recommendations made regarding the Population/Family Planning sector," including those from a health sector assessment carried out in 1990, implying the HIV program took advantage of lessons learned from population and family planning (USAID 1992a).

Family planning money even helped build the infrastructure for the research that established Senegal as a forerunner in the response to HIV. Specifically, Mboup and Ndoye, among others, argued that in order to effectively run family planning programs it would be necessary to have comprehensive knowledge of sexually transmitted infections among women. USAID agreed, and put funds towards increasing laboratory capacity, which ultimately supported the response to HIV (Poleykett 2012).

Most of USAID's initial HIV-related activities in Senegal were in fact channeled through their family planning grants. The Senegal Family Health and Population Project provided support for laboratories for testing for HIV and sexually transmitted infections, funded HIV information education and communication activities and condom distribution facilitated by the National AIDS Program, and incorporated information on HIV into the family planning training provided to medical personnel (USAID 1992a). The Family Health and Population Project also helped produce a widely distributed AIDS poster (Devres, Inc. 1991).

As in Malawi and Nigeria, USAID's social marketing programs were an easy point of transfer between family planning and HIV. The social marketing of Protec condoms that began in 1995 through the SOMARC program was a part of USAID's Family Planning and Child Survival project (SOMARC/The Futures Group International 1997). Donors intended Protec to be used for both family planning and HIV, and similar to Malawi, advertising emphasized protection of the family and birth spacing, in part to help reduce the negative association between condoms and promiscuity (Stephens and Ba 1996). Initial advertising included no mention of AIDS, only sexually transmitted infections, and to convince Senegalese consumers of its respectability and quality, Protec was available only through pharmacies (Stephens and Ba 1996). A review published a year after the launch concluded that "Now that [the social marketing program] has been successful in demystifying and establishing the credibility of the condom by focusing primarily on child spacing, the groundwork has been laid to target STD/HIV prevention" (Stephens and Ba 1996: 23; Wickstrom, Diagne, and Smith 2006). Thus family planning programs and their technologies formed the backbone of many early HIV interventions.

Other organizations first worked on family planning in Senegal, and then incorporated HIV into their portfolios. Family Health International, as a major USAID implementing partner in Senegal just as elsewhere, worked on family planning in Senegal from the early 1980s onwards, and then on HIV starting in the late 1980s (Family Health International 2002). The World Bank also first funded population activities in Senegal, particularly the 1988 population policy, and then began to support AIDS activities in 1991 as a small part of a US-$35 million loan to Senegal's Population and Health program (USAID 1999b). In 1988, very early in the HIV epidemic, the Ford Foundation gave thirteen AIDS grants to just four countries, three of which had field offices, including Senegal, and which were focused on women, especially sex workers (Brier 2009). Had Ford not already been working on family planning in Senegal, it is unlikely that Senegal would have benefitted from these early AIDS resources.

Many local NGOs existed prior to the advent of AIDS, and those that worked on family planning shifted their services once HIV appeared. USAID noted in its 1992 project authorization for the AIDSCAP-Senegal program that indigenous NGOs in Senegal were already promoting condoms for child spacing, and thus facilitating the reduction of sexually transmitted infections and HIV (USAID 1992a: 58). ASBEF, the long-time family planning organization, was founded more than ten years before the first AIDS case was discovered, and incorporated HIV prevention activities as early as 1990. As described above, ASBEF was involved in a number of activities that aimed to create dialogue with Islamic leaders about population, which may have established a formula for similar interactions around HIV. Since that time, its HIV-related activities have expanded to include large-scale condom distribution through its nation-wide network of clinics, HIV testing, and prevention of mother-to-child transmission of HIV. Some have even argued that ASBEF has turned so far towards HIV that its family planning activities have suffered (Wickstrom, Diagne, and Smith 2006).

While ASBEF is the largest local family planning NGO that transferred significant resources from pregnancy prevention to HIV prevention, other NGOs also shifted their portfolios. Africa Consultants International, founded just before HIV emerged, worked first in reproductive health, and then more explicitly on HIV. Other family planning organizations that came into existence soon after the advent of HIV, such as the Agence pour la Promotion des Activités de Population-Senegal (Agency for the Promotion of Population Activities in Senegal), founded in 1989, originally focused on population and reproductive health, but then expanded their work to include HIV in order to be able to obtain funding. The Groupe Pour l'Etude et l'Enseignement de la Population (Group for the Study and Teaching of Population) came into being during the AIDS era, in 1994, but initially focused primarily on family planning and population. Their mandate eventually expanded to incorporate HIV, and their early population education programming, supported by UNFPA, may have forged initial pathways that later helped introduce AIDS education into schools. These examples illustrate that organizational resources, even those funded after AIDS emerged, have facilitated Senegal's response.

As described above, a number of religious organizations helped connect the government to religious leaders to communicate about both family planning and HIV. The willingness of Senegalese religious leaders to engage with the government and other NGOs regarding intimate interventions is noteworthy, particularly compared to Malawi and Nigeria, where outreach certainly occurred, but with less intention and structure. While practice with such endeavors gained in the effort to promote family planning may have proved helpful when doing the same for HIV, respondents mentioned connections with religious leaders more frequently when describing HIV activities than family planning ones.

Transfers from family planning to HIV thus occurred particularly through resources and strategies associated with transnational and political factors. Donor organizations as well as local organizations that had worked in family planning readily turned their eye towards HIV. In addition, open communication between government and religious leaders was particularly important to both family planning and HIV prevention.

Where Transfers between Intimate Interventions Did Not Occur

As in Malawi and Nigeria, bureaucratic structures prevented knowledge gained from pregnancy prevention from transferring to HIV prevention, even in the face of support for integrating the two. Senegal also has experienced the same, broader challenges as Malawi and Nigeria in integrating family planning with HIV prevention.

Indeed, much support for integration has existed in Senegal. Early on Ibrahim Ndoye, as head of the National AIDS Committee, called for integration of information, education, and communication about HIV, sexually transmitted infections, and family planning because the target population – those who were sexually active – was the same (Devres, Inc. 1991). USAID's 1990 assessment of the population sector also suggested integrating family planning with other health interventions, including HIV and sexually transmitted infections (USAID 1992b). And Senegal's health decentralization plan required a district-level integrated health package that included both family planning and HIV/AIDS, which USAID strongly supported (USAID 2002).

But after HIV first appeared in 1986, it was placed under the sexually transmitted infection division of the Ministry of Health, not the family health division focused on pregnancy prevention, initially the Maternal and Child Health Division, which in 2001 became the Reproductive Health Division (République du Sénégal 2005). At the time of field-work in 2010 these two divisions appeared to have good relations – the sexually transmitted infection division had even channeled money back to the reproductive health division – but were physically separated, at opposite ends of Avenue Blaise Diagne in Dakar. In addition, the Maternal and Child Health Division, although involved with the provision of contraception, was distinct from the National Family Planning Program, which donors leery of working within existing health structures had set up as its own, vertical program. Furthermore, HIV ultimately came under the purview of a separate bureaucratic entity, the National AIDS Program. Both it and the National Family Planning Program, however, were mandated to respond to AIDS, creating bureaucratic confusion that resulted in a lack of collaboration through the 1990s (Devres, Inc. 1991; Wilson 1998). These separations isolated most women from screening for sexually transmitted infections, which generally focused on sex workers. For example, a review conducted in 1995 found that counseling sessions on HIV were "practically non-existent" as a part of family planning service delivery (Ministry of Health and Social Action, National Family Planning Program of Senegal and Population Council 1995: 1).

At lower levels, integrating family planning with other reproductive health services also proved challenging as family planning was often located in a separate building, and some staff were reticent to discuss sexually transmitted infections with family planning clients (Hardee et al. 1998). Respondents felt that even if a connection between pregnancy prevention and HIV prevention could be achieved through service delivery, it could not be mirrored at higher levels precisely because of bureaucratic structures, and in some cases, because of turf. As a respondent explained,

"HIV and family planning really function independently. There are indirect links through condoms but not a real strong institutional link. Our organization integrates things at a district level, but it's more difficult to integrate at a political level – programs have their own means and turf. It's not just the government to blame, but also the donors. It's much easier to integrate at an operational level, and the donors are more supportive of that."[31]

---

[31] S26, international NGO.

For those who wish to better integrate family planning with HIV prevention activities, these bureaucratic divisions will be a major hurdle. Most respondents saw the connection between pregnancy prevention and HIV prevention as a current-day issue, and in particular understood the link to be best made through the HIV side of the equation, specifically through prevention of mother-to-child transmission of HIV, but also through service-delivery more generally. As one respondent described, "It's systematic to hear about family planning if you come in for HIV testing – this is the only time to talk to people."[32]

Thus even in a case like Senegal where the preexisting family planning infrastructure strongly supported the HIV response, donor preference for vertical programs, other bureaucratic structures, and to a certain extent turf all undermined at least some of the potential transfer of resources, broadly defined, between pregnancy prevention and HIV prevention.

Conclusion

In Senegal, as with Malawi and Nigeria, transnational and political factors best explain responses to HIV. In particular, Senegal's open relationship with the international community and technocratic leadership proved vital to the country's rapid and comprehensive response to HIV. Organizational resources for pregnancy prevention transferred to HIV prevention within international organizations working in Senegal as well as within national organizations. But perhaps more than direct borrowing from one intimate intervention to another, Senegal's experience reveals that openness to the outside world and a long history of the existence of, and respect for, technocratic leadership mattered independently to each intervention.

We will never know whether the response to HIV in Senegal actually helped prevent a worse HIV epidemic. Certainly Senegal started from an advantaged position, with almost universal circumcision and a less-virulent form of HIV (type 2). Regardless of the causality between the input and the outcome, there is no doubt the Senegalese government took all the "right" steps as defined by the global AIDS field, and even helped define those right steps. The case of Senegal demonstrates par excellence that leadership in the response to AIDS can come in many

[32] S23, local NGO.

different forms, including political but also technocratic. The government's willingness to respond to HIV stemmed in no small part from the ability of technocratic leaders (Mboup, Ndoye, and Seck) to have a voice from the very beginning. It was thus a different type of leadership that mattered in Senegal, unlike a personalist ruler in Uganda, or an inward-looking authoritarian in Malawi.

Although HIV rates remain low among the general population in Senegal, a recent increase in hostility towards homosexuals has hampered support for men who have sex with men, one of the populations at greatest risk for HIV. Senegal penalizes homosexuality, and HIV prevalence among men who have sex with men was 18.5 percent in 2013 (Conseil National de Lutte Contre le Sida 2014). A backlash began in 2008, when a popular magazine, *Icône*, published photos of a gay wedding that had occurred several years prior. Following the publication, some of the individuals shown in the photographs were arrested, and although all those arrested were ultimately released (BBC News 2008), the publication of those pictures fomented a further series of events. Later in 2008, the director of AIDES Sénégal, an NGO engaged in HIV prevention for men who have sex with men, was arrested in his home along with eight other men, likely all participating in an activity related to the NGO's work. The men were sentenced to eight years in prison on charges of indecent conduct and unnatural acts, but the sentencing was overturned on appeal within several months (Grew 2009).

Hostility towards gays, in particular conjunction with HIV, continued. Later in 2009 the body of Madieye Diallo, an activist and a leader of a gay organization called And Ligay, was dragged out of his grave several hours after being buried and dumped on his parents' doorstep. Diallo was HIV-positive but had stopped taking his medication following the publication of his photo in *Icône*, leading to his presumably premature death (Callimachi 2010). Jamra, the same organization so crucial to garnering the initial support of Islamic leaders in the response to AIDS, has been actively involved in the public discussion of these events, condemning homosexuality, and thus eroding Islamic support for the response to HIV (BBC News 2009). Periodic attacks against gays have continued since then. The worsening climate undermines prevention among one of the most-at-risk populations in Senegal, and has caused some tension between Senegal and Western allies, with President Macky Sall bluntly stating in the presence of Barack Obama that he would not work to decriminalize homosexuality (Fisher 2013).

The unraveling of what had otherwise been a relatively tolerant context for men who have sex with men, and with it some of the positive relationship between the state and Islamic NGOs, demonstrates that even though history influences current-day outcomes, it does not solely determine them. Path dependent forces pushing a country down a "good" path do not ensure that path continues to be taken, just as it is also possible to exit less productive paths. Such an exit is demonstrated by Senegal's recent rapid increases in the contraceptive prevalence rate, likely resulting from intensive donor efforts to correct supply chain issues combined with some increased demand.

Senegal's good relationships with the international community broadly, as well as with the global population and AIDS fields specifically, are themselves a form of path dependence, and one that has created positive policy feedback loops. The valence of the relationship with the international community predated either family planning or HIV programs, but each intimate intervention provided an opportunity for Senegal to demonstrate a good relationship, and in so doing, reinforce it. There was thus no long shadow of population control as in Malawi, and no need for leaders to tag elements of either intimate intervention as anti-Western, thus removing what has been a major barrier to program implementation in other countries.

7 | Conclusion: The Implications of Intimate Interventions for Global Health

In the preceding chapters, I have argued that understanding the history of intimate interventions – programs, policies, and organizational actions that aim to change sexual behavior in the name of the individual or collective good – helps to explain countries' differential responses to the HIV epidemic. Looking across sub-Saharan African countries as well as at the individual experiences of Malawi, Nigeria, and Senegal, I used the model developed in Chapter 1 to parse the different possible explanations. This model focused on the transnational, political, socio-cultural, and economic factors driving variation in country-level behavior. The cross-national analysis and case studies showed that transnational and political factors explained most of the differences in country-level responses to HIV, with many of the resources, discourses, and strategies associated with family planning programs ultimately affecting HIV prevention interventions and outcomes.

The book's main contribution is to demonstrate that policies and programs have histories that shape their contours and influence their outcomes. Such a claim is not radical, and yet it departs significantly from the conclusions of many scholars who have studied health interventions in developing countries because, not surprisingly, scholars and their findings are themselves the result of disciplinary tendencies. These disciplinary tendencies have in turn limited a deep analysis of policy and programmatic history. Specifically, that public health scholars have carried out so much research on intimate interventions has led to a focus on the individual, rather than social, political, and structural factors. At the same time, historians and anthropologists – those most likely to consider history or to use the ethnographic techniques that would readily reveal its importance – have not been the primary actors investigating broad-scale health interventions in sub-Saharan Africa. Political scientists, although they have developed an extensive study of political processes in Africa, have only just recently turned their eye to health interventions. And sociologists have studied wealthier countries or focused extensively on norm transmission. The book bridges many of these divides by juxtaposing both macro- and meso-level perspectives with social, political, and historical factors in order to understand the drivers of variation in intimate interventions across sub-Saharan Africa. The main conclusion is that policy and programmatic histories, while not the only forces influencing interventions, do so in important ways.

In this concluding chapter, I summarize how transnational, political, sociocultural, and economic factors explain variation in intimate interventions, with a particular eye to the transfers between pregnancy prevention and HIV prevention. Specifically, I synthesize the findings from the exploration of the transfer of resources, discourses, and strategies from pregnancy prevention to HIV prevention at the global level (Chapter 2), the analysis of variation in HIV prevention across all sub-Saharan African countries (Chapter 3), and the experiences of the three case study countries (Chapters 4–6). The analysis demonstrates that treating pregnancy prevention as an example of an intimate intervention that preceded HIV allows us to better understand countries' responses to HIV. Pregnancy prevention efforts alone do not explain variation in HIV prevention efforts, but nor does any other single factor. I relate these conclusions to two broader areas. First, I use them to discuss field theory. Second, I apply them to the case of maternal mortality mitigation in Malawi, Nigeria, and Senegal to demonstrate the wider applicability of the book's findings to a different health intervention.

Transnational Factors

Setting the stage for the importance of transnational factors to the experiences of individual countries, Chapter 2 describes where the global AIDS field borrowed, learned, and took from the global population field. In particular, resources in the form of donor funding, organizational activities, and human capital transferred from family planning to HIV prevention. Advocates within both the population and AIDS fields used many of the same discursive frames to promote their agendas. These organizations also took strategies originally developed for family planning – social marketing, entertainment-education, and community-based programs to distribute commodities and information – and applied them to HIV. Despite these connections, however, major barriers between the population and AIDS fields complicated collaboration and inhibited learning. In particular, many in the population field were hesitant to take on the stigmatized issue of HIV when they already had spent so much political capital prioritizing family planning. Because of the overwhelming involvement of donor organizations in intimate interventions, many of the transfers that occurred at the global level were reflected at the country level.

The extent and nature of relationships with external actors were the transnational factors that mattered most to variation in country-level responses to HIV, and also where experiences with family planning clearly transferred to HIV prevention. Specifically, funding relationships with donors developed in relation to family planning persisted through to HIV interventions. The cross-national analysis of all sub-Saharan African countries in Chapter 3 demonstrated that even after controlling for level of HIV, those countries that had received more donor attention for family planning also received higher levels of HIV funding. Similarly, documents from early donor HIV programs in the three case study countries explicitly referenced elements of extant family planning programs. Reflecting this overall trend, the case studies illustrate that the valence of relationships between individual countries and external actors strongly impacted intimate interventions. In Malawi, President Banda's relationship with the West inhibited both family planning programs and HIV prevention, with the history of family planning ultimately casting a "long shadow" onto HIV prevention (Kaler 2004). Nonetheless, donor organizations initially involved in family planning programs incorporated HIV into their work, and borrowed many strategies from family planning. In Nigeria, donor organizations actively shaped intimate interventions with family planning strategies flowing into HIV activities, and local NGOs initially focused on family planning became major players in the response to HIV. And in Senegal, not only did the same transfers occur within donor organizations as in Malawi and Nigeria, but a long and durable history of extremely positive relationships with the international community strongly facilitated the response to HIV.

Political Factors

Both civil society and technocratic leadership influenced family planning and HIV activities, and were a point of transfer between intimate interventions. The sub-Saharan African cross-national analysis shows that countries with older family planning NGOs received more funding for HIV. In addition, countries with family planning NGOs founded prior to the diagnosis of AIDS cases experienced greater declines in HIV prevalence during the 2000s, and those countries with a population policy experienced greater declines in HIV incidence during the 2000s, as well as had more extensive antiretroviral coverage for prevention of mother-to-child HIV transmission. The analysis of intimate interventions in Senegal demonstrates that being the kind of country that has many NGOs is as good for the response to HIV as are the actions of NGOs themselves. More generally, the three case studies clearly demonstrate that NGOs created to provide contraception went on to engage in HIV prevention work, and that technocratic leadership is hugely important to intimate interventions. In Malawi, the primary family planning NGO – Banja la Mtsogolo – went on to incorporate HIV activities into its country-wide network of clinics and outreach programs. But President Banda's legacy of squashing civil society and creating a hostile environment for intellectuals led to a real absence of both local organizations and technocratic leaders, negatively impacting intimate interventions and leaving fewer family planning resources available for the response to HIV. In Nigeria, three local family planning NGOs – the Association for Reproductive and Family Health, the Planned Parenthood Federation of Nigeria, and the Society for Family Health – ultimately became very important to the response to HIV, and the technocratic leadership of Minister of Health Ransome-Kuti both firmly supported family planning and ultimately the response to HIV. Other technocratic leaders, some with roots in family planning, also shaped HIV interventions. Finally, in Senegal, both the main family planning NGO, ASBEF, as well as a host of other NGOs that predated the HIV epidemic reoriented their activities towards HIV once it became an issue. In addition, three technocrats – Soulemayne Mboup, Ibrahim Ndoye, and Awa Marie Coll-Seck – provided real leadership in the response to HIV, legitimizing government action and facilitating relationships with outside actors. In all three countries, however, bureaucratic structuring within the Ministry of Health hampered some transfers from family planning to HIV prevention.

Sociocultural and Economic Factors

The impact of ethnic fractionalization on HIV interventions is most visible when examining all sub-Saharan African countries. Across all countries, those with more ethnically and linguistically diverse populations had lower antiretroviral coverage rates. In Malawi, the association between HIV and one minority ethnic and religious group, the Yao, appears to have complicated the implementation of medical male circumcision for HIV prevention, but there is no strong evidence that fractionalization overall prevented the government from responding to HIV. In Nigeria, ethnic and religious fractionalization challenges the overall process of governing, and in particular religious fractionalization drove some of the negative response to the population policy. Based on fieldwork, however, there was little evidence that Nigerians interpreted HIV as being caused by similar divides, or that relatively weak HIV prevention was driven by us-versus-them politics that allowed leaders to attribute HIV to groups other than their own. Finally, although Senegal has long possessed relative ethnic and religious harmony that has in turn facilitated overall stability, a direct link to intimate interventions is hard to discern. The government's willingness to engage with religious leaders on the subject of HIV appears to have been mediated through NGOs, and perhaps better reflects good government-civil society relationships more than a lack of ethnic fractionalization. Thus while sociocultural differences among the three case study countries, in particular varying degrees of ethnic and religious fractionalization, may have contributed to intimate interventions, transnational and political factors mattered more.

As with ethnic fractionalization, the role of economic factors was more evident in the cross-national analysis than the individual case studies. Richer countries experienced significantly greater declines in HIV incidence during the 2000s, as well as provided a greater percentage of their populations with antiretroviral therapy. Malawi, Nigeria, and Senegal are all supported by massive amounts of donor funding, so the effect of economics translates into roughly the same outcome: intensive donor involvement. Of the three countries, Nigeria has probably received the most concentrated donor gaze given the size of its economy and magnitude of its debt, but Malawi and Senegal's economic woes have left them strongly connected to international financial institutions. This donor involvement promoted the adoption of population policies. Nigeria is the only country, because of its significant oil reserves, that could have been expected to use its own resources in any substantial way for either family planning or HIV prevention, but chose not to do so, reflecting corruption and a low prioritization of the social sectors more broadly. Again, however, although economic factors explain some of the variation in responses to HIV, transnational and political factors explain more.

From the Population Field to the AIDS Field

As described in Chapter 1, a field consists of a set of individual and/or collective actors who interact with one another with a shared understanding of the purposes, relationships within, and rules of the field (Fligstein and McAdam 2011). One of the larger debates within the sociological research on fields is whether fields are static (Jepperson 1991), or dynamic (Fligstein and McAdam 2011). The analysis presented in this book offers a unique opportunity to engage this question as AIDS emerged as a new problem in the 1980s, and with it, a new field developed. The population field already existed, and as this book shows, the new AIDS field at the global level, as well as within individual countries, drew heavily from the population field. In particular, global and local AIDS fields borrowed (and some might say "took") organizations, strategies, and resources from parallel population fields. Organizations that had focused on providing contraception prior to AIDS incorporated HIV prevention into their activities, and in some cases shifted almost entirely to AIDS-related work. Programmers deployed strategies developed to provide contraception – such as social marketing, entertainment-education, and community-based distribution – in their quest to curb the spread of AIDS. And in many cases organizations redirected resources towards HIV that had previously gone towards family planning. These transfers illustrate the dynamism of fields and support a number of points made by Fligstein and McAdam (2011).

First, new fields emerge nearby closely related fields. Of course, global and local AIDS fields developed elements *de novo* as new organizations were founded at global, national, and local levels and new resources were generated, but the proximity to population fields shaped the contours of AIDS fields. Second, the emergence of AIDS was exactly the type of exogenous shock likely to change existing fields, in particular the population field. In many ways, the global population field initially resisted change associated with AIDS. Because members of the population field had fought so many battles to ensure access to contraception and reproductive health services, they were reticent to take on yet another stigmatized issue. In addition, the bureaucratic structure of the United Nations, with specific agencies for specific problems, already had a "slot" for AIDS in the form of the World Health Organization, and then later, UNAIDS. But the population field could not ignore the shock of AIDS forever. As resources began to trickle away and the concept of reproductive health gained prominence, discussion in the population field increased regarding integration of HIV into family planning and reproductive health services, and population organizations staked greater claims to HIV/AIDS. In short, the population field changed because of the (new) AIDS field.

Even after AIDS entered the scene, the impact of changes within the AIDS field on the population field demonstrate the broader dynamism of fields. Specifically, there was a slightly more than ten-year lag between the identification of AIDS and the availability of treatment. The lag was actually closer to fifteen years in sub-Saharan Africa given that affordable antiretroviral treatment, with the donor funding to back it, did not become available until the founding of the Global Fund and PEPFAR. The availability of treatment, however, radically changed both the AIDS and the population fields. In the AIDS field, it provided new energy, a way to quantify the success of interventions, and a morally unquestionable justification for attention to AIDS. Buoyed by the new major funders, new international organizations came into being as did local organizations within affected countries. At the same time, actors in the AIDS field turned their attention away from prevention because it seemed inherently harder to achieve, and was certainly harder to measure. Measurement became increasingly salient as the era of the Millennium Development Goals dawned, the one in which we still live, which requires demonstrable impact, prioritizes randomized control trials, and emphasizes quantification at the expense of understanding the complex interplay between politics, economics, culture, and history that this book strives to interrogate. Just as the AIDS field changed, so too did the population field, which finally started to better integrate HIV into its activities.

The dynamics of the AIDS and population fields also support Fligstein and McAdam's (2011) contention that the logic of fields, in particular their rules, continuously readjusts, rather than persists in a taken-for-granted manner that many scholars of institutions have assumed. Within the AIDS field, there is no taken-for-granted logic (or at least any one logic that lasts for a very long time). Instead, common understandings of the factors that drive HIV prevalence, and thus how HIV interventions should work, constantly evolve and bifurcate. For example, within the context of sub-Saharan Africa, the people perceived to fuel the AIDS epidemic have gone from the "at-risk" populations of sex workers, men who have sex with men, members of the military, and truck drivers to the married couples that make up the general population, and back again to those very same at-risk, or "key," populations. Similarly, the interventions to address HIV have gone from targeting at-risk populations to "mainstreaming" AIDS prevention into the activities of all organizations and back to the at-risk populations. These changes have occurred parallel to an increasing biomedicalization of HIV interventions, away from largely nontechnical methods to change sexual behavior towards medical male circumcision and the provision of antiretroviral therapy. Each shift in interpretation and intervention privileges different actors in the field, and is also influenced by the differential power of those actors.

The population field has also transformed over time, with evolving logics and framing principles. Initially many programmers, donors, and demographers believed that family planning programs alone could motivate people to change their fertility desires. When fertility failed to decline, or declined only slightly, despite massive influxes of funding and the same programs were criticized for coercion and excessive focus on targets, the field's goal shifted from providing contraception to providing reproductive health. The reproductive health concept permitted more actors in the field to come to the table, but despite the benefits of its fuzzy articulation to building consensus, may have ultimately distracted actors at both global and local levels from the very real need to provide contraception to those who desire it. Even though many in the population field feel that the AIDS field has taken away its resources and momentum, the AIDS field has also generated more funding for population activities writ large. The population field, and the broader health field, may now begin to benefit from these new resources as realization grows that the substantial resources generated for HIV/AIDS must confer benefits to health and society more broadly.

Perhaps more so than anything else, the population and AIDS fields demonstrate how fields overlap. Indeed, there are overlaps across levels, topics, and key actors. The global population and AIDS fields intersect directly at the local level of implementation, connected to higher levels via webs of funding, organizations, and ideas. Prevention of mother-to-child transmission of HIV really does require contraception, and preventing sexually transmitted infections, including HIV, really is part of reproductive health. Despite power differentials and spatial and cultural distance, ideas can and do flow in both directions, and the book shows that resources, discourses, and strategies connect both fields.

In short, taking a field perspective helps in interpreting the evolution of the population and AIDS fields, as well as the actions of the actors within each field. At the same time, the analysis of intimate interventions illustrates the ways in which new fields emerge, the dynamic and contingent nature of fields, and the dependence of fields on one another.

Considering Maternal Mortality

To what extent can the findings from this analysis be applied to other health and development problems in sub-Saharan Africa? The model from Chapter 1 identifies the sets of factors likely to drive variation in responses to a number of different health and development problems. The relative weight of each set of factors, however, will depend on the problem at hand and the structure of the related field(s). In particular, transnational factors will come into play when the international community particularly cares about an issue. That the two health areas explored in this book required *intimate* interventions influences the conclusions only in that we should expect a denser transfer of resources, discourses, and strategies between family planning and HIV interventions than between health interventions that are more peripherally related. Similarly, by virtue of being intimate interventions addressing private, sometimes stigmatized, behaviors, pregnancy prevention and HIV prevention required governments and other organizations to overcome more obstacles than do many health interventions. Thus they make a good "extreme" case of what drives variation in the intensity of health interventions.

The experience of maternal mortality interventions is productive in comparison to the conclusions from the story of family planning and HIV prevention across sub-Saharan Africa. Although many poor countries have high maternal mortality, the majority of global maternal deaths occur in sub-Saharan Africa (World Health Organization et al.

2012). They occur here because of high fertility, poor health systems, and lack of access to safe abortion. The exact magnitude of maternal mortality in sub-Saharan Africa did not become fully known until the early 1980s, as it was not until 1984 that the World Health Organization released country-level estimates of maternal mortality for the first time (International Women's Health Program n.d.). Thus, although those working in the health field – and women and their families – certainly knew earlier that maternal mortality was high, the overall and relative magnitude of the problem became much more publically visible starting only in the early 1980s. In conjunction with the availability of these statistics, the World Health Organization held a high-level meeting on maternal mortality in 1985, which was followed by another meeting in Nairobi in 1987 that led to the Safe Motherhood Initiative, the first coordinated global effort to reduce maternal mortality (Starrs 2006).

The race to achieve the Millennium Development Goals has increased global attention towards maternal mortality in recent years, in part because a large portion of maternal mortality has a relatively technological fix: increased contraceptive usage.[1] The plight of women dying in childbirth has never been hugely successful at garnering a major response in either individual countries or in the global community, most likely because it has been impossible to frame the issue in the terms most able to grab people's attention. Maternal mortality does not threaten security, as women do not make up the bulk of armies, nor are they generally even combatants. Furthermore, maternal mortality is a problem that has always existed, and so is difficult to turn into an "emergency" like the population bomb or the specter of AIDS.

Among the three case study countries, estimates of maternal mortality in 2008 varied greatly: 1140 maternal deaths per 100,000 live births in Malawi, 608 in Nigeria, and 401 in Senegal (Hogan et al. 2010). Given its population size and high fertility, however, Nigeria experiences a greater number of maternal deaths than the other two countries combined. According to the histories of intimate interventions in the three case study countries, we should expect an initially weak response from Malawi followed by a donor-supported technological

---

[1] The attention to maternal mortality is likely to continue in the era of the Sustainable Development Goals, given that reducing maternal mortality is the first target under goal three: Ensure Healthy Lives and Promote Well-Being for All at All Ages.

intervention, a response from Nigeria that matches the extent of donor interest, and a strong response from Senegal that follows global field recommendations. The existing literature suggests that the three countries responded in exactly these ways.

Malawi's response to maternal mortality resembles many aspects of its family planning programs and HIV interventions. Here, maternal mortality rose rapidly through the 1980s and 1990s due in large part to increasing HIV rates (Hogan et al. 2010). Although the government justified the 1982 decision to increase availability of modern contraception as a means to reduce maternal mortality, it was not until the mid-1990s, largely after the transition to democracy, that the government took some formal action in response to maternal mortality, including a Safe Motherhood Taskforce in 1993, and a number of donor-funded programs (Family Care International 2007). Then, in the 2000s, Malawi prioritized reducing maternal mortality, spurred by the push to achieve the Millennium Development Goals. Malawi was one of the first eight countries to launch the African Union's 2009 Campaign to Accelerate the Reduction in Maternal Mortality in Africa (CARMMA). After Joyce Banda assumed the presidency of Malawi in 2012, she made multiple statements about the need to center health and development programming around women, and strongly promoted reducing maternal mortality (e.g., CSIS Staff 2013). Malawi's response to maternal mortality thus resembles the histories of pregnancy prevention and HIV prevention in its relative lateness, but also in its demonstration of the capacity to implement donor-supported technological solutions. As with increased contraceptive prevalence and HIV treatment, and in particular Option B+, Malawi ultimately prioritized maternal mortality.

Nigeria's response to maternal mortality has also been similar to family planning and HIV prevention. Specifically, technocratic leaders have facilitated progress in the presence of otherwise distracting political and economic disarray. Olikoye Ransome-Kuti, the Minister of Health so important to the adoption of the 1988 population policy (itself justified in part as a means to reduce maternal mortality) and who also helped build the country's early HIV response, led a 1992 effort to liberalize Nigeria's abortion laws in the name of reducing maternal mortality and morbidity. Although the bill was written, it never passed due to extreme opposition from religious as well as women's groups (Oye-Adeniran, Long and Adewole 2004). The government then put forward very little effort towards reducing maternal mortality until the return to democracy in 1999 (Shiffman and Okonofua 2007). As with family planning and population policy, pressure from individuals in positions of relative power as well as global interest, particularly in relation to the Millennium Development Goals, led to maternal mortality reduction becoming a goal in numerous policies adopted from the early 2000s onwards (Bankole et al. 2009; Shiffman and Okonofua 2007). Nigeria's experience with maternal mortality thus parallels both pregnancy prevention and HIV prevention: early action driven by technocratic leaders, followed by higher-level national emphasis prompted by international actors but also facilitated by the return to democracy.

Senegal's efforts to reduce maternal mortality were early and followed the global maternal health field's guidelines. The Senegalese government requested assistance from the United Nations Development Programme in 1986 to develop and implement a safe motherhood program (Kimball et al. 1988), prior even to the launch of the international Safe Motherhood Initiative in 1987. Such progressive steps made Senegal one of the first, if not *the* first, country to embrace the new global emphasis on reducing maternal mortality. Almost twenty years later, Senegal again took concrete action towards improving maternal health, seeking to achieve Millennium Development Goal 5, but this time through a model that deviated from most donors' neoliberal emphasis on fee-for-service health care. In 2005, Senegal adopted the Free Delivery and Caesarean Policy which made delivery in a health facility free in the poorest five of Senegal's then-eleven regions (Witter, Armar-Klemesu, and Dieng 2008). The following year, the policy was expanded to deliveries at regional hospitals in all but one of Senegal's regions (Ministerial Leadership Initiative 2010). Senegal's response to maternal mortality parallels that of other intimate interventions: an early response that followed global field guidelines and that was technologically oriented.

The response to maternal mortality in the three cases thus reflects many of the patterns observed in pregnancy prevention and HIV prevention. More broadly this example demonstrates the power of the Millennium Development Goals, and likely now the Sustainable Development Goals, to spur action on issues that are not politically sensitive and have technological "fixes." Given that contraceptive use is a primary mechanism for maternal mortality interventions (in addition to attempts to improve quality of services and access to them), maternal mortality programs may have positive externalities for pregnancy prevention.

Conclusion

Overall, the evidence presented in the book demonstrates that policy and program histories are important determinants of the contours and even success of health interventions. These findings make possible several additional broad conclusions. First, relationships with global actors in addition to local institutional and organizational structures and histories are important to understanding responses to health problems. Thus transnational factors – the nature of countries' interactions with the global community and the extent of donor organization involvement – as well as political factors – including the strength and composition of civil society and the existence of technocratic leadership – influenced variation in both family planning and HIV prevention efforts. The resources, discourses, and strategies of family planning that manifested through transnational and political factors in turn structured responses to HIV.

The analyses at the global and national levels presented in the preceding chapters demonstrate that path dependence and policy feedback are important elements to consider when studying health interventions as any response to existing or new health problems will flow through the organizations, people, and resource chains associated with previous interventions. The outcomes of such path dependence and policy feedback may be either positive or negative. The more intimate the new health problem, the more the particular history of intimate interventions will influence the response, but the new health problem does not need to be intimate to draw from, or be influenced by, the experiences of previous health interventions. While resources associated with family planning in many cases benefitted HIV interventions, programs across sectors may fail because of a country's history with population interventions (cf. Nigeria's challenges with polio eradication), and new programs can bear undesirable marks of previous programs. The analyses also show that factors beyond history matter, and that history can be overcome. Indeed, family planning programs were not the sole determinant of HIV prevention interventions, and countries that have not always been hugely successful in one area can change: contraceptive prevalence has increased markedly in both Malawi and

Senegal, and Malawi has gained a reputation globally for implementing Option B+ to provide antiretroviral therapy to all HIV-positive mothers for life.

That global forces have so strongly shaped intimate interventions raises concerns about the relevance of these interventions at the local level. Although local organizations translate globally mandated interventions and are extremely important to local responses, what ultimately transfers from the global to the local may not fit very well, or may have unintended consequences (Esacove 2010; Esacove 2016; McDonnell 2016; Swidler and Watkins 2017; Tawfik and Watkins 2007). Any additional funding for HIV in sub-Saharan Africa, or for health more broadly, will filter through these relationships, and the dependence of local organizations on external resources may compromise their ability to act independently. As this book has shown, local organizations and their capacity matter hugely to the course of the response to health problems and emergencies. Future research needs to understand what types of organizations are most resilient, which are most nimble in task shifting, and how to ensure a diverse population of organizations in very different country settings. Carrying out such research in turn will require much better data on organizations and across multiple countries.

Relatedly, the comparison of intimate interventions shows that there will continue to be countries that are "winners" in the international aid game, and even regions within one country that receive more aid because of a well-placed local NGO, independent of their actual need for resources or the severity of the problem at hand. That local family planning NGOs came to work on HIV was as much about resource constraints and trends in the global population and AIDS fields as it was about individuals in those organizations realizing that they could and/or wanted to take action on HIV. Similarly, because human capital is always limited, and particularly so in sub-Saharan Africa, once a particular sector has captured it, that sector will disproportionately benefit. The population and AIDS fields, as well as the global community more broadly, needs to consider correcting some of those inequities in human resource distribution that have emerged through historical and path dependent processes.

Finally, the book demonstrates that despite weak states and extreme poverty, African organizations persist, function, and can have profound positive effects. Strong organizations developed to assist with one health problem will be at the ready to respond to the next problem. Again, they will likely be most productive in responding to similar types of problems, but they will be resources nonetheless. For this reason, donors should not shy away from investing in organizations on the grounds that such investments are "unsustainable": anything that can be done to help create strong organizations will increase the ability of countries to respond effectively to continuing and new health issues, be they noncommunicable or emergent infectious diseases.

References

Abu, Bala Dan. 1988. "God's Gift as a Problem: Federal Government's Population Policy Draws the Flak Nation-Wide." *Newswatch* February 29:14–19.

Acemoglu, Daron, Simon Johnson, and James A. Robinson. 2001. "The Colonial Origins of Comparative Development: An Empirical Investigation." *The American Economic Review* 91(5):1369–401.

Adam, Barry D. 2011. "Epistemic Fault Lines in Biomedical and Social Approaches to HIV Prevention." *Journal of the International AIDS Society* 14(Suppl 2):S2.

Adeokun, Lawrence, Joanne E. Mantell, Eugene Weiss, Grace Ebun Delano, Temple Jagha, Jumoke Olatoregun, Dora Udo, Stella Akinso, and Ellen Weiss. 2002. "Promoting Dual Protection in Family Planning Clinics in Ibadan, Nigeria." *International Family Planning Perspectives* 28(2):87–95.

Ahlberg, Beth Maina. 1991. *Women, Sexuality and the Changing Social Order: The Impact of Government Policies on Reproductive Behavior in Kenya*. Amsterdam: Gordon and Breach.

AIDS Analysis Africa. 1995. "New Figures Show Growing Epidemic in the Sahel." 5(6):1.

AIDS Prevention Initiative Nigeria. n.d.-a. "Collaboration between Harvard University (USA) and Université Cheikh Ante Diop (Senegal)." Available from: www.apin.harvard.edu/senegal.html. [1/21/2015].

———. n.d.-b. "An Endangered Nation: Nigeria Confronts an Escalating Epidemic." Boston, MA: Harvard School of Public Health.

Ainsworth, Martha, and Mead A. Over. 1997. *Confronting AIDS: Public Priorities in a Global Epidemic*. Washington, DC: World Bank.

Alesina, Alberto, Arnaud Devleeschauwer, William Easterly, Sergio Kurlat, and Romain Wacziarg. 2003. "Fractionalization." *Journal of Economic Growth* 8(2):155–94.

Allen, Tim, and Suzette Heald. 2004. "HIV/AIDS Policy in Africa: What Has Worked in Uganda and What Has Failed in Botswana?" *Journal of International Development* 16(8):1141–54.

Altman, Dennis. 1994. *Power and Community: Organizational and Cultural Responses to AIDS*. London: Taylor and Francis.

Alubo, Ogoh. 2002. "Breaking the Wall of Silence: AIDS Policy and Politics in Nigeria." *International Journal of Health Services* 32(3):551–66.

Anderson, Benedict. 1991. *Imagined Communities: Reflections on the Origin and Spread of Nationalism*. London: Verso.

Angotti, Nicole, Agatha Bula, Lauren Gaydosh, Eitan Zeev Kimchi, Rebecca L. Thornton, and Sara E. Yeatman. 2009. "Increasing the Acceptability of HIV Counseling and Testing with Three C's: Convenience, Confidentiality and Credibility." *Social Science & Medicine* 68(12):2263–70.

Angotti, Nicole, Margaret Frye, Amy Kaler, Michelle Poulin, Susan Cotts Watkins, and Sara Yeatman. 2014. "Popular Moralities and Institutional Rationalities in Malawi's Struggle Against AIDS." *Population and Development Review* 40(3):447–73.

Ansari, David A., and Allyn Gaestel. 2010. "Senegalese Religious Leaders' Perceptions of HIV/AIDS and Implications for Challenging Stigma and Discrimination." *Culture, Health & Sexuality* 12(1):1–16.

Arthur, W. Brian. 1994. *Increasing Returns and Path Dependence in the Economy*. Ann Arbor: University of Michigan Press.

Ashforth, Adam, and Susan Cotts Watkins. 2015. "Narratives of Death in Rural Malawi in the Time of AIDS." *Africa* 85(2):245–68.

Association for Reproductive and Family Health. n.d. "The ARFH Story." Available from: http://arfh-ng.org/about-us/. [5/17/2016].

Association Sénégalaise pour le Bien-être Familial. n.d. "Bienvenue sur le Site Web de l'ASBEF." Available from: www.asbef.sn/. [1/4/2016].

Atkinson, Brice, and Rukarangira Wa Nkera. 1993. *Logistics Systems and Contraceptive Supply Status Review: Malawi Child Spacing and AIDS Control Programs*. Arlington, VA: Family Planning Logistics Management Project.

Atkinson, Brice. 1992. *Logistics Systems and Contraceptive Supply Status Review: Malawi Child Spacing and AIDS Control Programs*. Arlington, VA: Family Planning Logistics Management Project.

Atzili, Boaz. 2012. *Good Fences, Bad Neighbors: Border Fixity and International Conflict*. Chicago: University of Chicago Press.

Auerbach, Judith D., Justin O. Parkhurst, and Carlos F. Cáceres. 2011. "Addressing Social Drivers of HIV/AIDS for the Long-Term Response: Conceptual and Methodological Considerations." *Global Public Health* 6(Suppl 3): S293–309.

Auvert, Bertran, Dirk Taljaard, Emmanuel Lagarde, Joelle Sobngwi-Tambekou, Remi Sitta, and Adrian Puren. 2005. "Randomized, Controlled Intervention Trial of Male Circumcision for Reduction of HIV Infection Risk: The ANRS 1265 Trial." *Plos Medicine* 2(11):1112–22.

Avong, Helen Nene. 2000. "Perception of and Attitudes toward the Nigerian Federal Population Policy, Family Planning Program and Family Planning in Kaduna State, Nigeria." *African Journal of Reproductive Health / La Revue Africaine de la Santé Reproductive* 4 (1):66–76.

Awondo, Patrick, Peter Geschiere, and Graeme Reid. 2012. "Homophobic Africa?: Towards a More Nuanced View." *African Studies Review* 55(3):115 68.

Babalola, Stella, S. B. Babalola, Niyi Adesina, and Yemi Arogbofa. 1992. *Analysis of the Nigerian Beneficiaries of the FHS Project: 1988–1992.* Washington, DC: USAID.

Badge, Edmond, Gary Engelberg, and Fatou Sarr. 1997. *Longue Quete d'Un Dialogue: l'Expérience du Projet AIDSCAP au Sénégal dans l'Implication des Leaders d'Opinion dans la Lutte contre le SIDA.* Dakar: Africa Consultants International.

Baird, Sarah J., Richard S. Garfein, Craig T. McIntosh, and Berk Özler. 2012. "Effect of a Cash Transfer Programme for Schooling on Prevalence of HIV and Herpes Simplex Type 2 in Malawi: A Cluster Randomised Trial." *The Lancet* 379(9823):1320–29.

Bakare, Idowu. 1996. *AIDS: Prevention through Education.* Ibadan: Spectrum Books Limited.

Baldwin, Peter. 2005. *Disease and Democracy: The Industrialized World Faces AIDS.* Berkeley, Los Angeles, London, and New York: University of California Press and Milbank Memorial Fund.

Banda, Mavbuto. 2015. "Global Fund Redirects $574 Million from Malawi AIDS Council." *Reuters-US.* Available from: www.reuters.com/article/us-malawi-aids-globalfund-idUSKBN0ML1FP20150325. [10/27/2015].

Banja la Mtsogolo. 2009. *BLM 2008 Annual Report.* Blantyre, Malawi: Banja la Mtsogolo.

n.d. "Our Impact." Available from: www.banja.org.mw/our-impact. [9/8/2014].

Bankole, Akinrinola, Gilda Sedgh, Friday Okonofua, Collins Imarhiagbe, Rubina Hussain, and Deirdre Wulf. 2009. *Barriers to Safe Motherhood in Nigeria.* New York: Guttmacher Institute.

Bankole, Akinrinola. 1994. *The Role of Mass Media in Family Planning Promotion in Nigeria.* Calverton, MD: Macro International, Inc.

Barker, Kriss. 2009. "Sex, Soap, and Social Change: The Sabido Methodology of Behavior Change Communication." Pp. 368–81 in *HIV AIDS: Global Frontiers in Prevention/Intervention,* edited by Cynthia Pope, Renee T. White, and Robert Malow. New York and London: Routledge.

Barnes, Carolyn, Dan Blumhagen, and Douglas Huber. 2010. *Malawi Community-Based Family Planning and HIV & AIDS Services Project: Mid-Term Evaluation*. Washington, DC: The Global Health Technical Assistance Project.

Barnett, Barbara. 2004. "Emma Says." *Feminist Media Studies* 4(2):111–28.

Barnett, Tony, and Alan Whiteside. 2006. *AIDS in the Twenty-First Century*. Basingstoke: Palgrave Macmillan.

Barnett, Tony, and Gwyn Prins. 2006. "HIV/AIDS and Security: Fact, Fiction and Evidence; A Report to UNAIDS." *International Affairs* 82(2):359–68.

Barrett, Deborah, and Amy Ong Tsui. 1999. "Policy as Symbolic Statement: International Response to National Population Policies." *Social Forces* 78(1):213–34.

Barrett, Deborah, and David John Frank. 1999. "Population Control for National Development: From World Discourse to National Policies." Pp. 198–221 in *Constructing World Culture: International Nongovernmental Organizations Since 1875*, edited by John Boli and George M. Thomas. Stanford, CA: Stanford University Press.

Barrett, Deborah, Charles Kurzman, and Suzanne Shanahan. 2010. "For Export Only: Diffusion Professionals and Population Policy." *Social Forces* 88(3):1183–207.

Barrett, Deborah. 1995. "Reproducing Persons as a Global Concern: The Making of an Institution." PhD Dissertation, Department of Sociology: Stanford University.

Bayart, Jean-François. 1993. *The State in Africa: The Politics of the Belly*. New York, NY: Longman.

——— 2000. "Africa in the World: A History of Extraversion." *African Affairs* 99:217–67.

Bayer, Ronald, and Claire Edington. 2009. "HIV Testing, Human Rights, and Global AIDS Policy: Exceptionalism and Its Discontents." *Journal of Health Politics, Policy & Law* 34(3):301–23.

BBC News. 2008. "Senegal 'Gay Wedding' Men Freed." Available from: http://news.bbc.co.uk/2/hi/africa/7233159.stm. [1/5/2016].

——— 2009. "Shock at Senegal Gay Jail Terms." Available from: http://news.bbc.co.uk/2/hi/africa/7817100.stm. [10/20/2010].

Becker, Charles, and René Collignon. 1999. "A History of Sexually Transmitted Diseases and AIDS in Senegal: Difficulties in Accounting for Social Logics in Health Policy." Pp. 65–96 in *Histories of Sexually Transmitted Diseases and HIV/AIDS in Sub-Saharan Africa*, edited by Philip W. Setel, Milton Lewis, and Maryinez Lyons. Westport, CT: Greenwood Press.

Behrman, Greg. 2004. *The Invisible People: How the US Has Slept Through the Global AIDS Pandemic, the Greatest Humanitarian Catastrophe of Our Time*. New York: Free Press.

Bendavid, Eran, Charles B. Holmes, Jay Bhattacharya, and Grant Miller. 2012. "HIV Development Assistance and Adult Mortality in Africa." *Journal of the American Medical Association* 307(19):2060–67.

Benton, Adia. 2015. *HIV Exceptionalism: Development through Disease in Sierra Leone*. Minneapolis: University of Minnesota Press.

Blanc, Ann K., and Amy O. Tsui. 2005. "The Dilemma of Past Success: Insiders' Views on the Future of the International Family Planning Movement." *Studies in Family Planning* 36(4):263–76.

Blankenship, Kim M., Sarah J. Bray, and Michael H. Merson. 2000. "Structural Interventions in Public Health." *AIDS* 14:S11–21.

Boli, John, and George M. Thomas. 1997. "World Culture in the World Polity: A Century of International Non-Governmental Organization." *American Sociological Review* 62:171–90.

Bollinger, Lori, and Adebiyi Adesina. 2013. *Cost-Effectiveness of Integrating PMTCT and MNCH Services: An Application of the LiST Model for Malawi, Mozambique, and Uganda*. DHS Occasional Paper No. 7. Calverton, MD: ICF International.

Bollinger, Lori, John Stover, and Idrissa Diop. 1999. *The Economic Impact of AIDS in Senegal*. Washington, DC: The Futures Group International.

Bollinger, Lori, John Stover, and O. Nwaorgu. 1999. *The Economic Impact of AIDS in Nigeria*. Washington, DC: The POLICY Project.

Bonga, Violet M. 1999. "The Question of Relevance in AIDS Education in Malawi." Pp. 177–84 in *AIDS and Development in Africa: A Social Science Perspective*, edited by Kempe Ronald Hope Sr. New York: The Haworth Press.

Bongaarts, John, Priscilla Reining, Peter Way, and Francis Conant. 1989. "The Relationship between Male Circumcision and HIV Infection in African Populations." *AIDS* 3(6):373–78.

Bongaarts, John, Thomas Buettner, Gerhard Heilig, and Francois Pelletier. 2008. "Has the HIV Epidemic Peaked." *Population and Development Review* 34(2):199–224.

Bongaarts, John, W. Parker Mauldin, and James F. Philips. 1990. "The Demographic Impact of Family Planning Programs." *Studies in Family Planning* 21(6):299–310.

Bongaarts, John. 2007. "Late Marriage and the HIV Epidemic in Sub-Saharan Africa." *Population Studies* 61(1):73–83.

Boohene, Esther, and Thomas E. Dow. 1987. "Contraceptive Prevalence and Family Planning Program Effort in Zimbabwe." *International Family Planning Perspectives* 13(1):1–7.

Boone, Catherine, and Jake Batsell. 2001. "Politics and AIDS in Africa: Research Agendas in Political Science and International Relations." *Africa Today* 48(2):3–33.

Bor, Jacob. 2007. "The Political Economy of AIDS Leadership in Developing Countries: An Exploratory Analysis." *Social Science & Medicine* 64(8):1585–99.

Boseley, Sarah. 2011. "Taming the Wild West of Family Planning." *The Guardian*. Available from: www.guardian.co.uk/lifeandstyle/2011 /dec/02/taming-wild-west-family-planning-senegal.

Boss, Susan, and Terrence W. Robinson. 1994. *The USAID Family Planning Program within the Nigerian Context*. Washington, DC: USAID.

Bradley, Sarah E.K., Trevor N. Croft, Joy D. Fishel, and Charles F. Westoff. 2012. *Revising Unmet Need for Family Planning*. Calverton, Maryland: ICF International.

Brandt, Allan M. 1988. "AIDS in Historical Perspective: Four Lessons from the History of Sexually Transmitted Diseases." *American Journal of Public Health* 78(4):367–71.

Brass, Jennifer N. 2016. *Allies or Adversaries: NGOs and the State in Africa*. New York: Cambridge University Press.

Bratton, Michael. 1989. "The Politics of Government-NGO Relations in Africa." *World Development* 17(4):569–87.

Brier, Jennifer. 2009. *Infectious Ideas: US Political Responses to the AIDS Crisis*. Chapel Hill: University of North Carolina Press.

Brown, Jeannie. 1994. *Evaluation of the Impact of the Protector Condom Campaign in Malawi*. SOMARC Occasional Paper No. 19. Washington, DC: USAID.

Browner, Carole H., and Carolyn F. Sargent. 2011. "Toward Global Anthropological Studies of Reproduction: Concepts, Methods, Theoretical Approaches." Pp. 1–17 in *Reproduction, Globalization, and the State*, edited by Carole H. Browner and Carolyn F. Sargent. Durham and London: Duke University Press.

Bryceson, Deborah Fahy, and Jodie Fonseca. 2006. "Risking Death for Survival: Peasant Responses to Hunger and HIV/AIDS in Malawi." *World Development* 34(9):1654–66.

Burchardt, Marian, Amy S. Patterson, and Louise Mubanda Rasmussen. 2013. "The Politics and Anti-politics of Social Movements: Religion and HIV/AIDS in Africa." *Canadian Journal of African Studies/La Revue canadienne des études africaines* 47(2):171–85.

Bureau for Africa. 2012. *Three Successful Sub-Saharan Africa Family Planning Programs: Lessons for Meeting the MDGs*. Washington, DC: USAID.

Busby, Joshua W. 2010. *Moral Movements and Foreign Policy*. Cambridge: Cambridge University Press.

Butler, A. 2005. "South Africa's HIV/AIDS Policy, 1994–2004: How Can It Be Explained?" *African Affairs* 104(417):591–614.

Caldwell, John C. 2000. "Rethinking the African AIDS Epidemic." *Population and Development Review* 26(1):117–35.

Caldwell, John C., and Fred T. Sai. 2007. "Family Planning in Ghana." Pp. 379–91 in *The Global Family Planning Revolution*, edited by Warren C. Robinson and John A. Ross. Washington, DC: The World Bank.

Caldwell, John C., and Pat Caldwell. 1996. "Toward an Epidemiological Model of AIDS in Sub-Saharan Africa." *Social Science History* 20(4):559–91.

Caldwell, John C., I. O. Orubuloye, and Pat Caldwell. 1992, "Fertility Decline in Africa: A New Type of Transition?" *Population and Development Review* 18(2):211–42.

Callimachi, Rukmini. 2010. "Even After Death, Abuse Against Gays Continues." *TheWorldPost*. Available from: www.huffingtonpost .com/huff-wires/20100412/af-senegal-gay-violence/. [10/20/2010].

Campbell, Catherine, Flora Cornish, and Morten Skovdal. 2012. "Local Pain, Global Prescriptions? Using Scale to Analyse the Globalisation of the HIV/AIDS Response." *Health & Place* 18(3):447–52.

Canning, David, Sangeeta Raja, and Abdo S. Yazbeck (Eds.). 2015. *Africa's Demographic Transition: Dividend or Disaster?* Washington, DC: World Bank and Agence Française de Développement.

Cassidy, Rebecca, and Melissa Leach. 2009. "Science, Politics, and the Presidential AIDS 'Cure'." *African Affairs* 108(433):559–80.

Center for Strategic and International Studies. n.d. "Peter Lamptey." Available from: www.smartglobalhealth.org/about/commissioners/ peter-lamptey/. [9/19/2014].

Central Intelligence Agency. 2014. "Senegal." *World Factbook*. Available from: www.cia.gov/library/publications/the-world-factbook/geos/sg .html. [9/12/2014].

Chabal, Patrick, and Jean-Pascal Daloz. 1999. *Africa Works: Disorder as Political Instrument*. Bloomington, IN: Indiana University Press.

Chabikuli, Nzapfurundi O, Dorka D Awi, Ogo Chukwujekwu, Zubaida Abubakar, Usman Gwarzo, Mohammed Ibrahim, Mike Merrigan, and Christoph Hamelmann. 2009. "The Use of Routine Monitoring and Evaluation Systems to Assess a Referral Model of Family Planning and HIV Service Integration in Nigeria." *AIDS* 23:S97–103.

Chafer, Tony. 2002. *The End of Empire in French West Africa: France's Successful Decolonization?* Oxford and New York: Berg.

2012. "Senegal." Pp. 38–56 in *Exit Strategies and State Building*, edited by Richard Caplan. New York: Oxford University Press.

Chigwedere, Pride, George R. Seage III, Sofia Gruskin, Tun-Hou Lee, and Max Essex. 2008. "Estimating the Lost Benefits of Antiretroviral Drug Use in South Africa." *JAIDS Journal of Acquired Immune Deficiency Syndromes* 49(4):410–15.

Chimbiri, Agnes M. 2007. "The Condom Is an 'Intruder' in Marriage: Evidence from Rural Malawi." *Social Science & Medicine* 64(5):1102–15.

Chimbwete, Chiweni, Susan Cotts Watkins, and Eliya Msiyaphazi Zulu. 2005. "The Evolution of Population Policies in Kenya and Malawi." *Population Research and Policy Review* 24(1):85–106.

Chin, James. 2007. *The AIDS Pandemic: The Collision of Epidemiology with Political Correctness*. Seattle: Radcliffe Publishing.

Chiona, J., F. Mkhori, M.A. Chimole, A. Assolari, A. Chamgwera, G. M Chisendera, and J. Roche. 1992. *Living Our Faith: Pastoral Letter of the Catholic Bishops of Malawi*. Balaka: Montfort Missionaries Press.

Chiphangwi, J., G. Liomba, H. M. Ntaba, H. Schmidt, F. Deinhardt, J. Eberle, G. Frosner, L. Gurtler, and G. Zoulek. 1987. "Human Immunodeficiency Virus Infection Is Prevalent in Malawi." *Infection* 15(5):363–63.

Chirwa, Isaac. 1993. "AIDS Epidemic in Malawi: Shaking Cultural Foundations." *Network* 13(4):31–32.

Chirwa, Wiseman Chijere. 1998. "Aliens and AIDS in Southern Africa: The Malawi-South Africa Debate." *African Affairs* 97(386):53–79.

1999. "Sexually Transmitted Diseases in Colonial Malawi." Pp. 143–66 in *Histories of Sexually Transmitted Diseases and HIV/AIDS in Sub-Saharan Africa*, edited by Philip W. Setel, Milton Lewis, and Maryinez Lyons. Westport, CT and London: Greenwood Press.

Choices. 2000. "Development Strategies Suffer Until We Address Population Issues." Pp. 4–9 in *Choices*.

Clapham, Christopher S. 1996. *Africa and the International System: the Politics of State Survival*. Cambridge: Cambridge University Press.

Clark, Benjamin Y. 2009. "Policy Adoption in Dynamic International Environments: Evidence from National AIDS Programs." *Public Administration and Development* 29(5):362–73.

2013. "Multilateral, Regional, and National Determinants of Policy Adoption: The Case of HIV/AIDS Legislative Action." *International Journal of Public Health* 58(2):285–93.

Cleland, John, and Mohamed M. Ali. 2006. "Sexual Abstinence, Contraception, and Condom Use by Young African Women: A Secondary Analysis of Survey Data." *The Lancet* 368(9549):1788–93.

Cleland, John, and Susan Cotts Watkins. 2006a. "Sex without Birth or Death: A Comparison of Two International Humanitarian Movements." Pp. 207–24 in *Social Information Transmission and Human Biology*, edited by Johnathan CK Wells, Simon Strickland, and Kevin Laland. Boca Raton, FL: CRC Taylor and Francis.

2006b. "The Key Lesson of Family Planning Programmes for HIV/AIDS Control." *AIDS* 20(1):1–3.

Cleland, John, Stan Bernstein, Alex Ezeh, Anibal Faundes, Anna Glasier, and Jolene Innis. 2006. "Family Planning: The Unfinished Agenda." *The Lancet* 368(9549):1810–27.

Clemens, Elisabeth S. 2007. "Toward a Historicized Sociology: Theorizing Events, Processes, and Emergence." *Annual Review of Sociology* 33:527–49.

Cohen, Barney. 2000. "Family Planning Programs, Socioeconomic Characteristics, and Contraceptive Use in Malawi." *World Development* 28(5):843–60.

Cohen, Jon. 2008. "The Great Funding Surge." *Science* 321(5888):512–19.

Collier, Paul, and Anke Hoeffler. 2004. "Greed and Grievance in Civil War." *Oxford Economic Papers* 56(4):563–95.

Conly, Shanti R., and Joanne E. Epp. 1997. *Falling Short: The World Bank's Role in Population and Reproductive Health*. Washington, DC: Population Action International.

Connelly, Matthew. 2008. *Fatal Misconception: The Struggle to Control World Population*. Cambridge and London: Belknap.

Conseil National de Lutte contre le Sida. 2002. *Plan Strategique 2002–2006 de Lutte contre le SIDA*. Dakar: Conseil National de Lutte contre le Sida.

2007. *Plan Strategique de Lutte contre le Sida 2007–2011*. Dakar: Conseil National de Lutte contre le Sida.

2014. *Rapport de Situation sur la Riposte Nationale à l'Épidémie de VIH/SIDA Sénégal: 2012–2013*. Dakar: Conseil National de Lutte contre le Sida, ONUSIDA.

Coulon, Christian, and Donal B. Cruise O'Brien. 1989. "Senegal." Pp. 145–64 in *Contemporary West African States*, edited by Donal B. Cruise O'Brien, John Dunn, and Richard Rathbone. New York: Cambridge University Press.

Crane, Barbara B. 1993. "International Population Institutions: Adapting to a Changing World Order." Pp. 351–96 in *Institutions for the Earth*, edited by Peter M. Haas, Robert O. Keohane, and Marc A. Levy. Cambridge, MA: MIT Press.

Crane, Johanna Taylor. 2013. *Scrambling for Africa: AIDS, Expertise, and the Rise of American Global Health Science*. Ithaca: Cornell University Press.

CSIS Staff. 2013. "President Joyce Banda: New Focus on Women's Health and Empowerment in Malawi." [Blog] *Smart Global Health Blog*. Available from: www.smartglobalhealth.org/blog/entry/president-joyce-banda-new-focus-on-womens-health-and-empowerment-in-malawi/. [1/9/2013].

Daly, John L. 2001. "AIDS in Swaziland: The Battle from Within." *African Studies Review* 44(1):21–35.

Danart, Arthur, William Mackie, Cindie Cisek, Neema Kondoole, and Nyson Chizani. 2004. *Midterm Evaluation of Population Services International's Improving Health through Social Marketing Project.* Lilongwe: USAID.

De Cock, Kevin M., and Anne M. Johnson. 1998. "From Exceptionalism to Normalisation: A Reappraisal of Attitudes and Practice around HIV Testing." *BMJ* 316(7127):290–3.

de Jong, Ferdinand. 2005. "A Joking Nation: Conflict Resolution in Senegal." *Canadian Journal of African Studies / Revue Canadienne des Etudes Africaines* 39(2):389–413.

De Sweemer, Cecile C., and Tom Lyons. 1975. "Nigeria." *Studies in Family Planning* 6(8):291–93.

de Waal, Alex. 2006. *AIDS and Power: Why There Is No Political Crisis – Yet.* London: Zed Books.

Decoteau, Claire Laurier. 2013. *Ancestors and Antiretrovirals: The Biopolitics of HIV/AIDS in Post-Apartheid South Africa.* Chicago: University of Chicago Press.

Delaunay, Karine, A Didier Blibolo, and Katy Cissé-Wone. 1999. "Des ONG et des Associations: Concurrences et Dépendances sur un "Marché du Sida" Émergent (Cas Ivoirien et Sénégalais)." Pp. 69–89 in *Organiser la Lutte contre le Sida: Une Étude Comparative sur les Rapports État/Société Civile en Afrique (Cameroun, Congo, Côte-d'Ivoire, Kenya, Sénégal),* edited by Marc-Eric Gruénais. Paris: Institut de Recherche pour le Développement.

Delaunay, Karine, and Jocelyne Quinio. 1999. "Les Acteurs Non Gouvernementaux au Sénégal: Une Présence Massive mais une Intervention Difficile à Évaluer" Pp. 187–203 in *Organiser la Lutte contre le Sida: Une Étude Comparative sur les Rapports État/Société Civile en Afrique (Cameroun, Congo, Côte-d'Ivoire, Kenya, Sénégal),* edited by Marc-Eric Gruénais. Paris: Institut de Recherche pour le Développement.

Dembele, Demba Moussa. 2003. *Debt and Destruction in Senegal: A Study of Twenty Years of IMF and World Bank Policies.* London: World Development Movement.

Desclaux, Alice. 2004. "Equity in Access to AIDS Treatment in Africa: Pitfalls among Achievements." Pp. 115–32 in *Unhealthy Health Policy: A Critical Anthropological Examination,* edited by Arachu Castro and Merrill Singer. Walnut Creek, CA: Altamira Press.

Devres, Inc. 1991. *Final Evaluation of USAID/Senegal's Family Health and Population Project.* Dakar: USAID.

Dibua, Jeremiah I. 2004. "Collapse of Purpose: Ibrahim Babangida, 1985–1993." Pp. 207–35 in *Troubled Journey: Nigeria Since the Civil War*, edited by Levi A. Nwachuku and G.N. Uzoigwe. Lantham, MD: University Press of America.

Dickinson, Elizabeth. 2010. "The Long Emergency." *Foreign Policy*. Available from: http://foreignpolicy.com/2010/06/25/the-long-emergency/. [5/15/2015].

Dickson, Kim E., Nhan T. Tran, Julia L. Samuelson, Emmanuel Njeuhmeli, Peter Cherutich, Bruce Dick, Tim Farley, Caroline Ryan, and Catherine A. Hankins. 2011. "Voluntary Medical Male Circumcision: A Framework Analysis of Policy and Program Implementation in Eastern and Southern Africa." *PLoS Med* 8(11):e1001133.

Dionne, Kim Yi, and Michelle Poulin. 2013. "Ethnic Identity, Region and Attitudes towards Male Circumcision in a High HIV-Prevalence Country." *Global Public Health* 8(5):607–18.

Dionne, Kim Yi, Patrick Gerland, and Susan Watkins. 2013. "AIDS Exceptionalism: Another Constituency Heard From." *AIDS and Behavior* 17(3):825–31.

Dionne, Kim Yi. 2011. "The Role of Executive Time Horizons in State Response to AIDS in Africa." *Comparative Political Studies* 44(1):55–77.
   2012. "Local Demand for a Global Intervention: Policy Priorities in the Time of AIDS." *World Development* 40(12):2468–77.

Diop, Biram. 2013. "Civil-Military Relations in Senegal." Pp. 236–56 in *Military Engagement: Influencing Armed Forces Worldwide to Support Democratic Transitions, Volume II (Regional and Country Studies)*, edited by Dennis Blair. Washington, DC: Brookings Institution Press.

Diouf, Daouda. 2007. *HIV/AIDS Policy in Senegal*. New York: Open Society Institute.

Diouf, Mamadou. 1998. "The French Colonial Policy of Assimilation and the Civility of the Originaires of the Four Communes (Senegal): A Nineteenth Century Globalization Project." *Development and Change* 29(4):671–96.

Dixon-Mueller, Ruth, and Adrienne Germain. 1994. "Population Policy and Feminist Action in Three Developing Countries." *Population and Development Review* 20(Supplement: The New Politics of Population: Conflict and Consensus in Family Planning):197–219.

Dixon-Mueller, Ruth. 1993. "The Sexuality Connection in Reproductive Health." *Studies in Family Planning* 24(5):269–82.

Do Espirito Santo, Maria Eugênia G., and Gina D. Etheredge. 2004. "And then I Became a Prostitute ... Some Aspects of Prostitution and Brothel Prostitutes in Dakar, Senegal." *The Social Science Journal* 41(1):137–46.

Dobbin, Frank, Beth Simmons, and Geoffrey Garrett. 2007. "The Global Diffusion of Public Policies: Social Construction, Coercion, Competition, or Learning?" *Annual Review of Sociology* 33(1):449–72.

Dodoo, F. Nii-Amoo, and Ashley E. Frost. 2008. "Gender in African Population Research: The Fertility/Reproductive Health Example." *Annual Review of Sociology* 34:431.

Donaldson, Peter. 1990. *Nature Against Us*. Chapel Hill and London: University of North Carolina Press.

Donnelly, John. 2003. "In Africa, Hope Emerges: Senegal's Aggressive AIDS Strategy Saves Thousands from Infection." *Boston Globe*. Available from: www.boston.com/news/specials/lives_lost/senegal/. [3/16/2012].

———. 2012. "The President's Emergency Plan For AIDS Relief: How George W. Bush and Aides Came to 'Think Big' on Battling HIV." *Health Affairs* 31(7):1389–96.

Dorward, Andrew, Ephraim Chirwa, and T. S. Jayne. 2011. "Malawi's Agricultural Input Subsidy Program Experience over 2005–09." Pp. 289–317 in *Yes Africa Can: Success Stories from a Dynamic Continent*, edited by Punam Chuhan-Pole and Manka Angwafo. Washington, DC: World Bank.

Doyle, Shane. 2013. *Before HIV: Sexuality, Fertility and Mortality in East Africa, 1900–1980*. Oxford: Oxford University Press for the British Academy.

Dozon, Jean-Pierre, and Didier Fassin. 1989. "Raison Épidémiologique et Raisons d'État. Les Enjeux Socio-Politiques du SIDA en Afrique." *Sciences Sociales et Santé* 7(1):21–36.

Dugger, Cynthia. 2007. "Ending Famine, Simply by Ignoring the Experts." *The New York Times*. Available from: www.nytimes.com/2007/12/02/world/africa/02malawi.html?_r=1&scp=1&sq=malawi%20fertilizer&st=cse. [5/23/2012].

Dunkle, Kristin L., Rob Stephenson, Etienne Karita, Elwyn Chomba, Kayitesi Kayitenkore, Cheswa Vwalika, Lauren Greenberg, and Susan Allen. 2008. "New Heterosexually Transmitted HIV Infections in Married or Cohabiting Couples in Urban Zambia and Rwanda: An Analysis of Survey and Clinical Data." *The Lancet* 371(9631):2183–91.

Easterly, William, and Ross Levine. 1997. "Africa's Growth Tragedy: Policies and Ethnic Divisions." *The Quarterly Journal of Economics* 112(4):1203–50.

Ebigbola, Joshua Akinola. 2000. "National Population Policy: A Viable Option to Human Development." Pp. 3–23 in *Population and Development Issues: Ideas and Debates: Essays in Honor of Professor P.O. Olusanya*, edited by Joshua A. Ebigbola and Elisha P. Renne. Ibadan: African Book Builders.

Ebin, Victoria. 2000. "Sex Workers Promote AIDS Awareness in Senegal." *Population Reference Bureau*. Available from: www.prb.org/Publi cations/Articles/2000/SexWorkersPromoteAIDSAwarenessinSenegal .aspx. [1/5/2016].

Eboko, Fred. 2005. "Patterns of Mobilization: Political Culture in the Fight Against AIDS." Pp. 37–58 in *The African State and the AIDS Crisis*, edited by Amy S. Patterson. Aldershot: Ashgate.

Echenberg, Myron. 2006. "Historical Perspectives on HIV/AIDS: Lessons from South Africa and Senegal." Pp. 89–96 in *The HIV/AIDS Epidemic in Sub-Saharan Africa in a Historical Perspective*, edited by Philippe Denis and Charles Becker. Dakar: Reseau Senegal: Droit, Ethique et Sante.

Economic Commission for Africa. 1988. *Social, Cultural and Legislative Factors Affecting Family Formation and Fertility in Selected African Countries*. Addis Ababa: Economic Commission for Africa, Population Division.

2004. *Scoring African Leadership for Better Health*. Addis Ababa: Economic Commission for Africa.

Edström, Jerker, and Hayley MacGregor. 2010. "The Pipers Call the Tunes in Global Aid for AIDS: The Global Financial Architecture for HIV Funding as Seen by Local Stakeholders in Kenya, Malawi and Zambia." *Global Health Governance* 4(1).

Ehrlich, Paul. 1969. *The Population Bomb*. San Francisco: Sierra Club.

Ehusani, George Omaku. 1994. *The Politics of Population Control*. Zaria, Nigeria: Ahmadu Bello University Press.

Elbe, Stefan. 2006. "Should HIV/AIDS Be Securitized? The Ethical Dilemmas of Linking HIV/AIDS and Security." *International Studies Quarterly* 50(1):119–44.

Engelberg, Gary. 2005. "Question Success: Did Senegal Do the Right Thing, or Is the Worst of AIDS Yet to Come?" *WorldView* 18(2):75–78.

EngenderHealth. n.d. "Nigeria." Available from: www.engenderhealth.org/ our-countries/africa/nigeria.php. [3/9/2015].

England, Roger. 2006. "Coordinating HIV Control Efforts: What To Do with the National AIDS Commissions." *The Lancet* 367(9524):1786–9.

2007. "Are We Spending Too Much on HIV?" *British Medical Journal* 334(7589):344.

Englebert, Pierre. 2000. *State Legitimacy and Development in Africa*. Boulder, CO: Lynne Rienner.

Englund, Harri. 2006. *Prisoners of Freedom: Human Rights and the African Poor*. Berkeley: University of California Press.

Epstein, Helen, and Martina Morris. 2011. "Concurrent Partnerships and HIV: An Inconvenient Truth." *Journal of the International AIDS Society* 14(1):13.

Esacove, Anne W. 2010. "Love Matches." *Gender & Society* 24(1):83–109.

2013. "Good Sex/Bad Sex: The Individualised Focus of US HIV Prevention Policy in Sub-Saharan Africa, 1995–2005." *Sociology of Health & Illness* 35(1):33–48.

2016. *Modernizing Sexuality: U.S. HIV Prevention in Sub-Saharan Africa.* New York: Oxford University Press.

Essex, Max, Souleymane Mboup, Phyllis J. Kanki, Richard G. Marlink, and Sheila G. Tlou (Eds.). 2002. *AIDS in Africa, Second Edition.* New York: Kluwer Academic Publishers.

Fair, Molly. 2008. *From Population Lending to HNP Results: The Evolution of the World Bank's Strategies in Health, Nutrition and Population.* Washington, DC: World Bank.

Falobi, Omololu, and Olayide Akanni (Eds.). 2004. *Slow Progress: An Analysis of Implementation of Policies and Action on HIV/AIDS Care and Treatment in Nigeria.* Lagos: Journalists Against AIDS Nigeria.

Falobi, Omololu. 1999. "New AIDS Policy in Nigeria Raises the Stakes – but Optimism Remains Scarce." *AIDS Analysis Africa* 9(5):10–11.

Falola, Toyin, and Matthew M. Heaton. 2008. *A History of Nigeria.* Cambridge: Cambridge University Press.

Family Care International. 2007. *Safe Motherhood, A Review: The Safe Motherhood Initiative 1987–2005.* New York: Family Care International.

Family Health International. 1997. *Family Health International AIDS Control and Prevention Project Final Report, Volume 1.* Arlington, VA: Family Health International.

2002. "Senegal Program Overview." Available from: http://web.archive .org/web/20020616091730/http://www.fhi.org/en/cntr/africa/senegal/ senegalofc.html. [1/14/2015].

2007a. *Nigeria Final Report.* Arlington, VA: Family Health International.

2007b. *Senegal Final Report.* Arlington, VA: Family Health International.

2010. *Four Decades of Improving Lives Worldwide: 2010 Annual Report.* Durham, NC and Arlington, VA: Family Health International.

n.d. *Strengthening Capacity to Develop Local Responses to Critical Needs.* Abuja: Family Health International.

Fan, Victoria, Denizhan Duran, Rachel Silverman, and Amanda Glassman. 2013. *HIV/AIDS Intervention Packages in Five Countries: A Review of Budget Data.* Washington, DC: Center for Global Development.

Faruq, Alhaji Sheikh Usman. 1989. *Family Planning: Islamic Viewpoint.* Lagos and Kano, Nigeria: Paragon.

Fasawe, Olufunke, Carlos Avila, Nathan Shaffer, Erik Schouten, Frank Chimbwandira, David Hoos, Olive Nakakeeto, and Paul De Lay. 2013.

"Cost-Effectiveness Analysis of Option B+ for HIV Prevention and Treatment of Mothers and Children in Malawi." *PLoS ONE* 8(3):e57778.

Fatusi, Adesegun O., and Akin Jimoh. 2006. "The Roles of Behavior Change Communication and Mass Media." Pp. 323–48 in *AIDS in Nigeria: A Nation on the Threshold*, edited by Olusoji Adeyi, Phyllis J. Kanki, Oluwole Odutolu, and John A. Idoko. Cambridge, MA: Harvard University Press.

Federal Ministry of Health. 2007. *National Programmatic Assessment for Family Planning and HIV Counseling and Testing Integration in Nigeria*. Abuja: Global HIV/AIDS Initiative Nigeria.

Federal Republic of Nigeria. 1988. *National Policy on Population for Development, Unity, Progress, and Self-Reliance*. Lagos: Federal Ministry of Health/Department of Population Activities.

2001. *National Reproductive Health Policy and Strategy to Achieve Quality Reproductive & Sexual Health for All Nigerians*. Abjua: Federal Ministry of Health.

2004. *National Policy on Population for Sustainable Development*. Abuja: National Population Commission.

2008. *National HIV/AIDS and Reproductive Health Survey, 2007 (NARHS Plus)*. Abuja: Federal Ministry of Health.

Ferguson, James. 2006. *Global Shadows: Africa in the Neoliberal World Order*. Durham and London: Duke University Press.

Feyisetan, Bamikale James. 1998. *Implementation of Policies, Programmes and Laws Related to Reproductive Health and Reproductive Rights in Selected African Countries*. Addis Ababa: Economic Commission for Africa.

FHI 360. 2012. "FHI 360's Journey toward an AIDS-Free Generation." Available from: www.fhi360.org/news/fhi-360s-journey-toward-aids-free-generation. [5/17/2012].

Finger, William R. 1991. "Clinic-Based Intervention Projects: STD and Family Planning Programs Get Involved." *Network* 12(1):11, 13–14.

Fisher, Max. 2013. "From Colonialism to 'Kill the Gays': The Surprisingly Recent Roots of Homophobia in Africa." [Blog] *WorldViews*. Available from: www.washingtonpost.com/blogs/worldviews/wp/2013/06/27/from-colonialism-to-kill-the-gays-the-surprisingly-recent-roots-of-homophobia-in-africa/.

Fisher, William F. 1997. "Doing Good? The Politics and Antipolitics of NGO Practices." *Annual Review of Anthropology* 26:439–64.

Fligstein, Neil, and Doug McAdam. 2011. "Toward a General Theory of Strategic Action Fields." *Sociological Theory* 29(1):1–26.

Folayan, Morenike. 2004. "HIV/AIDS: The Nigerian Response." Pp. 85–104 in *The Political Economy of AIDS in Africa*, edited by Nana K. Poku and Alan Whiteside. Aldershot: Ashgate.

Foley, Ellen E. 2009. *Your Pocket Is What Cures You: The Politics of Health in Senegal.* New Brunswick, NJ: Rutgers University Press.

Foley, Ellen E., and Anne Hendrixson. 2011. "From Population Control to AIDS: Conceptualising and Critiquing the Global Crisis Model." *Global Public Health* 6(Suppl 3):S310–22.

Foley, Ellen E., and Rokhaya Nguer. 2010. "Courting Success in HIV/AIDS Prevention: The Challenges of Addressing a Concentrated Epidemic in Senegal." *African Journal of AIDS Research* 9(4):325–36.

Fonner, Virginia A, Julie Denison, Caitlin E Kennedy, Kevin O'Reilly, and Michael Sweat. 2012. "Voluntary Counseling and Testing (VCT) for Changing HIV-Related Risk Behavior in Developing Countries." *Cochrane Database Systematic Reviews* 9:CD001224.

Forbes, Ann Armbrecht. 1999. "The Importance of Being Local: Villagers, NGOs, and the World Bank in the Arun Valley, Nepal." *Identities-Global Studies in Culture and Power* 6(2–3):319–44.

Forman, Lisa. 2011. "Global AIDS Funding and the Re-Emergence of AIDS Exceptionalism " *Social Medicine* 6(1):45–51.

Forster, Peter G. 1994. "Culture, Nationalism, and the Invention of Tradition in Malawi." *The Journal of Modern African Studies* 32(3):477–97.

2001. "AIDS in Malawi: Contemporary Discourse and Cultural Continuities." *African Studies* 60(2):245–61.

Fortson, Jane G. 2008. "The Gradient in Sub-Saharan Africa: Socioeconomic Status and HIV/AIDS." *Demography* 45(2):303–22.

Foster, Gregory D., Alan Ned Sabrosky, and William J. Taylor. 1989. "Global Demographic Trends to the Year 2010: Implications for U.S. Security." *The Washington Quarterly* 12(2):5–24.

Foucault, Michel. 1978. *The History of Sexuality: An Introduction.* New York: Vintage.

Fox, Ashley M. 2014. "AIDS Policy Responsiveness in Africa: Evidence from Opinion Surveys." *Global Public Health* 9(1–2):224–48.

Fox, Ashley M., Allison B. Goldberg, Radhika J. Gore, and Till Bärnighausen. 2011. "Conceptual and Methodological Challenges to Measuring Political Commitment to Respond to HIV." *Journal of the International AIDS Society* 14(2):1–13.

Frank, Odile, and Geoffrey McNicoll. 1987. "An Interpretation of Fertility and Population Policy in Kenya." *Population and Development Review* 13(2):209–43.

Garbus, Lisa. 2003. *HIV/AIDS in Malawi.* San Francisco: AIDS Research Institute/AIDS Policy Research Center.

Garenne, Michel, Alain Giami, and Christophe Perrey. 2013. "Male Circumcision and HIV Control in Africa: Questioning Scientific

Evidence and the Decision-Making Process." Pp. 185–210 in *Global Health in Africa: Historical Perspectives on Disease Control*, edited by Tamara Giles-Vernick and Jr. James L.A. Webb. Athens, OH: Ohio University Press.

Garrett, Laurie. 1994. *The Coming Plague: Newly Emerging Diseases in a World out of Balance*. New York: Penguin.

Gauri, Varun, and Evan S. Lieberman. 2006. "Boundary Institutions and HIV/AIDS Policy in Brazil and South Africa." *Studies in Comparative International Development* 41(3):47–73.

Gellar, Sheldon. 1995. *Senegal: An African Nation Between Islam and the West (second edition)*. Boulder, CO: Westview Press.

2005. *Democracy in Senegal: Tocquevillian Analytics in Africa*. New York: Palgrave Macmillan.

Gellman, Barton. 2000. "Death Watch: The Global Response to AIDS in Africa." *The Washington Post*. Available from: www.washingtonpost.com/wp-dyn/content/article/2006/06/09/AR2006060901326.html. [7/24/2014].

Gibbon, Peter. 1992. "Population and Poverty in the Changing Ideology of the World Bank." Pp. 133–45 in *Population and the Development Crisis in the South*, edited by Mikael Hammarskjold, Bertil Egero, and Staffan Lindberg. Bastad, Sweden: Programme on Population and Development in Poor Countries.

Gibbs, Andrew, Samantha Willan, Alison Misselhorn, and Jaqualine Mangoma. 2012. "Combined Structural Interventions for Gender Equality and Livelihood Security: A Critical Review of the Evidence from Southern and Eastern Africa and the Implications for Young People." *Journal of the International AIDS Society* 15(Suppl 1):17362.

Gibney, Alex. 2014. *Finding Fela!* New York: Kino Lorber.

Gilman, Lisa. 2009. *The Dance of Politics: Gender, Performance, and Democratization in Malawi*. Philadelphia: Temple University Press.

Ginsburg, Faye, and Rayna Rapp. 1991. "The Politics of Reproduction." *Annual Review of Anthropology* 20:311–43.

Gisselquist, David, John J. Potterat, Stuart Brody, and Francois Vachon. 2003. "Let It Be Sexual: How Health Care Transmission of AIDS in Africa Was Ignored." *International Journal of STD & AIDS* 14(3):148–61.

Gisselquist, David. 2008. *Points to Consider: Responses to HIV/AIDS in Africa, Asia, and the Caribbean*. London: Adonis & Abbey.

Global Fund to Fight AIDS, Tuberculosis and Malaria. n.d.-a. "Grant Portfolio." Available from: www.theglobalfund.org/en/portfolio/. [5/16/2016].

n.d.-b. "History of the Global Fund." Available from: www.theglobalfund.org/en/history/. [5/16/2016].

n.d.-c "Scale-up of Comprehensive HIV and AIDS Treatment, Care and Support in Nigeria." Available from: www.theglobalfund.org/en/portfolio/country/grant/?grant=NGA-506-G09-H. [12/15/2015].

Goldberg, Allison B., Ashley M. Fox, Radhika J. Gore, and Till Bärnighausen. 2012. "Indicators of Political Commitment to Respond to HIV." *Sexually Transmitted Infections* 88(2):e1.

Goldenberg, Suzanne. 2011. "Focus on HIV-AIDS Cost Family Planning a Decade, Says UN Population Chief." *The Guardian*. Available from: www.guardian.co.uk/environment/2011/oct/24/population-hiv-aids-mistake-un. [10/27/2011].

Goldstone, Jack A. 2010. "The Four Megatrends that Will Change the World "*Foreign Affairs* 89 (1):31–43.

Goldstone, Jack A., Eric P. Kaufmann, and Monica Duffy Toft (Eds.). 2012. *Political Demography: How Population Changes Are Reshaping International Security and National Politics*. Boulder, CO and Oxford: Paradigm Publishers and Oxford University Press.

Gomez-Perez, Muriel. 2011. "Des Élites Musulmanes Sénégalaises dans l'Action Sociale: Des Expériences de Partenariats et de Solidarités." *Bulletin de l'APAD* 33.

Gordenker, Leon, Roger A. Coate, Christer Jonsson, and Peter Soderholm. 1995. *International Cooperation in Response to AIDS*. London and New York: Pinter.

Gordon, April A. 2003. *Nigeria's Diverse Peoples*. Santa Barbara, CA: ABC-CLIO.

Gordon, Colin. 1991. "Governmental Rationality: An Introduction." Pp. 1–51 in *The Foucault Effect: Studies in Governmentality*, edited by Graham Burchell, Colin Gordin, and Peter Miller. Chicago: University of Chicago Press.

Gordon, David F. 2002. *The Next Wave of HIV/AIDS: Nigeria, Ethiopia, Russia, India, and China*. Washington, DC: National Intelligence Council.

Gordon, Gill, and Tony Klouda. 1989. *Preventing a Crisis: AIDS and Family Planning Work*. London: Macmillan Publishers for International Planned Parenthood Federation.

Gore, Radhika J., Ashley M. Fox, Allison B. Goldberg, and Till Bärnighausen. 2014. "Bringing the State Back In: Understanding and Validating Measures of Governments' Political Commitment to HIV." *Global Public Health* 9(1–2):98–120.

Government of Malawi. 1986. *Workshop on Family Spacing for Child Survival and Development*. Lilongwe: UNICEF.

1994. *National Population Policy*: Office of the President and Cabinet, Department of Economic Planning and Development.

1996. *Family Planning Policy and Contraceptive Guidelines, Second Edition*. Lilongwe: Ministry of Health and Population and National Family Welfare Council of Malawi.

2002. *Reproductive Health Policy*. Lilongwe: Ministry of Health and Population.

2011. *Guidelines for Family Planning Communication*. Lilongwe: Ministry of Health, Health Education Unit.

2012a. *2012 Global AIDS Response Progress Report for Malawi*. Lilongwe: Government of Malawi.

2012b. *National Population Policy*. Lilongwe: Ministry of Economic Planning and Development.

Gow, Jeff. 2002. "The HIV/AIDS Epidemic in Africa: Implications for US Policy." *Health Affairs* 21(3):57–69.

Goyder, Hugh. 2003. *Report of the Final Evaluation of Umoyo Network Malawi*. Washington, DC: NGO Networks for Health.

Gray, Peter B. 2004. "HIV and Islam: Is HIV Prevalence Lower among Muslims?" *Social Science & Medicine* 58(9):1751–56.

Grebe, Eduard. 2011. "The Treatment Action Campaign's Struggle for AIDS Treatment in South Africa: Coalition-building Through Networks." *Journal of Southern African Studies* 37(4):849–68.

Greeley, Edward H. 1988. "The Role of Non-Governmental Organizations in AIDS Prevention: Parallels to African Family Planning Activity." Pp. 131–44 in *AIDS in Africa: The Social and Policy Impact*, edited by Norman Miller and Richard C. Rockwell. Lewiston, NY and Queenston, ON: The Edwin Mellen Press.

Green, Edward C. 1994. *AIDS and STDs in Africa: Bridging the Gap between Traditional Healing and Modern Medicine*. Boulder, CO: Westview Press.

2003. *Rethinking AIDS Prevention*. Westport, CT: Praeger.

2011. *Broken Promises: How the AIDS Establishment Has Betrayed the Developing World*. Sausalito, CA: PoliPoint Press.

Green, Edward C., Daniel T. Halperin, Vinand Nantulya, and Janice A. Hogle. 2006. "Uganda's HIV Prevention Success: The Role of Sexual Behavior Change and the National Response." *AIDS and Behavior* 10(4):335–46.

Green, Edward C., Phoebe Kajubi, Allison Ruark, Sarah Kamya, Nicole D'Errico, and Norman Hearst. 2013. "The Need to Reemphasize Behavior Change for HIV Prevention in Uganda: A Qualitative Study." *Studies in Family Planning* 44(1):25–43.

Greene, Margaret E., and Ann E. Biddlecom. 2000. "Absent and Problematic Men: Demographic Accounts of Male Reproductive Roles." *Population and Development Review* 26(1):81–115.

Greenhalgh, Susan. 2003. "Science, Modernity, and the Making of China's One-Child Policy." *Population and Development Review* 29(2):163–96.

Gregson, Simon, Geoffrey P. Garnett, Constance A. Nyamukapa, Timothy B. Hallett, James J. C. Lewis, Peter R. Mason, Stephen K. Chandiwana, and Roy M. Anderson. 2006. "HIV Decline Associated with Behavior Change in Eastern Zimbabwe." *Science* 311(5761):664–66.

Gregson, Simon. 2003. "The Influence of HIV/AIDS on Demography and Demographic Research." Pp. 88–110 in *Learning from HIV/AIDS*, edited by George Ellison, Melissa Parker, and Catherine Campbell. Cambridge: Cambridge University Press.

Grew, Tony. 2009. "Senegalese AIDS Activist among Nine Men Jailed for Sodomy." *PinkNews*. Available from: www.pinknews.co.uk/2009/01/08/senegalese-gay-rights-activist-among-nine-men-jailed-for-sodomy/. [10/20/2010].

Grier, Sonya, and Carol A. Bryant. 2005. "Social Marketing in Public Health." *Annual Review of Public Health* 26(1):319–39.

Grosskurth, Heiner, Frank Mosha, James Todd, Ezra Mwijarubi, Arnoud Klokke, Kesheni Senkoro, Philippe Mayaud, John Changalucha, Angus Nicoll, Gina ka-Gina, James Newell, Kokugonza Mugeye, David Mabey, and Richard Hayes. 1995. "Impact of Improved Treatment of Sexually Transmitted Diseases on HIV Infection in Rural Tanzania: Randomised Controlled Trial." *The Lancet* 346(8974):530–36.

Grown, Caren. 2008. "Non-Governmental Organizations." *The New Palgrave Dictionary of Economics: Second Edition*, edited by Lawrence Blume and Steven Durlauf. London: Palgrave Macmillan.

Gruskin, Sofia. 2009. "Approaches to Sexual and Reproductive Health and HIV Policies and Programmes: Synergies and Disconnects." Pp. 124–39 in *Reproductive Health and Human Rights*, edited by Laura Reichenbach and Mindy Jane Roseman. Philadelphia: University of Pennsylvania Press.

Gueye, El Hadj Moustapha. 1995. *Questions et Reponses sur les Problemes de Population*. Dakar: Association National des Imams et Ulemas du Senegal.

Gupta, Geeta Rao, Justin O. Parkhurst, Jessica A. Ogden, Peter Aggleton, and Ajay Mahal. 2008. "Structural Approaches to HIV Prevention." *The Lancet* 372(9640):764–75.

Guyer, Jane I. 1995. "Wealth in People, Wealth in Things – Introduction." *The Journal of African History* 36(1):83–90.

Haacker, Markus. 2016. *The Economics of the Global Response to HIV/AIDS*. Oxford: Oxford University Press.

Halperin, Daniel T., and Helen Epstein. 2004. "Concurrent Sexual Partnerships Help to Explain Africa's High HIV Prevalence: Implications for Prevention." *The Lancet* 364(9428):4–6.

Halperin, Daniel T., Owen Mugurungi, Timothy B. Hallett, Backson Muchini, Bruce Campbell, Tapuwa Magure, Clemens Benedikt, and Simon Gregson. 2011. "A Surprising Prevention Success: Why Did the HIV Epidemic Decline in Zimbabwe?" *PLoS Med* 8(2):e1000414.

Hanenberg, Robert S., Wiwat Rojanapithayakorn, Prayura Kunasol, and David C. Sokal. 1994. "Impact of Thailand's HIV-Control Programme as Indicated by the Decline of Sexually Transmitted Diseases." *The Lancet* 344(8917):243–5.

Hardee, Karen, Kokila Agarwal, Nancy Luke, Ellen Wilson, Margaret Pendzich, Marguerite Farrell, and Harry Cross. 1998. *Post-Cairo Reproductive Health Policies and Programs: A Comparative Study of Eight Countries*. Washington, DC: The Futures Group.

Harman, Sophie. 2010. *The World Bank and HIV/AIDS: Setting a Global Agenda*. London and New York: Routledge.

Harries, Anthony D, Erik J Schouten, Simon D Makombe, Edwin Libamba, Henry N Neufville, Eliab Some, Godfrey Kadewere, and Douglas Lungu. 2007. "Ensuring Uninterrupted Supplies of Antiretroviral Drugs in Resource-Poor Settings: An Example from Malawi." *Bulletin of the World Health Organization* 85(2):152–55.

Hartmann, Betsy. 1995. *Reproductive Rights and Wrongs*. Boston, MA: South End Press.

Hayes, Richard, and Helen Weiss. 2006. "Understanding HIV Epidemic Trends in Africa." *Science* 311(5761):620–21.

Hayes, Richard, Deborah Watson-Jones, Connie Celum, Janneke van de Wijgert, and Judith Wasserheit. 2010. "Treatment of Sexually Transmitted Infections for HIV Prevention: End of the Road or New Beginning?" *AIDS* 24:S15–26.

Hearst, Norman, and Sanny Chen. 2004. "Condom Promotion for AIDS Prevention in the Developing World: Is It Working?" *Studies in Family Planning* 35(1):39–47.

Hellandendu, Joseph Muta'a. 2012. "Contributory Factors to the Spread of HIV/AIDS and It Impacts in Sub-Saharan African Countries." *European Scientific Journal* 8(14):144–56.

Heller, Jacob. 2008. *The Vaccine Narrative*. Nashville: Vanderbilt University Press.

Henisz, Witold J., Bennet A. Zelner, and Mauro F. Guillen. 2005. "The Worldwide Diffusion of Market-Oriented Infrastructure Reform, 1977–1999." *American Sociological Review* 70(6):871–97.

Hennink, Monique, Eliya Zulu, and Francis Dodoo. 2001. *Effective Delivery of Reproductive Health Services to Men: A Review Study in Kenya and Malawi*. Southampton, UK: University of Southampton.

Henry, Kathleen. 2000. "Breaking the Silence in Nigeria: An Appeal to Presidents." *IMPACT ON HIV* 2(2):16.

Herbst, Jeffrey. 2000. *States and Power in Africa*. Princeton, NJ: Princeton University Press.

Hodgson, Dennis, and Susan Cotts Watkins. 1997. "Feminists and Neo-Malthusians: Past and Present Alliances." *Population and Development Review* 23(3):469–523.

Hogan, Margaret C., Kyle J. Foreman, Mohsen Naghavi, Stephanie Y. Ahn, Mengru Wang, Susanna M. Makela, Alan D. Lopez, Rafael Lozano, and Christopher J. L. Murray. 2010. "Maternal Mortality for 181 Countries, 1980–2008: A Systematic Analysis of Progress towards Millennium Development Goal 5." *The Lancet* 375(9726):1609–23.

Holmen, Hans. 2010. *Snakes in Paradise: NGOs and the Aid Industry in Africa*. Sterling, VA: Kumarian Press.

Homaifar, Nazaneen, and Suzan Zuljani Wasik. 2005. "Interviews with Senegalese Commercial Sex Trade Workers and Implications for Social Programming." *Health Care for Women International* 26(2):118–33.

Homaifar, Nazaneen. 2006. "Taking a Step towards Prevention: Senegal's Policy of Legalizing the Sex Trade." *Exchange* 1:14–15.

Hunsmann, Moritz. 2009. "Political Determinants of Variable Aetiology Resonance: Explaining the African AIDS Epidemics." *International Journal of STD & AIDS* 20(12):834–38.

Hutchinson, Eleanor, Justin Parkhurst, Sam Phiri, Di Gibb, Nathaniel Chishinga, Benson Droti, and Susan Hoskins. 2011. "National Policy Development for Cotrimoxazole Prophylaxis in Malawi, Uganda and Zambia: The Relationship between Context, Evidence and Links." *Health Research Policy and Systems* 9(Suppl 1):S6.

Hyden, Goran. 1980. *Beyond Ujamma in Tanzania: Underdevelopment and an Uncaptured Peasantry*. Berkeley: University of California Press.

Idoko, John. 2012. "A Clinician's Experience with the President's Emergency Plan for AIDS Relief in Nigeria: A Transformative Decade of Hope." *Health Affairs* 31(7):1422–28.

Igoe, Jim, and Tim Kelsall. 2005. "Introduction: Between a Rock and a Hard Place." Pp. 1–33 in *Between a Rock and a Hard Place: African NGOs, Donors and the State*, edited by Jim Igoe and Tim Kelsall. Durham, NC: Carolina Academic Press.

Iliffe, John. 2006. *The African AIDS Epidemic: A History*. Athens, OH: Ohio University Press.

Information Project for Africa, Inc. 1991. *Population Control and National Security: A Review of US National Security Policy on Population Issues, 1970–1988*. Washington, DC: Information Project for Africa, Inc.

Ingram, Alan. 2010. "Governmentality and Security in the US President's Emergency Plan for AIDS Relief (PEPFAR)." *Geoforum* 41(4):607–16.

Institute for Health Metrics and Evaluation. 2014. *Financing Global Health 2013: Transition in an Age of Austerity* Seattle, WA: Institute for Health Metrics and Evaluation.

International HIV/AIDS Alliance, and Global Fund to Fight AIDS Tuberculosis and Malaria. 2008. *Civil Society Success on the Ground: Community Systems Strengthening and Dual-Track Financing*. Brighton and Geneva: International HIV/AIDS Alliance and Global Fund to Fight AIDS Tuberculosis and Malaria.

International HIV/AIDS Alliance. 1999. *Extracts from Sixth Annual Supporters Meeting Documentation 8th March 1999 – London*. London: International HIV/AIDS Alliance.

International Planned Parenthood Federation Africa Region. n.d. "Where We Work: Nigeria." Available from: www.ippfar.org/en/Where/NG.htm. [7/12/2011].

International Planned Parenthood Federation. 2002. *Learning from the Field: Experiences in HIV Prevention from Family Planning Associations Worldwide*. London: International Planned Parenthood Federation.

2009. *A World of Possibilities*. London: International Planned Parenthood Federation.

n.d.-a. "About IPPF." Available from: www.ippf.org/en/About/. [9/5/2014].

n.d.-b. "Financial." Available from: www.ippf.org/about-us/financial. [9/5/2014].

International Women's Health Program. n.d. "Safe Motherhood Timeline." Available from: http://iwhp.sogc.org/index.php?page=safe-motherhood-timeline&hl=en_US. [1/7/2013].

IRIN. 2012. "Senegal under President Wade." Available from: www.irinnews.org/report.aspx?reportid=94934. [1/14/2015].

Ita, Christian. 2006. "The Last of 'Kuti Original'." *OnlineNigeria*. Available from: http://nm.onlinenigeria.com/templates/?a=6935&z=12. [2/12/2011].

Jahn, Andreas, Sian Floyd, Amelia C Crampin, Frank Mwaungulu, Hazzie Mvula, Fipson Munthali, Nuala McGrath, Johnbosco Mwafilaso, Venance Mwinuka, Bernard Mangongo, Paul E M Fine, Basia Zaba, and Judith R Glynn. 2008. "Population-Level Effect of HIV on Adult

Mortality and Early Evidence of Reversal After Introduction of Antiretroviral Therapy in Malawi." *The Lancet* 371:1603–11.

Janowitz, Barbara, Jane Chege, Andrew Thompson, Naomi Rutenberg, and Rick Homan. 2000. "Community-Based Distribution in Tanzania: Costs and Impacts of Alternative Strategies to Improve Worker Performance." *International Family Planning Perspectives* 26(4):158–60+93–95.

Jepperson, Ronald L. 1991. "Institutions, Institutional Effects, and Institutionalism." Pp. 143–63 in *The New Institutionalism in Organizational Analysis*, edited by Walter W. Powell and Paul J. Dimaggio. Chicago and London: University of Chicago Press.

Jewkes, Rachel K., Mzikazi Nduna, Jonathan Levin, Nwabisa Jama, Kristin Dunkle, Adrian Puren, and Nata Duvvury. 2008. "Impact of Stepping Stones on Incidence of HIV and HSV-2 and Sexual Behaviour in Rural South Africa: Cluster Randomised Controlled Trial." *British Medical Journal* 337(7666).

John Snow, Inc. 1998. *Support to AIDS and Family Health Project: Final Report*. Lilongwe: USAID.

Johnson, Kiersten, Ilona Varallyay, and Paul Ametepi. 2012. *Integration of HIV and Family Planning Health Services in Sub-Saharan Africa: A Review of the Literature, Current Recommendations, and Evidence from the Service Provision Assessment Health Facility Surveys*. Calverton, Maryland: ICF International.

Johnson, Stanley. 1987. *World Population and the United Nations*. Cambridge: Cambridge University Press.

Johnson-Hanks, Jennifer. 2006. *Uncertain Honor: Modern Motherhood in an African Crisis*. Chicago: University of Chicago Press.

Jönsson, Christer, and Peter Söderholm. 1995. "IGO: NGO Relations and HIV/AIDS: Innovation or Stalemate?" *Third World Quarterly* 16(3):459–76.

Joshi, Shareen, and T. Paul Schultz. 2007. *Family Planning as an Investment in Development: Evaluation of a Program's Consequences in Matlab, Bangladesh*. Yale University Economic Growth Center Discussion Paper No. 951. New Haven, CT: Yale University Economic Growth Center.

Jurgens, Ralph, and Fatim Louise Dia. 2006. *Leadership in Action: A Case Study of the "Observatoire," A Group of NGOs in Senegal*. Hove, UK: International HIV/AIDS Alliance.

Kaiser Family Foundation, and UNAIDS. 2016. *Financing the Response to HIV in Low- and Middle-Income Countries: International Assistance from Donor Governments in 2015*. Menlo Park/Washington, DC: Kaiser Family Foundation.

Kaiser Family Foundation. 2015a. "The Global HIV/AIDS Timeline." Available from: www.kff.org/hivaids/timeline/hivtimeline.cfm. [5/16/2016].

2015b. *The U.S. President's Emergency Plan for AIDS Relief (PEPFAR)*. Menlo Park, CA: Kaiser Family Foundation.

Kaler, Amy. 2003. *Running After Pills: Politics, Gender, and Contraception in Colonial Zimbabwe*. Portsmouth, NH: Heinemann.

2004. "The Moral Lens of Population Control: Condoms and Controversies in Southern Malawi." *Studies in Family Planning* 35(2):105–15.

2009. "Health Interventions and the Persistence of Rumour: The Circulation of Sterility Stories in African Public Health Campaigns." *Social Science & Medicine* 68(9):1711–19.

Kalipeni, Ezekiel, and Njeri Mbugua. 2005. "A Review of Preventative Efforts in the Fight against HIV and AIDS in Africa." *Norwegian Journal of Geography* 59:26–36.

Kalipeni, Ezekiel. 1992. "Population Redistribution in Malawi since 1964." *Geographical Review* 82(1):13–28.

1997. "The AIDS Pandemic in Malawi: A Somber Reflection." Pp. 23–47 in *Issues and Perspectives on Health Care in Contemporary Sub-Saharan Africa*, edited by Ezekiel Kalipeni and Philip Thiuri. Lewiston, NY: Edwin Mellen Press.

Kanki, Phyllis J., and Olusoji Adeyi. 2006. "Introduction." Pp. 7–15 in *AIDS in Nigeria: A Nation on the Threshold*, edited by Olusoji Adeyi, Phyllis J. Kanki, Oluwole Odutolu, and John A. Idoko. Cambridge, MA: Harvard University Press.

Kanki, Phyllis, Pradeep Kakkattil, and Mariangela Simao. 2012. "Scaling Up HIV Treatment and Prevention Through National Responses and Innovative Leadership." *JAIDS Journal of Acquired Immune Deficiency Syndromes* 60:S27–30.

Kantner, John F., and Andrew Kantner. 2006. *International Discord on Population and Development*. New York: Palgrave Macmillan.

Karim, Quarraisha Abdool, and Salim S Abdool Karim. 2002. "The Evolving HIV Epidemic in South Africa." *International Journal of Epidemiology* 31(1):37–40.

Karim, Quarraisha Abdool, Cheryl Baxter, and Salim Abdool Karim. 2013. "Topical Microbicides – What's New?" *JAIDS Journal of Acquired Immune Deficiency Syndromes* 63:S144–49.

Kennedy, Barbara. 1984. *Malawi IBRD Population Sector Study*. Washington, DC: The World Bank.

Kerr, David, and Jack Mapanje. 2002. "Academic Freedom and the University of Malawi." *African Studies Review* 45(02):73–91.

Kimball, A.M., S. Cisse, G. Fayemi, S. Ericcson, S. Helfenbein, A. Nakoulima, N. T. Sene, and E. Papiernik. 1988. "Preliminary Report of an Identification Mission for Safe Motherhood, Senegal: Putting the M Back in M.C.H." *International Journal of Gynaecology and Obstetrics* 26(2):181–7.

King, Michael, and Elspeth King. 1992. *The Story of Medicine and Disease in Malawi: The 130 Years Since Livingstone.* Blantyre, Malawi: Montfort Press.

Kingdon, John W. 1995. *Agendas, Alternatives, and Public Policies.* Boston: Little, Brown & Company.

Kippax, Susan, and Martin Holt. 2009. *The State of Social and Political Science Research Related to HIV: A Report for the International AIDS Society.* Geneva: International AIDS Society.

Kiragu, Karungari, Susan Krenn, Bola Kusemiju, Joseph K. T. Ajiboye, Ibiba Chidi, and Otum Kalu. 1996. *Promoting Family Planning Through Mass Media in Nigeria: Campaigns Using a Public Service Announcement and a National Logo.* Baltimore, MD: Johns Hopkins Center for Communication Programs.

Kissling, Frances. 2010. "Close Your Eyes and Think of Rome." *Mother Jones* 35(3):44–45.

Knight, Lindsay. 2008. *UNAIDS: The First 10 Years 1996–2006.* Geneva: UNAIDS.

Kornfield, Ruth. 1996. *Quality of Family Planning Community-Based Distribution Services in Malawi.* Lilongwe: Support to AIDS and Family Health.

La Ferrara, Eliana, Alberto Chong, and Suzanne Duryea. 2008. *Soap Operas and Fertility: Evidence from Brazil.* Inter-American Development Bank Working Paper Series WP-633. Washington, DC: Inter-American Development Bank.

Leahy, Elizabeth. 2007. *The Shape of Things to Come.* Washington, DC: Population Action International.

LeVan, A. Carl. 2015. *Dictators and Democracy in African Development: The Political Economy of Good Governance in Nigeria.* New York: Cambridge University Press.

Lewis, David A. 2011. "HIV/Sexually Transmitted Infection Epidemiology, Management and Control in the IUSTI Africa Region: Focus on Sub-Saharan Africa." *Sexually Transmitted Infections* 87(Suppl 2):ii10–13.

Lewis, Peter M. 1992. "Political Transition and the Dilemma of Civil Society in Africa." *Journal of International Affairs* 46(1):31–54.

Li, Tania Murray. 2007. *The Will to Improve: Governmentality, Development, and the Practice of Politics.* Durham and London: Duke University Press.

Liagin, Elizabeth. 1996. *Excessive Force: Power, Politics, and Population Control*. Washington, DC: Information Project for Africa, Inc.

Lieberman, Evan S. 2007. "Ethnic Politics, Risk, and Policy-Making A Cross-National Statistical Analysis of Government Responses to HIV/AIDS." *Comparative Political Studies* 40(12):1407–32.

2009. *Boundaries of Contagion*. Princeton, NJ: Princeton University Press.

Lo, Nathan, Anita Lowe, and Eran Bendavid. 2016. "Abstinence Funding Was Not Associated with Reductions in HIV Risk Behavior in Sub-Saharan Africa." *Health Affairs*: 35(5): 856–63.

Locoh, Therese, and Yara Makdessi. 1996. *Population Policies and Fertility Decline in Sub-Saharan Africa*. Paris: Centre Français sur la Population et le Développement.

Lom, Mamadou Mika. 2001. "Senegal's Recipe for Success: Early Mobilization and Political Commitment Keep HIV Infections Low." *Africa Recovery* 15(1–2):24–25 +29.

Lordan, Grace, Kam Ki Tang, and Fabrizio Carmignani. 2011. "Has HIV/AIDS Displaced Other Health Funding Priorities? Evidence from a New Dataset of Development Aid for Health." *Social Science & Medicine* 73(3):351–55.

Low-Beer, Daniel, and Rand Stoneburner. 2004. "Uganda and the Challenge of HIV/AIDS." Pp. 165–90 in *The Political Economy of AIDS in Africa*, edited by Nana K. Poku and Alan Whiteside. Aldershot: Ashgate.

Lozano, Rafael, Mohsen Naghavi, Kyle Foreman, et al. 2012. "Global and Regional Mortality from 235 Causes of Death for 20 Age Groups in 1990 and 2010: A Systematic Analysis for the Global Burden of Disease Study 2010." *The Lancet* 380(9859):2095–128.

Luke, Nancy, and Susan Cotts Watkins. 2002. "Reaction of Developing Country Elites to International Population Policy." *Population and Development Review* 28(4):707–33.

Lund, Christian. 2006. "Twilight Institutions: Public Authority and Local Politics in Africa." *Development and Change* 37(4):685–705.

Lush, Louisiana, Gill Walt, John Cleland, and Susannah Mayhew. 2001. "The Role of MCH and Family Planning Services in HIV/STD Control: Is Integration the Answer?" *African Journal of Reproductive Health* 5(3):29–46.

Lwanda, John Lloyd Chipembere. 2002. "*Tikutha*: The Political Culture of the HIV/AIDS Epidemic in Malawi." Pp. 151–65 in *A Democracy of Chameleons: Politics and Culture in the New Malawi*, edited by Harri Englund. Uppsala, Sweden: Nordiska Afrikainstitutet.

2003. "The [In]visibility of HIV/AIDS in the Malawi Public Sphere." *African Journal of AIDS Research* 2(2):113–26.

248References

2004. "Politics, Culture, and Medicine: An Unholy Trinity? Historical Continuities and Ruptures in the HIV/AIDS Story in Malawi." Pp. 29–42 in HIV and AIDS in Africa: Beyond Epidemiology, edited by Ezekiel Kalipeni, Susan Craddock, Joseph R. Oppong, and Jayoti Ghosh. Oxford: Blackwell Publishing Ltd.

2011. ""EDZI Ndi Dolo" ("AIDS is Mighty"): Singing HIV/AIDS in Malawi, 1980–2008." Pp. 384–403 in The Culture of AIDS in Africa: Hope and Healing in Music and the Arts, edited by Gegory Barz and Judah M. Cohen. New York: Oxford University Press.

Macpherson, J. Muir, and Stephen Weymouth. 2012. "The Social Construction of Policy Reform: Economists and Trade Liberalization around the World." International Interactions 38(5):670–702.

Malarcher, Shawn. 2005. Family Planning Success Stories in Sub-Saharan Africa. Baltimore, MD: The INFO Project at the Johns Hopkins Bloomberg School of Public Health/Center for Communication Programs.

Manji, Firoze, and Carl O'Coill. 2002. "The Missionary Position: NGOs and Development in Africa." International Affairs 78(3):567–83.

Marlink, Richard, Phyllis Kanki, Ibou Thior, Karin Travers, Geoffrey Eisen, Tidiane Siby, Ibrahima Traore, Chung-Cheng Hsieh, Mamadou Ciré Dia, El-Hadji Gueye, James Hellinger, Aissatou Guèye-Ndiaye, Jean-Louis Sankalé, Ibrahima Ndoye, Souleymane Mboup, and Max Essex. 1994. "Reduced Rate of Disease Development after HIV-2 Infection as Compared to HIV-1." Science 265(5178):1587–90.

Masebu, Peter. 1997. "Effective STD Treatment Can Reduce HIV." Panafrican News Agency. Available from: http://allafrica.com/stories/199712090057.html. [3/16/2012].

1998. "Call For High Level Commitment To HIV Prevention." Panafrican News Agency. Available from: http://allafrica.com/stories/199806280020.html. [3/16/2012].

Mauldin, W. Parker, and John A Ross. 1991. "Family Planning Programs: Efforts and Results, 1982–89." Studies in Family Planning 22(6):350–67.

May, John F. 2012. World Population Policies: Their Origin, Evolution, and Impact. Dordrecht: Springer.

Mazzocco, K. 1988. "Nigeria's New Population Policy." International Health News 9(3):1, 12.

Mbodj, Fatou, and Bernard Taverne. 2004. "HAART's Impact on the Senegalese AIDS-Association Movement." Pp. 171–81 in The Senegalese Antiretroviral Drug Access Initiative. An Economic, Social, Behavioural and Biomedical Analysis, edited by Alice Desclaux, Isabelle Laniece, Ibra Ndoye, and Bernard Taverne.

Paris: Agence Nationale de Recherches sur le Sida, UNAIDS, World Health Organization.

Mbodj, Mohamed, Babacar Mané, and Waly Badiane. 1992. "Population et "Développement": Quelle Politique?" Pp. 177–204 in *Sénégal, Trajectoires d'un État* edited by Momar-Coumba Diop. Dakar: Codesria.

McDonnell, Terence E. 2016. *Best Laid Plans: Cultural Entropy and the Unraveling of AIDS Media Campaigns.* Chicago and London: University of Chicago Press.

McInnes, Colin, and Kelley Lee. 2012. "Framing and Global Health Governance: Key Findings." *Global Public Health* 7(Suppl 2):S191–98.

McInnes, Colin. 2006. "HIV/AIDS and Security." *International Affairs* 82(2):315–26.

McIntosh, William Alex, and John K. Thomas. 2004. "Economic and Other Societal Determinants of the Prevalence of HIV: A Test of Competing Hypotheses." *The Sociological Quarterly* 45(2):303–24.

McKenna, S. L., G. K. Muyinda, D. Roth, M. Mwali, N. Ngandu, A. Myrick, C. Luo, F. H. Priddy, V. M. Hall, A. A. vonLieven, J. R. Sabatino, K. Mark, and S. A. Allen. 1997. "Rapid HIV Testing and Counseling for Voluntary Testing Centers in Africa." *AIDS* 11:S103–10.

McNamara, Robert S. 1984. "Time Bomb or Myth: The Population Problem." *Foreign Affairs* 62(5):1107–31.

McNicoll, Geoffrey. 2006. "Policy Lessons of the East Asian Demographic Transition." *Population and Development Review* 32(1):1–25.

Mechai Viravaidya Foundation. n.d. "Biography: Mechai Viravaidya." Available from: www.mechaifoundation.org/biography.php. [5/16/2016].

Meda, Nicolas, Ibra Ndoye, Souleymane Mboup, Alpha Wade, Salif Ndiaye, Cheikh Niang, Fatou Sarr, Idrissa Diop, and Michel Carael. 1999. "Low and Stable HIV Infection Rates in Senegal: Natural Course of the Epidemic or Evidence for Success of Prevention?" *AIDS* 13:1397–405.

Medley, Amy, Caitlin Kennedy, Kevin O'Reilly, and Michael Sweat. 2009. "Effectiveness of Peer Education Interventions for HIV Prevention in Developing Countries: A Systematic Review and Meta-Analysis." *AIDS Education and Prevention* 21(3):181–206.

Menzies, Nick, Betty Abang, Rhoda Wanyenze, Fred Nuwaha, Balaarn Mugisha, Alex Coutinho, Rebecca Bunnell, Jonathan Mermini, and John M. Blandford. 2009. "The Costs and Effectiveness of Four HIV Counseling and Testing Strategies in Uganda." *AIDS* 23(3):395–401.

Meredith, Martin. 2005. *The Fate of Africa.* New York: Public Affairs.

Merry, Sally Engle. 2006. "Transnational Human Rights and Local Activism: Mapping the Middle." *American Anthropologist* 108(1):38–51.

Merson, Michael H., James W. Curran, Caroline Hope Griffith, and Braveen Ragunanthan. 2012. "The President's Emergency Plan for AIDS Relief: From Successes of the Emergency Response to Challenges of Sustainable Action." *Health Affairs* 31(7):1380–88.

Merson, Michael H., Jeffrey O'Malley, David Serwadda, and Chantawipa Apisuk. 2008. "HIV Prevention 1: The History and Challenge of HIV Prevention." *The Lancet* 372(9637):475–88.

Meyer, John W. 2004. "The Nation as Babbit: How Countries Conform." *Contexts* 3(3):42–47.

Meyer, John W., John Boli, George M. Thomas, and Francisco O. Ramirez. 1997. "World Society and the Nation-State." *American Journal of Sociology* 103(1):144–81.

Mhloyi, Marvellous M. 1995. "Racing Against Time." Pp. 13–25 in *HIV & AIDS: The Global Inter-Connection*, edited by Elizabeth Reid. Hartford, CT: Kumarian Press.

Migdal, Joel S. 2001. *State in Society: Studying How States and Societies Transform and Constitute One Another*. Cambridge: Cambridge University Press.

Miller, Grant, and Kimberly Singer Babiarz. 2014. *Family Planning: Program Effects*. NBER Working Paper No. 20586. Cambridge, MA: National Bureau of Economics Research.

Miller, Kate, Eliya Msiyaphazi Zulu, and Susan Cotts Watkins. 2001. "Husband-Wife Survey Responses in Malawi." *Studies in Family Planning* 32(2):161–74.

Ministere de la Santé Publique et de l'Action Social, Comite National de Lutte contre le SIDA, Association Nationale des Imams et Oulemas du Senegal, and Jamra. 1995. *Guide Islam et SIDA: Recueil de Sermons et Conferences*. Dakar: Ministere de la Santé Publique et de l'Action Social, Comite National de Lutte contre le SIDA.

Ministerial Leadership Initiative. 2010. "Reducing Financial Barriers to Reproductive Health Care: Senegal Spotlight." Washington, DC: Aspen Global Health and Development.

Ministry of Development Planning and Cooperation. 2010. *RAPID: Population and Development in Malawi*. Lilongwe, Malawi: Population Unit, Ministry of Development Planning and Cooperation.

Ministry of Health and Social Action, National Family Planning Program of Senegal, and Population Council. 1995. *Situation Analysis of the Family Planning Service Delivery System in Senegal – Condensed Report*. Dakar: Population Council.

Ministry of Health. n.d.-a. *Our Common Secret: An Information Booklet on Child Spacing*. Liliongwe: Health Education Section, Ministry of Health.

n.d.-b. *A Pictorial – Story Guide to Child Spacing.* Liliongwe: Health Education Section, Ministry of Health.

Mintrom, Michael, and Phillipa Norman. 2009. "Policy Entrepreneurship and Policy Change." *Policy Studies Journal* 37(4):649–67.

Mintrom, Michael. 1997. "Policy Entrepreneurs and the Diffusion of Innovation." *American Journal of Political Science* 41(3):738–70.

Mitchell, Maura. 2002. ""Living Our Faith:" The Lenten Pastoral Letter of the Bishops of Malawi and the Shift to Multiparty Democracy, 1992–1993." *Journal for the Scientific Study of Religion* 41(1):5–18.

Mkandawire, Paul, Isaac Luginaah, and Rachel Bezner-Kerr. 2011. "Deadly Divide: Malawi's Policy Debate on HIV/AIDS and Condoms." *Policy Sciences* 44(1):81–102.

Mojola, Sanyu A. 2014. *Love, Money, and HIV: Becoming a Modern African Woman in the Age of AIDS.* Berkeley, CA: University of California Press.

Moran, Dominque. 2004. "HIV/AIDS, Governance and Development: The Public Administration Factor." *Public Administration and Development* 24(1):7–18.

Morfit, N. Simon. 2011. ""AIDS Is Money": How Donor Preferences Reconfigure Local Realities." *World Development* 39(1):64–76.

Morris, Martina, and Mirjam Kretzschmar. 1997. "Concurrent Partnerships and the Spread of HIV." *AIDS* 11(5):641–48.

Mosley, Henry H., and Gladys Branic. 1989. "Population Policy in Sub-Saharan Africa: Agendas of International Agencies." Pp. 463–506 in *Population Policy in Sub-Saharan Africa: Drawing on International Experience.* Liege, Belgium: International Union for the Scientific Study of Population.

Moss, Kellie. 2015. *Foreign NGO Engagement in U.S. Global Health Efforts: Foreign NGOs Receiving USG Support Through USAID.* Menlo Park, CA: Kaiser Family Foundation.

Mousky, Stafford. 2002. "UNFPA's Role in the Population Field." Pp. 211–47 in *An Agenda for People: The UNFPA through Three Decades,* edited by Nafis Sadik. New York and London: New York University Press.

Mwaura, Peter. 1999. "Pioneers in the Control of HIV/AIDS." *Africa Recovery* 12(4):8.

Nathanson, Constance A. 2007. *Disease Prevention as Social Change.* New York: Russell Sage Foundation.

National Action Committee on AIDS. 2001. *HIV/AIDS Emergency Action Plan (HEAP).* Abuja: Federal Republic of Nigeria.

2005. *National Strategic Framework for Action (2005–2009).* Abuja: Federal Republic of Nigeria.

National Agency for the Control of AIDS. 2007. *Joint Midterm Review of the HIV/AIDS National Strategic Framework for Action 2005–2009.* Abuja: Federal Republic of Nigeria.

2008. *Global Fund Round 5 HIV/AIDS Programme: Annual Progress Report.* Abuja, Nigeria: National Agency for the Control of AIDS.

2009a. *National HIV/AIDS Policy Review Report.* Abuja: Federal Republic of Nigeria.

2009b. *National Policy on HIV/AIDS.* Abuja: Federal Republic of Nigeria.

2009c. *Nigeria National Response to HIV/AIDS Update.* Abuja: Federal Republic of Nigeria.

2014. *Global AIDS Response Country Progress Report* Abuja: National Agency for the Control of AIDS.

National Family Planning Council. 1998. *Family Planning Handbook for Community Based Distribution Agents in Malawi.* Lilongwe: Ministry of Health and Population.

National Family Welfare Council of Malawi. 1994. *The Malawi National Family Planning Strategy 1994–1998.*

National HIV/AIDS Database Project. 2000. *HIV/AIDS in Nigeria: Past, Present, Impacts.* Lagos: Nigerian Institute of Medical Research.

National Intelligence Council. 2000. *The Global Infectious Disease Threat and Its Implications for the United States.* Washington, DC: National Intelligence Council.

National Research Council. 1986. *Population Growth and Economic Development: Policy Questions.* Washington, DC: The National Academies Press.

National Statistical Office, and ICF Macro. 2011. *Malawi Demographic and Health Survey 2010.* Zomba, Malawi and Calverton, MD: National Statistical Office and ICF Macro.

Nattrass, Nicoli. 2006. "What Determines Cross-Country Access to Antiretroviral Treatment?" *Development Policy Review* 24(3):321–37.

2008. "Are Country Reputations for Good and Bad Leadership on AIDS Deserved? An Exploratory Quantitative Analysis." *Journal of Public Health* 30(4):398–406.

Ndoye, Ibra, Bernard Taverne, Alice Desclaux, Isabelle Lanièce, Marc Egrot, Eric Delaporte, Papa Salif Sow, Souleymane Mboup, Omar Sylla, and Mounirou Ciss. 2004. "The Senegalese Antiretroviral Access Initiative: An Introduction." Pp. 3–19 in *The Senegalese Antiretroviral Drug Access Initiative. An Economic, Social, Behavioural and Biomedical Analysis,* edited by Alice Desclaux, Isabelle Laniece, Ibra Ndoye, and Bernard Taverne. Paris: ANRS, UNAIDS, WHO.

Newland, Lynda. 2001. "The Deployment of the Prosperous Family: Family Planning in West Java." *National Women's Studies Association Journal* 13(3):22–48.

Newton, Gary. 1990. "USAID Support to the Health and Population Sector in Malawi." Paper presented to National Workshop on Population-Development Projects and Program Implementation, Lilongwe.

Ngalamulume, Kalala. 2004. "Keeping the City Totally Clean: Yellow Fever and the Politics of Prevention in Colonial Saint-Louis-du-Sénégal, 1850–1914." *The Journal of African History* 45(2):183–202.

——— 2011. "Prostitution and Disease in French Senegal, 1848–1920." Paper presented to African Studies Association, Washington, DC, November 17–19.

Nguyen, Vinh Kim. 2010. *The Republic of Therapy*. Durham and London: Duke University Press.

Niang, Cheikh Ibrahima, Amadou Moreau, Codou Bop, Cyrille Compaoré, and Moustapha Diagne. 2004. *Targeting Vulnerable Groups in National HIV/AIDS Programs: The Case of Men Who Have Sex with Men*. Washington, DC: World Bank.

Niang, Cheikh Ibrahima. 2001. "Culture and its Impact on HIV/AIDS Prevention and Care: Case Study on the Senegalese Experience." Paper presented to Sub-Reginal Workshop on the Cultural Approach to HIV/AIDS Prevention and Care for Sustainable Human Development, Dakar, August 6–8.

——— 2008. "Senegal: Rethinking HIV/AIDS and Democratic Governance." Pp. 331–72 in *The Political Cost of AIDS in Africa: Evidence from Six Countries*, edited by Kondwani Chirambo. Pretoria: IDASA.

Nichols, Douglas, Salif Ndiaye, Nadine Burton, Barbara Janowitz, Lamine Gueye, and Mouhamadou Gueye. 1985. "Vanguard Family Planning Acceptors in Senegal." *Studies in Family Planning* 16(5):271–78.

Noble, Kenneth B. 1990. "Nigeria Is Spared the Worst of AIDS, but Experts Wonder for How Long." *New York Times*. Available from: www.nytimes.com/1990/11/18/world/nigeria-is-spared-the-worst-of-aids-but-experts-wonder-for-how-long.html. [3/16/2012].

Nortman, Dorothy, and Ellen Hofstatter. 1980. *Population and Family Planning Programs : A Compendium of Data through 1978*. New York: Population Council.

Nugent, Paul. 2004. *Africa Since Independence: A Comparative History*. New York: Palgrave Macmillan.

Nyanda, Macleod E., and Wanderson R. Mmanga. 1990. "Focus Group Exploration of Condoms, Names, Packs and Concepts in Malawi."

Zomba: Centre for Social Research and Demographic Unit, University of Malawi.

O'Malley, J. 2004. "Can This Marriage Work? Linking the Response to AIDS with Sexual and Reproductive Health and Rights." Pp. 58–63 in *Countdown 2015: Sexual and Reproductive Health and Rights for All*, edited by Anuradha Bhattacharjee. Washington, DC: Population Action International.

Obetsebi-Lamptey, Jake, and Michael N. Thomas. 1981. *CSM Feasibility Study – Nigeria*. Washington, DC: USAID Office of Population.

Odimegwu, Clifford O. 1998. *An Appraisal of the National Population Policy for Development*. Ibadan: Development Policy Center.

Odutolu, Oluwole, Babatunde A. Ahonsi, Michael Gboun, and Oluwatoyin M. Jolayemi. 2006. "The National Response to HIV/AIDS." Pp. 241–79 in *AIDS in Nigeria: A Nation on the Threshold*, edited by Olusoji Adeyi, Phyllis J. Kanki, Oluwole Odutolu, and John A. Idoko. Cambridge, MA: Harvard University Press.

Ogbogu, Irene, and Omokhudu Idogho. 2006. "The Role of Civil Society Organizations in HIV/AIDS Control." Pp. 295–308 in *AIDS in Nigeria: A Nation on the Threshold*, edited by Olusoji Adeyi, Phyllis J. Kanki, Oluwole Odutolu, and John A. Idoko. Cambridge, MA: Harvard University Press.

Olukoya, 'Peju, and Jane Ferguson. 2003. "Obituary: Olikoye Ransome-Kuti." *The Lancet* 362:175.

Oluwaseun, Jawando. 2003. "Tribute to a Man of Valour." *Growing Up* 11(2):8.

Omran, Abdel-Rahim. 1992. *Family Planning in the Legacy of Islam*. New York: Routledge/United Nations Population Fund.

Ong, Aiwah, and Stephen J. Collier (Eds.). 2005. *Global Assemblages: Technology, Politics and Ethics as Anthropological Problems*. Oxford: Blackwell Publishing.

Opportunities and Choices Programme. n.d. *Characteristics of Users of BLM Reproductive Health Services in Lilongwe, Factsheet 17*. Southampton, UK: Opportunities and Choices Programme, Department of Social Statistics, University of Southampton.

Organization of the Petroleum Exporting Countries (OPEC). 2016. *OPEC Annual Statistical Bulletin*. Vienna: OPEC.

Orisasona, Sam, Toyin Akpan, and Pius Adejoh. 1996. *People's Perspectives on Family Planning and Population Policies in Nigeria*. Lagos: Empowerment and Action Research Centre.

Orubuloye, I. O. 1983. "Toward National Population Policy on Population." Pp. 170–78 in *Population and Development in Nigeria*, edited by I. O. Orubuloye and O.Y. Oyeneye. Ibadan, Nigeria: Nigerian Institute of Social and Economic Research.

Oster, Emily. 2012. "HIV and Sexual Behavior Change: Why Not Africa?" *Journal of Health Economics* 31(1):35–49.

Ostergard, Robert L., Jr., and Crystal Barcelo. 2005. "Personalist Regimes and the Insecurity Dilemma: Prioritizing AIDS as a National Security Threat in Uganda." Pp. 155–69 in *The African State and the AIDS Crisis*, edited by Amy S. Patterson. Aldershot: Ashgate.

Osuide, Simeon O. 1988. "The 1988 Nigerian Population Policy." *Habitat International* 12(4):119–23.

Oye-Adeniran, Boniface A., Carolyn M. Long, and Isaac F. Adewole. 2004. "Advocacy for Reform of the Abortion Law in Nigeria." *Reproductive Health Matters* 12(24):209–17.

Pachauri, Saroj. 1994. "Relationship between AIDS and Family Planning Programmes: A Rationale for Developing Integrated Reproductive Health Services." *Health Transition Review* 4(Suppl):321–47.

Packard, Randall M., and Paul Epstein. 1991. "Epidemiologists, Social Scientists, and the Structure of Medical Research on AIDS in Africa." *Social Science & Medicine* 33(7):771–94.

Pact Malawi. 2007. *The Response to HIV/AIDS in Malawi: A Civil Society Sector Study*. Lilongwe: Pact Malawi.

Parkhurst, Justin O., and Louisiana Lush. 2004. "The Political Environment of HIV: Lessons from a Comparison of Uganda and South Africa." *Social Science & Medicine* 59(9):1913–24.

Parkhurst, Justin, David Chilongozi, and Eleanor Hutchinson. 2015. "Doubt, Defiance, and Identity: Understanding Resistance to Male Circumcision for HIV Prevention in Malawi." *Social Science & Medicine* 135:15–22.

Patterson, Amy S. 2005. "Introduction: The African State and the AIDS Crisis." Pp. 1–16 in *The African State and the AIDS Crisis*, edited by Amy S. Patterson. Aldershot: Ashgate.

2006. *The Politics of AIDS in Africa*. Boulder, CO: Lynne Rienner Publishers.

2010. "Church Mobilisation and HIV/AIDS Treatment in Ghana and Zambia: A Comparative Analysis." *African Journal of AIDS Research* 9(4):407–18.

2011. *The Church and AIDS in Africa*. Boulder and London: First Forum Press.

2013. "Pastors as Leaders in Africa's Religious AIDS Mobilisation: Cases from Ghana and Zambia." *Canadian Journal of African Studies/La Revue canadienne des études africaines* 47(2):207–26.

Patton, Cindy. 1990. *Inventing AIDS*. New York and London: Routledge.

2002. *Globalizing AIDS*. Minneapolis, MN: University of Minnesota Press.

Paxton, Nathan A. 2012. "Political Science(s) and HIV: A Critical Analysis." *Contemporary Politics* 18(2):141–55.

Pearce, Tola Olu. 1995. "Women's Reproductive Practices and Biomedicine: Cultural Conflicts and Transformations in Nigeria." Pp. 195–208 in *Conceiving the New World Order: The Global Politics of Reproduction*, edited by Faye D. Ginsburg and Rayna Rapp. Berkeley, CA: University of California Press.

PEPFAR. 2014. *Tenth Annual Report to Congress*. Washington, DC: PEPFAR.

2015. *PEPFAR Country/Regional Operational Plan (COP/ROP) 2015 Guidance*. Washington, DC: PEPFAR.

Pepin, Jacques. 2011. *The Origins of AIDS*. Cambridge: Cambridge University Press.

Performance Needs Assessment Team. 2001. *Assessing the Performance of Family Planning Service at the Primary Care Level in Nigerian Local Government Area Health Centers and NGO Clinics*. Washington, DC: USAID.

Peters, Pauline E., Daimon Kambewa, and Peter A. Walker. 2010. "Contestations Over "Tradition" and "Culture" in a Time of AIDS." *Medical Anthropology* 29(3):278–302.

Pfeiffer, James. 2004. "Condom Social Marketing, Pentecostalism, and Structural Adjustment in Mozambique: A Clash of AIDS Prevention Messages." *Medical Anthropology Quarterly* 18(1):77–103.

Phillips, James F., Elizabeth F. Jackson, Ayaga A. Bawah, Bruce MacLeod, Philip Adongo, Colin Baynes, and John Williams. 2012. "The Long-Term Fertility Impact of the Navrongo Project in Northern Ghana." *Studies in Family Planning* 43(3):175–90.

Phillips, James F., Wayne S. Stinson, Shushum Bhatia, Makhlisur Rahman, and J. Chakraborty. 1982. "The Demographic Impact of the Family Planning–Health Services Project in Matlab, Bangladesh." *Studies in Family Planning* 13(5):131–40.

Phillips, James F., Wendy L. Greene, and Elizabeth F. Jackson. 1999. *Lessons from Community-based Distribution of Family Planning in Africa*. New York: Population Council.

Phoolcharoen, Wiput. 1998. "HIV/AIDS Prevention in Thailand: Success and Challenges." *Science* 280(5371):1873–74.

Pierson, Paul. 1993. "Review: When Effect Becomes Cause: Policy Feedback and Political Change." *World Politics* 45(4):595–628.

2000. "Increasing Returns, Path Dependence, and the Study of Politics." *The American Political Science Review* 94(2):251–67.

Pigg, Stacey Leigh, and Vincanne Adams. 2005. "Introduction: The Moral Object of Sex." Pp. 1–38 in *Sex in Development: Science, Sexuality, and Morality and Global Perspective*, edited by Vincanne Adams and Stacy Leigh Pigg. Durham and London: Duke University Press.

Pillai, Vijayan K., T. S. Sunil, and Rashmi Gupta. 2003. "AIDS Prevention in Zambia: Implications for Social Services." *World Development* 31(1):149–61.

Piot, Peter. 2012. *No Time to Lose: A Life in Pursuit of Deadly Viruses*. New York and London: WW Norton and Company.

Pisani, Elizabeth. 1999. *Acting Early to Prevent AIDS: The Case of Senegal*. Geneva: UNAIDS.

  2000. "AIDS in the 21st Century: Some Critical Considerations." *Reproductive Health Matters* 8(15):63–76.

  2008. *The Wisdom of Whores: Bureaucrats, Brothels, and the Business of AIDS*. New York and London: WW Norton and Company.

Planned Parenthood Federation of Nigeria. n.d. "About PPFN." Available from: www.ppfn.org/about.html. [7/12/2011].

Poleykett, Branwyn. 2012. "Intimacy, Technoscience, and the City: Regulating "Prostitution" in Dakar, 1946–2010." PhD Dissertation: London School of Economics.

  2015. "Molecular and Municipal Politics: Research and Regulation in Dakar." Pp. 237–56 in *Para-States and Medical Science: Making African Global Health*, edited by P. Wenzel Geissler. Durham and London: Duke University Press.

Polgreen, Lydia. 2005. "Nigeria in Deal to Pay Off Most of Its Foreign Debt." *New York Times*. Available from: www.nytimes.com/2006/04/22/world/22nigeria.html. [3/5/2015].

Population Council. 2013. *Big Ideas: Population Council 2013 Annual Report*. New York: Population Council.

Population Information Communication Branch. n.d. *A Nation's Population as an Asset, Not a Liability*. Apapa, Nigeria: Federal Ministry of Information and Culture.

Population Reference Bureau. 2015. *2015 World Population Data Sheet*. Washington, DC: Population Reference Bureau.

Population Services International. n.d.-a "Nigeria." Available from: www.psi.org/nigeria. [7/13/2011].

  n.d.-b "PSI At A Glance." Available from: www.psi.org/about/at-a-glance/. [5/18/2012].

Population Technical Assistance Project. 1988. *Contraceptive Social Marketing (CSM) Assessment*. Arlington, VA: International Science and Technology Institute, Inc.

Potts, Malcolm, Daniel T. Halperin, Douglas Kirby, Ann Swidler, Elliot Marseille, Jeffrey D. Klausner, Norman Hearst, Richard G. Wamai, James G. Kahn, and Julia Walsh. 2008. "Reassessing HIV Prevention." *Science* 320:749–50.

Potts, Malcolm, Eliya Zulu, Michael Wehner, Federico Castillo, and Courtney Henderson. 2013. *Crisis in the Sahel: Possible Solutions and the Consequences of Inaction.* Berkeley, CA: University of California, Berkeley and African Institute for Development Policy.

Poulin, Michelle, and Adamson S. Muula. 2011. "An Inquiry into the Uneven Distribution of Women's HIV Infection in Rural Malawi." *Demographic Research* 25(28):869–902.

Preston-Whyte, Eleanor. 2008. "Culture in Action: Reactions to Social Responses to HIV/AIDS in Africa." Pp. 255–75 in *AIDS, Culture, and Africa*, edited by Douglas A. Feldman. Gainesville: University Press of Florida.

Prins, Gwyn. 2004. "AIDS and Global Security." *International Affairs* 80(5):931–52.

Pritchett, Lant H. 1994. "Desired Fertility and the Impact of Population Policies." *Population and Development Review* 20(1):1–55.

Pritchett, Lant, and Michael Woolcock. 2004. "Solutions When the Solution is the Problem: Arraying the Disarray in Development." *World Development* 32(2):191–212.

Probst, Peter. 1999. "'Mchape' '95, or, the Sudden Fame of Billy Goodson Chisupe: Healing, Social Memory and the Enigma of the Public Sphere in Post-Banda Malawi." *Africa: Journal of the International African Institute* 69(1):108–37.

ProCon.org. 2015. "100 Countries and Their Prostitution Policies." Available from: http://prostitution.procon.org/view.resource.php?resourceID=000772. [5/17/2016].

Pronyk, Paul M., James R. Hargreaves, Julia C. Kim, Linda A. Morison, Godfrey Phetla, Charlotte Watts, Joanna Busza, and John D. H. Porter. 2006. "Effect of a Structural Intervention for the Prevention of Intimate-Partner Violence and HIV in Rural South Africa: A Cluster Randomised Trial." *The Lancet* 368(9551):1973–83.

Putzel, James. 2003. *Institutionalising an Emergency Response: HIV/AIDS and Governance in Uganda and Senegal.* London: Department for International Development.

2004. "The Global Fight Against AIDS: How Adequate Are the National Commissions?" *Journal of International Development* 16(8):1129–40.

2006. "A History of State Action: The Politics of AIDS in Uganda and Senegal." Pp. 171–84 in *The HIV/AIDS Epidemic in Sub-Saharan*

Africa in a Historical Perspective, edited by Philippe Denis and Charles Becker. Dakar: Réseau Sénégal: Droit, Éthique et Santé.

Quist-Arcton, Ofeibea. 2001. "Seven-Part Series on AIDS in Senegal." *AllAfrica*. Available from: http://allafrica.com/stories/200106260446.html. [3/16/2012].

Radelet, Steven. 2010. *Emerging Africa: How 17 Countries Are Leading the Way*. Washington, DC: Center for Global Development.

Raufu, Abiodun. 2001. "AIDS Scare Hits Nigerian military." *AIDS Analysis Africa* 11(5):14.

———. 2002. "Nigeria Promises Free Antiretroviral Drugs to HIV Positive Soldiers." *BMJ* 324(7342):870.

———. 2003. "Obituaries: Olikoye Ransome-Kuti." *British Medical Journal* 326 1400.

Reaves, Jessica. 2007. "What the Rest of Africa Could Learn about AIDS." *Chicago Tribune* April 22:2.1.

Reid, Elizabeth. 1995. *HIV and Development: The Lessons of Cairo*. New York: United Nations Development Programme.

Renaud, Michelle Lewis. 1997. *Women at the Crossroads: A Prostitute Community's Response to AIDS in Urban Senegal*. London: Routledge.

Renders, Marleen. 2002. "An Ambiguous Adventure: Muslim Organisations and the Discourse of 'Development' in Senegal." *Journal of Religion in Africa* 32(1):61–82.

Reniers, Georges, and Susan Watkins. 2010. "Polygyny and the Spread of HIV in Sub-Saharan Africa: A Case of Benign Concurrency." *AIDS* 24(2):299–307.

Renne, Elisha P. 1996. "Perceptions of Population Policy, Development, and Family Planning Programs in Northern Nigeria." *Studies in Family Planning* 27(3):127–36.

———. 2003. *Population and Progress in a Yoruba Town*. Ann Arbor: University of Michigan Press.

———. 2010. *The Politics of Polio in Northern Nigeria*. Bloomington: Indiana University Press.

———. 2016. "Interpreting Population Policy in Nigeria." Pp. 260–89 in *Reproductive States: Global Perspectives on the Invention and Implementation of Population Policy*, edited by Rickie Solinger and Mie Nakachi. New York: Oxford University Press.

République du Sénégal. 2005. "Loi n° 2005–18, du 5 Août 2005, Relative à la Santé de la Reproduction." Dakar: République du Sénégal.

Réseau Islam et Population. 1996. *La Déclaration de Politique de Population à la Lumière des Enseignements Islamiques*. Dakar: République du Sénégal/FUNUAP.

Richey, Lisa Ann, and Stefano Ponte. 2011. *Brand Aid: Shopping Well to Save the World*. Minneapolis, MN: University of Minnesota Press.

Richey, Lisa Ann. 2003. "HIV/AIDS in the Shadows of Reproductive Health Interventions." *Reproductive Health Matters* 11(22):30–35.

2004. "Construction, Control and Family Planning in Tanzania: Some Bodies the Same and Some Bodies Different." *Feminist Review* 78:56–79.

2005. "Uganda: HIV/AIDS and Reproductive Health." Pp. 95–126 in *Where Human Rights Begin: Health, Sexuality, and Women in the New Millennium*, edited by Wendy Chavkin and Ellen Chesler. New Brusnwick, NJ: Rutgers University Press.

2008. *Population Politics and Development: From the Policies to the Clinics*. New York: Palgrave Macmillan.

Robinson, Rachel Sullivan. 2010a. "Social Resources and Health Disparities: The Impact of NGOs on HIV Prevalence and Treatment in Sub-Saharan Africa." Paper presented to American Sociological Association, Atlanta, GA, August 14–17.

2010b. *UNFPA in Context: An Institutional History*. Washington, DC: Center for Global Development.

2011. "From Population to HIV: The Organizational and Structural Determinants of HIV Outcomes in Sub-Saharan Africa." *Journal of the International AIDS Society* 14(Suppl 2):1–13.

2012. "Negotiating Development Prescriptions: The Case of Population Policy in Nigeria." *Population Research and Policy Review* 31 (2):267–96.

2015. "Population Policy in Sub-Saharan Africa: A Case of Both Normative and Coercive Ties to the World Polity." *Population Research and Policy Review* 34(2):201–21.

2016. "Population Policy Adoption in Sub-Saharan Africa: An Interplay of Global and Local Forces." *Population Horizons* 13(1):1–9.

Rosenberg, Tina. 2014. "On AIDS: Three Lessons from Africa." [Blog] *Opinionator*. Available from: http://opinionator.blogs.nytimes.com/20 14/07/31.

Rosenfield, Allan G., and Caroline J. Min. 2007. "The Emergence of Thailand's National Family Planning Program." Pp. 221–33 in *The Global Family Planning Revolution*, edited by Warren C. Robinson and John A. Ross. Washington, DC: The World Bank.

Ross, John, and Ellen Smith. 2011. "Trends in National Family Planning Programs, 1999, 2004 and 2009." *International Perspectives on Sexual and Reproductive Health* 37(3):125–33.

Ruger, Jennifer Prah. 2005. "The Changing Role of the World Bank in Global Health." *American Journal of Public Health* 95(1):60–70.

Rushton, Simon. 2010. "Framing AIDS: Securitization, Development-ization, Rights-ization." *Global Health Governance* 4(1).

Rutenberg, Naomi, and Deborah Weiss. 2010. "Horizons: Looking Back, Moving Forward." *Public Health Reports* 125(2):269–71.

Sachs, Jeffrey D. 2012. "How Malawi Fed Its Own People." *The New York Times*. Available from: www.nytimes.com/2012/04/20/opinion/how-m alawi-fed-its-own-people.html?_r=2. [2/25/2015].

Sadik, Nafis (Ed.). 2002. *Agenda for People: The UNFPA Through Three Decades*. New York: New York University Press.

SAfAIDS, and Ford Foundation. n.d. *Success Story – Towards Universal Access to Comprehensive Sexual & Reproductive Health Services: Malawi's Implementation of the Maputo Plan of Action (MPoA) – The Milestones Achieved*. Harare: SAfAIDS and Ford Foundation.

Sai, Fred T. 1994. *Dr. Fred Sai Speaks Out*. London: International Planned Parenthood Federation.

Sai, Fred T., and Lauren A. Chester. 1990. "The Role of the World Bank in Shaping Third World Population Policy." Pp. 179–91 in *Population Policy: Contemporary Issues*, edited by Godfrey Roberts. New York: Praeger.

Sala-Diakanda, Daniel M. 1996. *Mission Report: Programme Review and Strategy Development (PRSD) Exercise in Nigeria*. Addis Ababa: Economic Commission for Africa.

Sanogo, Diouratié, Saumya RamaRao, Heidi Jones, Penda N'Diaye, Bineta M'Bow, and Cheikh Bamba Diop. 2003. "Improving Quality of Care and Use of Contraceptives in Senegal." *African Journal of Reproductive Health / La Revue Africaine de la Santé Reproductive* 7(2):57–73.

Sawers, Larry, and Eileen Stillwaggon. 2010. "Understanding the Southern African 'Anomaly': Poverty, Endemic Disease and HIV." *Development and Change* 41(2):195–224.

Sayagues, Mercedes. 2004. "Cardinals and Khalifs Unite Against AIDS." *Inter Press Service News Agency*. Available from: http://ipsnews.net/ new_nota.asp?idnews=24549. [3/14/2012].

Schindlmayr, Thomas. 2004. "Explicating Donor Trends for Population Assistance." *Population Research and Policy Review* 23:25–54.

Schneider, William H. 2013. "History of Blood Transfusion in Sub-Saharan Africa." *Transfusion Medicine Reviews* 27(1):21–8.

Schoepf, Brooke G. 2001. "International AIDS Research in Anthropology: Taking a Critical Perspective on the Crisis." *Annual Review of Anthropology* 30:335–61.

Schoffeleers, Matthew. 1999. "The AIDS Pandemic, the Prophet Billy Chisupe, and the Democratization Process in Malawi." *Journal of Religion in Africa* 29(4):406–41.

Seck, Mamadou Mansour. 2001. "Testimony of Ambassador Mamadou Mansour Seck from Senegal on HIV/AIDS: The Case of Senegal and USAID Support." Hearing to House Committee on International Relations, United States Congress, June 7.

Seckinelgin, Hakan. 2012. "The Global Governance of Success in HIV/AIDS Policy: Emergency Action, Everyday Lives and Sen's Capabilities." *Health & Place* 18(3):453–60.

Seeley, Janet, Charlotte H Watts, Susan Kippax, Steven Russell, Lori Heise, and Alan Whiteside. 2012. "Addressing the Structural Drivers of HIV: A Luxury or Necessity for Programmes?" *Journal of the International AIDS Society* 15(Suppl 1):17397.

Seidel, G. 1993. "The Competing Discourses of HIV/AIDS in Sub-Saharan Africa: Discourses of Rights and Empowerment vs Discourses of Control and Exclusion." *Social Science & Medicine* 36(3):175–94.

Sending, Ole Jacob, and Iver B. Neumann. 2006. "Governance to Governmentality: Analyzing NGOs, States, and Power." *International Studies Quarterly* 50(3):651–72.

Sène, Rokhaya. 2005. "La Problematique de la Population et de la Pauvrété au Sénégal dans un Contexte d'Ajustement Structurel." PhD Dissertation, Département de Géographie: Université Cheikh Anta Diop.

Sepúlveda, Jaime, and Christopher Murray. 2014. "The State of Global Health in 2014." *Science* 345(6202):1275–78.

Serieux, John E., Spy Munthali, Ardeshir Sepehri, and Robert White. 2012. "The Impact of the Global Economic Crisis on HIV and AIDS Programs in a High Prevalence Country: The Case of Malawi." *World Development* 40(3):501–15.

Setel, Philip W., Milton Lewis, and Maryinez Lyons (Eds.). 1999. *Histories of Sexually Transmitted Diseases and HIV/AIDS in Sub-Saharan Africa*. Westport, CT and London: Greenwood Press.

Shelton, James D. 2007. "Ten Myths and One Truth about Generalised HIV Epidemics." *The Lancet* 370(9602):1809–11.

Shiffman, Jeremy, and Ana Lucía Garcés del Valle. 2006. "Political History and Disparities in Safe Motherhood between Guatemala and Honduras." *Population and Development Review* 32(1):53–80.

Shiffman, Jeremy, and Friday E. Okonofua. 2007. "The State of Political Priority for Safe Motherhood in Nigeria." *British Journal of Obstetrics and Gynaecology* 114(2):127–33.

Shiffman, Jeremy, and Stephanie Smith. 2007. "Generation of Political Priority for Global Health Initiatives: A Framework and Case Study of Maternal Mortality." *The Lancet* 370(9595):1370–79.

Shiffman, Jeremy, David Berlan, and Tamara Hafner. 2009. "Has Aid for AIDS Raised All Health Funding Boats?" *JAIDS Journal of Acquired Immune Deficiency Syndromes* 52:S45–48.

Shiffman, Jeremy. 2008. "Has Donor Prioritization of HIV/AIDS Displaced Aid for Other Health Issues?" *Health Policy and Planning* 23:95–100.

Shircliff, Eric J., and John M. Shandra. 2011. "Non-Governmental Organizations, Democracy, and HIV Prevalence: A Cross-National Analysis." *Sociological Inquiry* 81(2):143–73.

Silliman, Jael Miriam. 1999. "Expanding Civil Society, Shrinking Political Spaces." Pp. 133–62 in *Dangerous Intersections*, edited by Jael Miriam Silliman and Ynestra King: South End Press.

Simmons, Ann M. 2001. "In AIDS-Ravaged Africa, Senegal Is a Beacon of Hope." *Los Angeles Times*. Available from: http://articles.latimes.com/ 2001/mar/09/news/mn-35429. [9/29/2014].

Simmons, George, and Rushikesh Maru. 1988. *The World Bank's Population Lending and Sector Review*. Washington, DC: Population and Human Resources Department, The World Bank.

Sinding, Steven W. 1991. *Strengthening the Bank's Population Work in the Nineties*. Washington, DC: Population and Human Resources Department, The World Bank.

Sinding, Steven, and Sara Seims. 2002. "Challenges Remain but Will Be Different." Pp. 137–50 in *An Agenda for People: The UNFPA through Three Decades*, edited by Nafis Sadik. New York and London: New York University Press.

Singh, Jyoti Shankar. 2002. "UNFPA and the Global Conferences." Pp. 152–74 in *An Agenda for People: The UNFPA through Three Decades*, edited by Nafis Sadik. New York and London: New York University Press.

Singh, Susheela, Jacqueline E. Darroch, and Lori S. Ashford. 2014. *Adding It Up: The Costs and Benefits of Investing in Reproductive Health for 2014*. New York: Guttmacher Institute and UNFPA.

Singhal, Arvind, and Everett M. Rogers. 2003. *Combating AIDS: Communication Strategies in Action*. Thousand Oaks: Sage.

Skocpol, Theda, and Edwin Amenta. 1986. "States and Social Policies." *Annual Review of Sociology* 12(1):131–57.

Skocpol, Theda. 1992. *Protecting Soldiers and Mothers: The Political Origins of Social Policy in the United States*. Cambridge, MA: Harvard University Press.

Smith, Daniel Jordan. 2004a. "Contradictions in Nigeria's Fertility Transition: The Burdens and Benefits of Having People." *Population and Development Review* 30(2):221–38.

2004b. "Premarital Sex, Procreation, and HIV Risk in Nigeria." *Studies in Family Planning* 35(4):223–35.

2007. *The Culture of Corruption*. Princeton, NJ: Princeton University Press.

2010. "Corruption, NGOs, and Development in Nigeria." *Third World Quarterly* 31(2):243–58.

2014. *AIDS Doesn't Show Its Face: Inequality, Morality, and Social Change in Nigeria*. Chicago: University of Chicago Press.

Smith, Julia H., and Alan Whiteside. 2010. "The History of AIDS Exceptionalism." *Journal of the International AIDS Society* 13(1):47–47.

Society for Women and AIDS in Africa Nigeria Chapter. n.d. "Welcome." Available from: www.swaa-nigeria.org/new/index.php. [3/11/2015].

Solo, Julie, Roy Jacobstein, and Deliwe Malema. 2005. *Repositioning Family Planning – Malawi Case Study: Choice, Not Chance*. New York: The ACQUIRE Project/EngenderHealth.

SOMARC/The Futures Group International. 1997. *SOMARC Country Workplans*. Washington, DC: SOMARC/The Futures Group International.

Starrs, Ann M. 2006. "Safe Motherhood Initiative: 20 years and Counting." *The Lancet* 368(9542):1130–32.

Stephens, Betsy, and Bineta Ba. 1996. *Evaluation of the Senegal Social Marketing Program*. Dakar: USAID.

Stillwaggon, Eileen. 2003. "Racial Metaphors: Interpreting Sex and AIDS in Africa." *Development and Change* 34(5):809–32.

2006. *AIDS and the Ecology of Poverty*. Oxford: Oxford University Press.

Stoler, Ann Laura. 1995. *Race and the Education of Desire*. Durham and London: Duke University Press.

2002. *Carnal Knowledge and Imperial Power: Race and the Intimate in Colonial Rule*. Berkeley, Los Angeles, and London: University of California Press.

Stover, John, Leanne Dougherty, and Margaret Ham. 2006. *Are Cost Savings Incurred by Offering Family Planning Services at Emergency Plan HIV/AIDS Care and Treatment Facilities?* Washington, DC: USAID.

Strachan, Molly, Akua Kwateng-Addo, Karen Hardee, Sumi Subramaniam, Nicole Judice, and Koki Agar. 2004. *An Analysis of Family Planning Content in HIV/AIDS, VCT, and PMTCT Policies in 16 Countries*. POLICY Working Paper Series No. 9. Washington, DC: POLICY Project.

Strand, Per. 2012. "Public Opinion as Leadership Disincentive: Exploring a Governance Dilemma in the AIDS Response in Africa." *Contemporary Politics* 18(2):174–85.

Stratton, Sara. 2015. "Senegal Celebrates Great Progress in Family Planning During National Review." [Blog] *Vital*. Available from: www.intra

health.org/blog/senegal-celebrates-great-progress-family-planning-dur ing-national-review#.VQn58o54pcQ. [2/25/2014].

Suberu, Rotimi T. 2001. *Federalism and Ethnic Conflict in Nigeria.* Washington, DC: United States Institute of Peace Press.

Sullivan, Rachel. 2007. "Leveraging the Global Agenda for Progress: Population Policies and Non-Governmental Organizations in Sub-Saharan Africa." PhD Dissertation, Graduate Group in Sociology and Demography: University of California, Berkeley.

Susser, Ida. 2009. *AIDS, Sex, and Culture: Global Politics and Survival in Southern Africa.* Chichester, West Sussex: Wiley-Blackwell.

Sweat, Michael D., Julie Denison, Caitlin Kennedy, Virginia Tedrow, and Kevin O'Reilly. 2012. "Effects of Condom Social Marketing on Condom Use in Developing Countries: A Systematic Review and Metaanalysis, 1990–2010." *Bulletin of the World Health Organization* 90(8):613–22.

Swidler, Ann, and Susan Cotts Watkins. 2017. *A Fraught Embrace: The Romance and Reality of AIDS Altruism in Africa.* Princeton and Oxford: Princeton University Press.

Taha, Taha E., Gina A. Dallabetta, Donald R. Hoover, John D. Chiphangwi, Laban A. R. Mtimavalye, George N. Liomba, Newton I. Kumwenda, and Paolo G. Miotti. 1998. "Trends of HIV-1 and Sexually Transmitted Diseases among Pregnant and Postpartum Women in Urban Malawi." *AIDS* 12(2):197–203.

Tarnoff, Curt. 1994. *Population and Development: The 1994 Cairo Conference.* Washington, DC: Congressional Research Service.

Tavory, Iddo, and Ann Swidler. 2009. "Condom Semiotics: Meaning and Condom Use in Rural Malawi." *American Sociological Review* 74(2):171–89.

Tawfik, Linda, and Susan Cotts Watkins. 2007. "Sex in Geneva, Sex in Lilongwe, and Sex in Balaka." *Social Science & Medicine* 64(5):1090–101.

The AIDS Support Organisation. n.d. "About TASO." Available from: www .tasouganda.org/index.php?option=com_content&view=article&i d=51&Itemid=61. [5/22/2012].

The Futures Group. 1983. *The Effects of Population Factors on Social and Economic Development.* Washington, DC: The Futures Group.

The Guardian. 1987. "Emphasis on Health Care Programme." *The Guardian* (Lagos) 1/1/87:1–2.

The Lancet. 2011. "HIV Treatment as Prevention – It Works." *The Lancet* 377(9779):1719.

The Washington Post. 2003. "Text of President Bush's 2003 State of the Union Address." Available from: www.washingtonpost.com/wp-srv/o npolitics/transcripts/bushtext_012803.html. [5/16/2012].

Thioye, Ismail Diene. 1998. *Barrières à la Distribution à Base Communautaire et à la Commercailisation Sociale des Contraceptifs au Sénégal*. Dakar: Direction de la Planification Des Ressources Humaines.

Thomas, Lynn M. 2003. *Politics of the Womb: Women, Reproduction, and the State in Kenya*. Berkeley and Los Angeles: University of California Press.

Thompson, Catherine. 1995. *Condom Initiative (Condoms, Contraception and Marriage): Report on Consultation Meeting*. Lilongwe: Support to AIDS and Family Health.

Tieu, Hong-Van, Morgane Rolland, Scott M. Hammer, and Magdalena E. Sobieszczyk. 2013. "Translational Research Insights from Completed HIV Vaccine Efficacy Trials." *JAIDS Journal of Acquired Immune Deficiency Syndromes* 63:S150–54.

Tilly, Charles. 2001. "Mechanisms in Political Processes." *Annual Review of Political Science* 4(1):21–41.

Timberg, Craig, and Daniel Halperin. 2012. *Tinderbox: How the West Sparked the AIDS Epidemic and How the World Can Finally Overcome*. New York: Penguin Press.

Timbs, Liz. 2011. "Lethal, Incurable, and Controversial: The Responses of American NGOs to the AIDS Epidemic in Southern Africa." MA Thesis, Department of History, George Washington University.

Tipping, Sharon. 1993. *The Marketing of CSM Condoms for AIDS Prevention*. Rosslyn, VA: USAID/Office of Population.

Torfing, Jacob. 2009. "Rethinking Path Dependence in Public Policy Research." *Critical Policy Studies* 3(1):70–83.

Trinitapoli, Jenny, and Alexander Weinreb. 2012. *Religion and AIDS in Africa*. New York: Oxford University Press.

Trussell, James. 2011. "Contraceptive Efficacy." Pp. 779–863 in *Contraceptive Technology:20th Revised Edition*, edited by Robert A. Hatcher, James Trussell, Anita L. Nelson, Willard Cates, Deborah Kowal, and Michael S. Policar. New York: Ardent Media.

TvT Associates. 2002. *HIV/AIDS in Nigeria: A USAID Brief*. Washington, DC: The Synergy Project.

TvT Associates/The Synergy Project. 2002. *USAID/Nigeria HIV/AIDS Strategy Assessment Report*. Washington, DC: TvT Associates.

Umeh, Davidson, and Florence Ejike. 2004. "The Role of NGOs in HIV/AIDS Prevention in Nigeria." *Dialectical Anthropology* 28(3):339–52.

UNAIDS Leadership Transition Working Group. 2009. *UNAIDS: Preparing for the Future*. Washington, DC: Center for Global Development.

UNAIDS, and Harvard School of Public Health. 1999. *Level and Flow of National and International Resources for the Response to HIV/AIDS, 1996–1997*. Geneva: UNAIDS.

UNAIDS, and World Health Organization. 2008. *Epidemiological Fact Sheet: Malawi.* Geneva: UNAIDS and WHO.

UNAIDS. 2008. *Report on the Global AIDS Epidemic.* Geneva: UNAIDS.

2009. "Leadership in Senegal's AIDS Response." Available from: www .unaids.org/en/KnowledgeCentre/Resources/FeatureStories/archive/20 09/20090409_Senegal.asp. [28 April 2010].

2010. *Report on the Global AIDS Epidemic.* Geneva: UNAIDS.

2011. *Countdown to Zero.* Geneva: UNAIDS.

2014. *The Gap Report.* Geneva: UNAIDS.

2016a. "Country Factsheets: Malawi, 2015." Available from: http://aid sinfo.unaids.org/. [12/29/16].

2016b. "Country Factsheets: Senegal, 2015." Available from: http://aid sinfo.unaids.org/. [12/29/16].

United Nations Development Programme. 2014. *Human Development Report 2014: Sustaining Human Progress – Reducing Vulnerabilities and Building Resilience.* New York: United Nations Development Programme.

United Nations Population Division. 2003. *National Responses to HIV/ AIDS: A Review of Progress.* New York: United Nations Population Division.

United Nations Population Fund (UNFPA). 1981. *Inventory of Population Projects in Developing Countries Around the World 1979/80.* New York: UNFPA.

1986. *Inventory of Population Projects in Developing Countries Around the World 1984/85.* New York: UNFPA.

2004. *Population, Reproductive Health and Gender Equity in Malawi: An Overview of UNFPA's Contribution 2002–2006.* Lilongwe: UNFPA.

2006. *Financial Resource Flows for Population Activities in 2004.* New York: UNFPA.

2009. *Financial Resource Flows for Population Activities in 2007.* New York: UNFPA.

2013. *Financial Resource Flows for Population Activities in 2011.* New York: UNFPA.

2014. *Financial Resource Flows for Population Activities in 2012.* New York: United Nations Population Fund.

n.d. "Preventing HIV Infection, Promoting Reproductive Health." Available from: www.unfpa.org/publications/preventing-hiv-infection-promoting-reproductive-health. [12/22/2014].

United Nations. 1988. *Case Studies in Population Policy: Nigeria.* New York: Department of International Economic and Social Affairs.

2003. *Networking: Directory of African NGOs, Second Edition.* New York: United Nations.

United States Agency for International Development (USAID) Africa Bureau. 1998. *Family Planning and Health Activities in Nigeria.* Washington, DC: USAID.

United States Agency for International Development (USAID). 1992a. *Project Authorization for the Senegal AIDS Control and Prevention Project.* Dakar: USAID.

1992b. *Senegal Child Survival/Family Planning (SCS/FP) Project – Project Paper.* Dakar: USAID.

1992c. *Support to AIDS and Family Health (STAFH) Project Paper, Volume I.* Washington, DC: USAID; emphasis in the original.

1994. *Nigeria Family Health Services: Project Paper.* Washington, DC: USAID.

1995. *Family Planning In Nigeria: The Human Costs Of Discontinuing USAID'S Family Planning Program.* Washington, DC: USAID.

1998. *Family Planning and Health Activities in Senegal.* Washington, DC: USAID Africa Bureau.

1999a. *Nigeria and HIV/AIDS: Key Talking Points.* Washington, DC: USAID.

1999b. *Senegal and HIV/AIDS: Key Talking Points.* Washington, DC: USAID.

2002. *USAID/Senegal HIV/AIDS Strategy 2002–2006 (Draft).* Washington, DC: USAID.

2003a. *Success Stories HIV/AIDS – Film Romance Persuades Nigerians to Practice Safe Sex.* Washington, DC: USAID.

2003b. *Senegal Country Profile, HIV/AIDS.* Washington, DC: USAID Bureau for Global Health.

2004a. *Directory of Associations of People Living with HIV/AIDS, Second Edition.* Washington, DC: USAID.

2004b. *Health Profile: Senegal – HIV/AIDS.* Dakar: USAID.

2013. "HIV and AIDS Timeline." Available from: www.usaid.gov/what-we-do/global-health/hiv-and-aids/technical-areas/hiv-and-aids-timeline. [5/16/2016].

n.d. "Nigeria." Available from: www.usaid.gov/our_work/global_health/aids/Countries/africa/nigeria.html. [1/20/2011].

Vaughan, Megan. 1994. "Health and Hegemony: Representation of Disease and the Creation of the Colonial Subject in Nyasaland." Pp. 173–201 in *Contesting Colonial Hegemony: State and Society in Africa and India,* edited by Dagmar Engles and Shula Marks. London: British Academic Press.

Vaughan, Peter W., and Everett M. Rogers. 2000. "A Staged Model of Communication Effects: Evidence from an Entertainment-Education Radio Soap Opera in Tanzania." *Journal of Health Communication* 5(3):203–27.

Vaughan, Peter W., Everett M. Rogers, Arvind Singhal, and Ramadhan M. Swalehe. 2000. "Entertainment-Education and HIV/AIDS Prevention: A Field Experiment in Tanzania." *Journal of Health Communication* 5(3):81–100.

Venter, Dennis. 1995. "*Malawi: The Transition to Multi-Party Politics.*" Pp. 152–92 in *Democracy and Political Change in Sub-Saharan Africa*, edited by John Wiseman. New York: Routledge.

Villalón, Leonardo A. 1995. *Islamic Society and State Power in Senegal: Disciples and Citizens in Fatick.* Cambridge: Cambridge University Press.

Walsh, Diana Chapman, Rima E. Rudd, Barbara A. Moeykens, and Thomas W. Moloney. 1993. "Social Marketing for Public Health." *Health Affairs* 12(2):104–19.

Wamai, Richard, Brian Morris, Stefan Bailis, David Sokal, Jeffrey Klausner, Ross Appleton, Nelson Sewankambo, David Cooper, John Bongaarts, Guy de Bruyn, Alex Wodak, and Joya Banerjee. 2011. "Male Circumcision for HIV Prevention: Current Evidence and Implementation in Sub-Saharan Africa." *Journal of the International AIDS Society* 14 (1):49.

Wangel, Anne-Marie. 1995. "AIDS in Malawi: A Case Study: A Conspiracy of Silence." Master's Dissertation, London School of Tropical Medicine and Hygiene.

Warwick, Donald P. 1982. *Bitter Pills.* Cambridge: Cambridge University Press.

Watkins, Susan Cotts, and Ann Swidler. 2013. "Working Misunderstandings: Donors, Brokers, and Villagers in Africa's AIDS Industry." *Population and Development Review* 38:197–218.

Watkins, Susan Cotts, Ann Swidler, and Thomas Hannan. 2012. "Outsourcing Social Transformation: Development NGOs as Organizations." *Annual Review of Sociology* 38:285–315.

Watkins, Susan Cotts. 2004. "Navigating the AIDS Epidemic in Rural Malawi." *Population and Development Review* 30(4):673–705.

Weber, Max. 1978. *Economy and Society: An Outline of Interpretive Sociology.* Berkeley, CA: University of California Press.

White, Richard G, Kate K Orroth, Judith R Glynn, Esther E Freeman, Roel Bakker, J Dik F Habbema, Fern Terris-Prestholt, Lilani Kumaranayake, Anne Buvé, and Richard J Hayes. 2008. "Treating Curable Sexually Transmitted Infections to Prevent HIV in Africa: Still an Effective Control Strategy?" *JAIDS Journal of Acquired Immune Deficiency Syndromes* 47(3):346–53.

Whiteside, Alan. 2008. *HIV/AIDS: A Very Short Introduction*. Oxford: Oxford University Press.

WHO Regional Office for Africa. 2014. *Implementation of Option B+ for Prevention of Mother-to-Child Transmission of HIV: The Malawi Experience*. Brazzaville: WHO Regional Office for Africa.

Wickstrom, Jane, Abdoulaye Diagne, and Alyson Smith. 2006. *Repositioning Family Planning – Senegal Case Study: Promising Beginnings, Uneven Progress*. New York: EngenderHealth/The ACQUIRE Project.

Wilcher, Rose, Theresa Hoke, Susan E. Adamchak, and Willard Cates. 2013. "Integration of Family Planning into HIV Services: A Synthesis of Recent Evidence." *AIDS* 27(1):S65–75.

Williams, Brian G., James O. Lloyd-Smith, Eleanor Gouws, Catherine Hankins, Wayne M. Getz, John Hargrove, Isabelle de Zoysa, Christopher Dye, and Bertran Auvert. 2006. "The Potential Impact of Male Circumcision on HIV in Sub-Saharan Africa." *Plos Medicine* 3(7):1032–40.

Williams, Eka, Kwame Asiedu, Barbara Riley, Joseph Nnorom, and Souleymaye Barry. 1995. *Re-Design of the AIDSCAP/Nigeria Program – Draft Proposal*. Washington, DC: USAID.

Williamson, Nancy, and Esther Boohene. 1990. "AIDS Prevention in Family Planning Programs." Pp. 203–10 in *The Handbook for AIDS Prevention in Africa*, edited by Peter Lamptey and Peter Piot. Durham, NC: Family Health International.

Wilmoth, John R., and Patrick Ball. 1992. "The Population Debate in American Popular Magazines, 1946–90." *Population and Development Review* 18(4):631–68.

Wilson, Anika. 2012. "Treating the Government Disease: AIDS Conspiracy Rumors, the Government of Malawi, and the Rhetoric of Accountability." *Contemporary Legend* 2(Series 3):57–84.

2013. *Folklore, Gender, and AIDS in Malawi: No Secret Under the Sun*. New York: Palgrave Macmillan.

Wilson, David, and Joy de Beyer. 2008. *Male Circumcision: Evidence and Implications*. Washington, DC: World Bank.

Wilson, Ellen. 1998. *Reproductive Health Case Study: Senegal*. Washington, DC: The Futures Group International.

Witter, Sophie, Margaret Armar-Klemesu, and Thierno Dieng. 2008. "National Fee Exemption Schemes for Deliveries: Comparing the Recent Experiences of Ghana and Senegal." Pp. 167–99 in *Reducing the Financial Barriers to Access to Obstetric Care*, edited by Fabienne Richard, Sophie Witter, and Vincent De Brouwere. Antwerp: ITG Press.

Wone, Katy Cissé. 1996. *Analyse Situationnelle du Sida au Sénégal: Rapport Préliminaire*. Dakar: Programme National de Lutte contre le Sida.

Woodberry, Robert D. 2012. "The Missionary Roots of Liberal Democracy." *The American Political Science Review* 106(2):244–74.

Woodling, Marie, Owain D. Williams, and Simon Rushton. 2012. "New Life in Old Frames: HIV, Development and the 'AIDS Plus MDGs' Approach." *Global Public Health* 7(Suppl 2):S144–58.

Woolcock, Michael, Simon Szreter, and Vijayendra Rao. 2011. "How and Why Does History Matter for Development Policy?" *Journal of Development Studies* 47(1):70–96.

World Bank. 1986. *Population Growth and Policies in Sub-Saharan Africa.* Washington, DC: World Bank.

1989. *Report of the Africa Region Task Force on Population FY 90–92.* Washington, DC: World Bank.

1992. *Population and the World Bank: Implications from Eight Studies.* Washington, DC: World Bank.

1996. *Senegal Integrated Health Sector Development Project – Project Information Document.* Washington, DC: World Bank.

2001. *Senegal-HIV/AIDS Prevention and Control Project – Project Information Document.* Washington, DC: World Bank.

2014. *World Development Indicators.* Washington, DC: World Bank.

n.d. "Health Project (01)." Available from: http://www.worldbank.org/projects/P002058/health-project-01?lang=en. [6/11/2008].

World Health Organization, and UNAIDS. 2007. *Male Circumcision: Global Trends and Determinants of Prevalence, Safety and Acceptability.* Geneva: World Health Organization.

World Health Organization, United Nations Children's Fund, United Nations Population Fund, and The World Bank. 2012. *Trends in Maternal Mortality: 1990 to 2010 Estimates.* Geneva: World Health Organization.

World Health Organization. 2000. *Health: A Key to Prosperity.* Geneva: World Health Organization.

2014. "Global Health Observatory Data Repository: Antiretroviral Therapy Coverage Data by Country." Available from: http://apps.who.int/gho/data/node.main.626. [10/3/2014].

Wright, Stephen. 1998. *Nigeria: Struggle for Stability and Status.* Boulder, CO: Westview Press.

Wroe, Daniel. 2012. "Donors, Dependency, and Political Crisis in Malawi." *African Affairs* 111(442):135–44.

Yaqub, Nuhu O. 1997. "Population Policy in Nigeria." Pp. 33–64 in *Women's Health, Population Policy and Family Planning Programmes in Nigeria,* edited by Empowerment and Action Research Center. Lagos: Empowerment and Action Research Center.

Yin, Sandra. 2007a. "In the News: Results Trickle Out from the Nigerian Census." *Population Reference Bureau.* Available from: www.prb .org/Articles/2007/ResultsFromNigerianCensus.aspx. [7/7/2011].

2007b. "Objections Surface Over Nigerian Census Results." *Population Reference Bureau.* Available from: www.prb.org/Articles/2007/Object ionsOverNigerianCensus.aspx. [7/7/2011].

Zaba, Basia, Ties Boerma, and Tanya Marchant. 1998. *Family Planning in the Era of AIDS: A Social Science Research Agenda.* Liege, Belgium: International Union for the Scientific Study of Population.

Zaggi, Hassan. 2013. "Rivers Govt Protests 2012 HIV Survey." *Daily Independent.* Available from: http://dailyindependentnig.com/2013/ 12/rivers-govt-protests-2012-hiv-survey/. [5/19/2015].

Zimbabwe National Statistics Agency, and ICF International. 2012. *Zimbabwe Demographic and Health Survey 2010–11.* Calverton, Maryland: ZIMSTAT and ICF International Inc.

Zimmerman, Margot, Carol Larivee, Rebeca Quiroga, CY Gopinath, Karen Ringheim, Siri Wood, Anne Wilson, Patricia Daunas, Linda Bruce, and Philip Sedlak. 2002. *Developing Materials on HIV/ AIDS/STIs for Low-Literate Audiences: A Guide.* Seattle, WA: PATH.

Zogby International, and Schneidman & Associates International. 2003. *National Perceptions of the Official Response to the HIV and AIDS Pandemic in Malawi.* Lilongwe: National AIDS Commission and UNAIDS.

Index

Page numbers in italics refer to figures and tables.

Multi-Country AIDS Program
(MAP), 50, 93, 184
Nigeria and, 33, 138, 143, 147, 155,
167
population and, 25, 49,
77–78
Senegal and, 175, 177, 184,
188, 199
World Fertility Survey, 47, 51
World Health Organization, 215
family planning and, 51, 139

Global Programme on AIDS, 39, 40,
51, 93
HIV and, 32, 38–39, 59, 93, 184, 212

Yao, 104, 130, 210

Zambia, 98n.10, 114
Zaire, *see* Democratic Republic of the
Congo
Zimbabwe, 25n.5, 26, 27, 75, 83,
99n.13, 110

For EU product safety concerns, contact us at Calle de José Abascal, 56–1°, 28003 Madrid, Spain or eugpsr@cambridge.org.

www.ingramcontent.com/pod-product-compliance
Ingram Content Group UK Ltd.
Pitfield, Milton Keynes, MK11 3LW, UK
UKHW020305140625
459647UK00005B/44